OTHER PMIC TITLES OF INTE

MEDICAL REFERENCE AND CLI?

Anesthesiology: Problems in Primary Care
Cardiology: Problems in Primary Care
Drugs of Abuse
Gastroenterology: Problems in Primary Care
Medical Care of the Adolescent Athlete
Medical Procedures for Referral
Neurology: Problems in Primary Care
Orthopaedics: Problems in Primary Care
Patient Care Emergency Handbook
Patient Care Flowchart Manual
Patient Care Procedures for Your Practice
Pulmonary Medicine: Problems in Primary Care
Questions & Answers on AIDS
Sexually Transmitted Diseases
Urology: Problems in Primary Care

PRACTICE MANAGEMENT

365 Ways to Manage the Business Called Private Practice
Achieving Profitability with a Medical Office System
Choosing and Using a Medical Office Computer
Computerizing Your Medical Office
Designing and Building Your Professional Office
Doctor Business
Encyclopedia of Practice and Financial Management
Getting Paid for What You Do
Health Information Management
Managing Medical Office Personnel
Managing the Physician's Office Laboratory
Marketing Strategies for Physicians
Medical Marketing Handbook
Medical Practice Handbook
Medical Software, Systems & Services Directory
Medical Staff Privileges
Negotiating Managed Care Contracts
New Practice Handbook
Patient Satisfaction
Patients Build Your Practice
Physician's Office Laboratory
Professional and Practice Development
Promoting Your Medical Practice
Starting in Medical Practice
Spanish/English Handbook for Medical Professionals

AVAILABLE FROM YOUR LOCAL MEDICAL BOOKSTORE
OR CALL 1-800-MED-SHOP

OTHER PMIC TITLES OF INTEREST

DICTIONARIES AND OTHER REFERENCE

Drug Interactions Index
Isler's Pocket Dictionary
Medical Acronyms, Eponyms and Abbreviations
Medical Phrase Index
Medical Word Building
Medico-Legal Glossary
Medico Mnemonica

CODING AND REIMBURSEMENT

CPT Coders Choice®, Thumb Indexed
CPT TimeSaver®, Ring Binder, Tab Indexed
CPT & HCPCS Coding Made Easy!
HCPCS Coders Choice®
Health Insurance Carrier Directory
ICD-9-CM, Coders Choice®, Thumb Indexed
ICD-9-CM, TimeSaver®, Ring Binder, Tab Indexed
ICD-9-CM Coding For Physicians Offices
ICD-9-CM Coding Made Easy!
Medicare Rules & Regulations
Physician Fees Guide
Reimbursement Manual for the Medical Office
Working with Insurance and Managed Care Plans

FINANCIAL MANAGEMENT

Accounts Receivable Management for the Medical Practice
Business Ventures for Physicians
Financial Planning Workbook for Physicians
Financial Valuation of Your Practice
Pension Plan Strategies
Physician Financial Planning in a Changing Environment
Securing Your Assets
Selling or Buying a Medical Practice

RISK MANAGEMENT

Law, Liability and Ethics for Medical Office Personnel
Malpractice Depositions
Malpractice: Managing Your Defense
Medical Risk Management
Testifying in Court

AVAILABLE FROM YOUR LOCAL MEDICAL BOOKSTORE
OR CALL 1-800-MED-SHOP

HEALTH & MEDICINE ON THE INTERNET

EDITED BY JAMES B. DAVIS

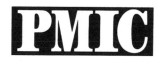

Health and Medicine on the Internet

ISBN #1-57066-065-4

Disclaimer

The publisher's best efforts have gone into creating this book, and great care has been taken to maintain the accuracy of the information contained in this book. However, the publisher does not guarantee the accuracy, adequacy or completeness of any information and is not responsible for any errors or omissions or any consequences arising from the use of the information contained in this book. Also, the publisher specifically disclaims, without limitation, any implied warranties of merchantability and fitness for a particular purpose with respect to listings on the book. In no event shall the publisher be responsible or liable for any loss of profit or other commercial damages, including but not limited to special, incidental, consequential or any other damages in connection with or arising out of furnishing, performance, or use of this book.

All information contained in this book is subject to change. Mention of a specific product or company does not imply an endorsement. The information you find on the internet should never replace the advice of a trained health professional. If you have any questions about your health, you should always consult a qualified health professional.

All of the images in this book have been obtained from online sources. The caption accompanying each illustration identifies its online source. Text and images available over the internet and other online services may be subject to copyright and other rights owned by third parties. Online availability of text and images does not imply that they may be reused without the permission of rights holders, although the Copyright Act does permit certain unauthorized reuse as fair use under 17 U.S.C. §107. Care should be taken to ensure that all necessary rights are cleared prior to reusing material distributed over the internet and other online services. Information about reuse is available from the institutions that make their materials available online.

Trademarks

The words in this book for which we have reason to believe trademark, service mark, or other proprietary rights may exist have been designated as such by use of initial capitalization. However, no attempt has been made to designate as trademarks or service marks all personal-computer words or terms in which proprietary rights might exist. The inclusion, exclusion, or definition of a word or term is not intended to affect, or to express any judgement on, the validity or legal status of any proprietary right which may be claimed in that word or term.

Practice Management Information Corporation
4727 Wilshire Blvd., Suite 300
Los Angeles, California 90010 U.S.A.
1-800-MED-SHOP

http://www.medicalbookstore.com

Printed in the United States of America

TABLE OF CONTENTS

INTRODUCTION

The fast growth of the internet and the enormous amount of information available online, as well as the potential power of this communication tool are unprecedented and, to the newcomer, perhaps intimidating. We have attempted to scope out simply one region of the vast online terrain, health and medicine. In doing so, we have discovered that it is in fact much more spectacular than originally anticipated. Even as we breath, it is expanding in both predictable and surprising ways.

Entering cyberspace is exciting, but without some direction it can also be exhausting and time-consuming. In an effort to aid physicians and other health care professionals to locate the areas of information and communities of support relevant to their interests, we have created this guide, *Health and Medicine on the Internet*.

For the purposes of this book, we presume that the reader already has a working knowledge of how to access and "surf" the internet. It is also assumed that the reader's primary interest is to tap into a specific pocket of information accessible on the internet, as easily and as quickly as possible. Frankly, you don't have time to waste determining which web sites are commercial, which are geared to patients, which are for students, and which may be out-dated. Instead, you want to go directly to a page that speaks to health care professionals like yourself, a page that is full of relevant, accurate, intelligent and up-to-date information. This book can point you to the sites best suited to your needs.

The World Wide Web and the personal computer are not typically considered to be medical tools but, used to their potential, they can enhance your career and help you to deliver superior medical services to your patients. Some of the most beneficial uses of the internet include 1) acquiring new medical knowledge; 2) networking through academic and professional organizations online; 3) sharing your opinions and soliciting the opinions of your peers; 4) fulfilling CME requirements and, in general, refreshing your medical knowledge base; 5) observing patients' needs and concerns to learn how you can best help them; and 6) gathering material that can be distributed to patients for a better understanding of their health and medical conditions.

Specific features of the internet make it particularly appealing to applications in health and medicine. For instance, the ability to transmit images digitally allows timely second- or third-opinions on significant patient radiographs to be given by experts who are located at sites far from the patient, possibly even across the world (i.e., telemedicine). Similarly, indeterminate or unusual patient results can be shared and discussed with large numbers of physicians, several of whom may have had similar cases. In addition, interactive simulations of patient encounters help physicians to conveniently develop their diagnostic skills. Database, library and information clearinghouse access is also convenient and immediate via the internet, and this permits the distribution and sharing of helpful statistical data and analysis. Finally, the hypertext nature of the medium allows physicians to consider innovative or alternative lines of medical investigation, some of which they may not even have realized existed.

Clinical textbooks, online professional journals, job and equipment postings, medical glossaries, drug references, databases of diseases, patient education sheets, photographic and radiographic images, diagrams, videos, audio files, interactive tours, quizzes and links to related topics... the material you can obtain from the internet takes many forms, is usually free, and instantly arrives on your computer screen as you sit at home or at the office.

Naturally, care must be taken when following advice given on the internet. Even though a site may appear professional or a discussion group may assert that it is moderated or "controlled," consider all information to be supplementary. Make sure that you can identify and trust the source of any information, and verify any medical or health advice through other mediums and with your own experience.

Health and Medicine on the Internet is divided into 69 sections, beginning with *Abuse* and ending with *Women's Health*. Each section is broken down into several subtopics that are arranged alphabetically. Every site listed includes the World Wide Web address (also known as the URL or Universal Resource Locator) and often a brief description of what you will find there. Illustrations of selected sites give you an idea of what they look like. At the beginning of each section, we've listed related topics, other sections where you might find additional information of interest to you. Finally, an index is provided at the end of this book in case you are not sure of where to start looking.

Although browsing on the net is certainly recommended, *Health and Medicine on the Internet* was designed so that you would not have to "stumble" upon a site that is of relevance to you. Rather, by using this book, you can identify it quickly, type the address into your computer, and visit it in moments.

While we have checked out every site in this book to verify its address and contents, there may be cases where the web site has moved or been discontinued.

Usually, a message will appear on your screen to tell you what has happened and, if the site has moved, to tell you the new URL or provide a link that takes you there. Because URLs can be rather cryptic, make sure you have typed it accurately. Capitalization and spelling are important. If you still do not get where you are trying to go, type just the beginning part of the address, which will take you to the domain, or computer, which acts as home to the web page of interest. From that point, you can often work your way down to arrive at the site that caught your eye.

For instance, the correct address to reach the National Institutes of Health page on grants funding opportunities is *http://www.nih.gov/grants/funding/funding.htm.* If you type in *http://www.nih.gov/*, you will arrive at the home page for the National Institutes of Health. Selecting "Grants and Contracts" with a click of your mouse takes you to *http://www.nih.gov/grants/*, from which you can choose "Grants" to reach the Grants Page of the Office of Extramural Research *(http://www.nih.gov/grants/oer.htm.* With just one more click, select "Funding Opportunities" and you will arrive at "Funding Opportunities: Grants."

There are over 2,500 different web sites listed in this book. In order to keep up with the rapid growth of the internet and the progress of medicine, we will update and add to this book annually, to provide you with the most accurate and helpful information around.

ABUSE

Covered in this section: *Child Abuse; Domestic Violence; Elder Abuse; General Topics; Recovery from Abuse; Sexual Abuse.*

Related section: *Children's Health/Pediatrics.*

Child Abuse

See also: Children's Health/Pediatrics.

Center for Children in Crisis

http://www.shadow.net/~cpt/

Child Abuse: A Handbook for Staff

http://www.fcbe.edu.on.ca/www/pubs/cah/cah_summary.html

Child Abuse and Neglect Clearinghouse

http://www.calib.com/nccanch/

Child Abuse Statistics, Research and Resources

http://www.jimhopper.com/abstats/

Child Neglect and Munchausen Syndrome by Proxy

http://ncjrs.org/txtfiles/chnegmun.txt

This site describes this form of abuse which involves a parent intentionally making his or her child critically ill. Prepared by the Department of Justice. PDF files available at:

http://ncjrs.org/pdffiles/chnegmun.pdf.

Child Sexual Abuse

http://www.cs.utk.edu/~bartley/sacc/childAbuse.html

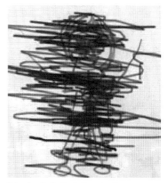

Linda Cain's Information on Child Sexual Abuse.
http://www.commnet.edu/QVCTC/student/LindaCain/sexabuse.html

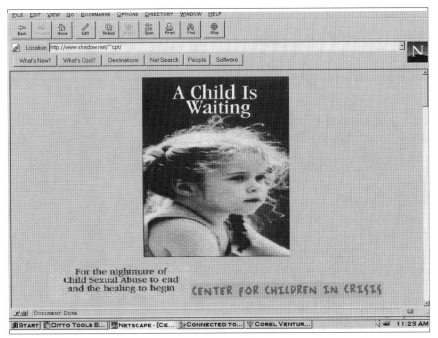

Center for Children in Crisis. *http://www.shadow.net/~cpt/*

Children and Sexual Assault: Important Information
http://www.lib.uchicago.edu/~loakleaf/child.html

Children's Safety Network: National Injury and Violence Prevention Resource Center
http://www.edc.org/HHD/csn/

Provides assistance to organizations seeking to reduce unintentional injuries and violence to children and adolescents. Offers online publications and publications available through the mail, as well as resources and links.

Factitious Disorder by Proxy/Munchausen by Proxy Syndrome Home Page
http://www.mindspring.com/~louisalasher/

Includes a quiz to check your knowledge of the syndrome and the potential for treatment.

Just in Case

http://www.discribe.ca/childfind/educate/jic/victim.hte

Parental guidelines, just in case your child is the victim of sexual abuse or exploitation.

Linda Cain's Information on Child Sexual Abuse

http://www.commnet.edu/QVCTC/student/LindaCain/sexabuse.html

Mothers Against Munchausen Syndrome by Proxy Allegation

http://www.msbp.com/

Munchausen by Proxy Syndrome

http://home.coqui.net:80/myrna/munch.htm

Research and Training Center in Rehabilitation and Childhood Trauma

http://www.nemc.org/rehab/homepg.htm

Sexual Assault Information Page: Incest and Child Sexual Abuse

http://www.cs.utk.edu/~bartley/index/
childSexualAbuse/

This site provides many links for survivors of incest and child sexual abuse. It includes statistics, research, recovery resources and support.

The Survivors' Voice

http://www.billboards.com/billboards/tsv/

Newsletter addressing issues of child abuse.

Domestic Violence

Cancer in Our Homes: Domestic Violence

http://www.mlode.com/~ra/ra8/index.html

Domestic Violence

http://www.en.com/users/allison/dvpage.html

Domestic Violence - Sites and Information
http://www.cs.utk.edu/~bartley/index/domesticViolence/

Men and Domestic Violence Index
http://www.vix.com/pub/men/domestic-index.html

SafetyNet: Domestic Violence Resources
http://www.cybergrrl.com/dv.html

Elder Abuse
See also: Aging/Gerontology.

Elder Abuse
http://www.calregistry.com/resources/eldabpag.htm
> How to know if you or someone else is the victim of elder abuse; links.

Elder Abuse Prevention: Information and Resource Guide
http://www.aimnet.com/~oaktree/elder/home.shtml

National Center on Elder Abuse
http://www.interinc.com/NCEA

General Topics
See also: Mental Health - Personality Disorders, Trauma.

Abuse/Sexual Abuse/Incest Resources
http://www.infi.net/~susanf.ablinks2.htm
> Many links, arranged alphabetically with brief descriptions.

Assault Prevention Information Network
*http://galaxy.einet.net/galaxy/Community/Safety/Assault-Prevention/apin/
APINindex.html*

Blain Nelson's Abuse Pages
http://www.pacificrim.net/~blainn/abuse

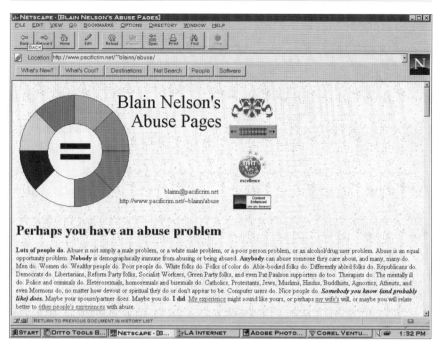

Blain Nelson's Abuse Pages. *http://www.pacificrim.net/~blainn/abuse*

Discord's Abuse Survivors' Resources
http://www.tezcat.com/~tina/psych.shtml

Links to websites addressing sexual, physical, emotional and ritual abuse and its effects. Newsgroups, FAQs and information sources offered. For survivors of abuse, their friends, families, and other concerned individuals.

Hopeful Hands
http://www.CoachCenter.com/hopeful.html

Karra's Korner
http://www.xroads.com/rainbow/karra.html

Abuse links.

REAL MEN Work to End Violence Against Women
http://www.cs.utk.edu/~bartley/other/realMen.html

Ritual Abuse and Healing Home Page
http://www.xroads.com/rahome/

SANCTUARY Home Page

http://avocado/wustl.edu/~chack/sanct/sanctuary.html

Survivor Ship

http://www.xroads.com/rainbow/svship/

An international forum discussing issues relevant to survivors of ritualistic abuse, torture, and mind control.

Recovery from Abuse

Sidran Foundation

http://www.access.digex.net/~sidran/

For those who have witnessed violent or traumatic events, the results of which have often been that they suffer symptoms of severe stress that may be disabling. The Sidran Foundation is devoted to education, advocacy and research to help these individuals. Includes *The Sidran Bookshelf on Trauma and Dissociation*, an annotated bibliography, and resources on dissociation disorder information, traumatic memories, sexual and child abuse, and issues related to survivors of trauma.

Wounded Healer Journal

http://idealist.com/wounded_healer/

For psychotherapists and survivors of abuse.

Sexual Abuse

Anonymous Sexual Abuse Recovery

http://www.worldchat.com/public/asarc/commsymp.htm

Common symptoms; abuse-related illnesses.

ASARian.org

http://www.asarian.org/

Free services to survivors of sexual abuse.

Men and Abuse, Rape

http://www.vix.com/pub/men/abuse/abuse.html

RAINN

http://www.rainn.org/
> RAINN = Rape, Abuse and Incest National Network.

Rape Prevention Education Program

http://pubweb.ucdavis.edu/Documents/RPEP/rpep.htm

Sexual Assault Information Page

http://www.cs.utk.edu/~bartley/saInfoPage.html

Lots of information, from acquaintance rape to pornography, to women's resources links.

Survivors' Page

http://www.wwns.com/~lara/survs.html
> Issues relating to sexual abuse.

ADDICTION & RECOVERY

Covered in this section: *Alcoholism; Drug Abuse; General Topics; Humor & Addiction; Internet Addiction; Nicotine; Recovery/Support; Research.*

Related section: *Mental Health.*

Alcoholism

Adult Children of Alcoholics
http://www.recovery.org/acoa/acoa.html

Al-Anon/Alateen
http://solar.std.utk.edu/~Al-Anon/
Text available in eight different languages.

Alcoholics Anonymous Information
http://www.csic.com/aa/

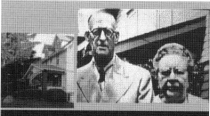
Dr. Bob's Home.
http://www.drbobs.com/index.html

Alcoholics Anonymous World Services
http://www.alcoholics-anonymous.org/

Alcoholics Victorious
http://www.iugm.org/av/
Christian support group for recovering alcoholics.

Big Book of Alcoholics Anonymous
http://www.recovery.org/aa/bigbook/ww/index.html

Dr. Bob's Home
http://www.drbobs.com/index.html
View the founder of Alcoholic Anonymous' home. Site not affiliated with AA.

Drinkwise
http://www.med.umich.edu/drinkwise/

National Association for Children of Alcoholics
http://www.health.org/nacoa/

Online AA Resources
http://www.recovery.org/aa/

Information about Alcoholics Anonymous, including its history, regional resources, online meeting information, bibliography. AA resources also available for non-English speakers.

Online Intergroup of Alcoholics Anonymous
http://aa-intergroup.org/

Online meeting information.

Online Recovery Resources (Non-AA)
http://www.recovery.org/rec2.html

Because AA may not be for everybody.

Physicians' Guide to Helping Patients with Alcohol Problems
http://www.niaaa.nih.gov/publications/physicn.htm

From the National Institute on Alcohol Abuse and Alcoholism.

Project Cork Institute and Database
http://www.dartmouth.edu/dms/cork/

Quizzes to Help Determine Alcohol Dependency
http://www.recovery.org/aa/aa-related/quizzes.txt

(Unofficial) Alcoholics Anonymous Page
http://www.halcyon.com/carrick/aa/aa-home.html

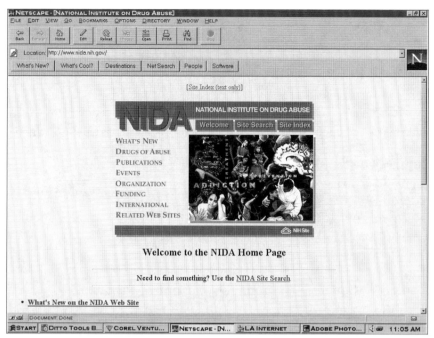

National Institute on Drug Abuse. *http://www.nida.nih.gov/*

Drug Abuse

Cocaine Anonymous
http://www.ca.org/

International Harm Reduction Association
http://www.drugtext.nl/ihra/default.htm

The International Harm Reduction Association is a professional association of individuals and organizations from around the world who are concerned about the development of drug policies to reduce the harmful consequences of drug use and current drug policies.

IRC Group of Narcotics Anonymous Home Page
http://www.csra.net/zeppr/irc-na.htm

Real-time chat group for Narcotics Anonymous (NA).

Narcotics Anonymous (NA)
http://www.wsoinc.com/

Narcotics Anonymous Local Area and Regional Information
http://www.nitehawk.com/never_alone/lists.html

National Institute on Drug Abuse
http://www.nida.nih.gov/

Part of the National Institutes of Health, the National Institute on Drug Abuse offers links and information about drugs of abuse, publications and research.

Other NA-Related Links
http://www.csra.net/zeppr/NA-Links.htm

Recovery on AOL and the Net
http://www.recovery.org/aa/meetings/online/aol-net.html

Meetings online.

United Nations International Drug Control Program
http://www.undcp.or.at/

General Topics

Addiction, Recovery and Prevention
http://www.idir.net/~irvcohen/

Addictions and Life Page
http://www.addictions.org/

Addictions Newsletter
http://www.kumc.edu/addictions_newsletter/

Published by Division 50 of the American Psychological Association.

Adult Children Online Resource Page
http://www.intac.com/%7Ewoy/drwoititz/source.htm

Alcohol and Drugs - General Information
http://www.wellesley.edu/Counseling/selfcare/alcdrug_info.html

American Society of Addiction Medicine
http://members.aol.com/asamoffice/index.html

Bureau of Alcohol, Tobacco and Firearms Home Page
http://www.atf.treas.gov/

Center for Substance Abuse Prevention Home Page
http://www.covesoft.com/csap.html

Dual Diagnosis Website
http://www.erols.com/ksciacca/

Co-occurring mental illness, drug addiction, and/or alcoholism. Information and resources for providers, addicts, their families and the general public.

Emotions Anonymous
http://www.dna.lth.se/home/Peter_Moller/EA /General_Info.html

HabitSmart
http://www.cts.com/crash/habtsmrt/

Information and resources to fight addictions, ranging from alcohol to drugs to cigarettes.

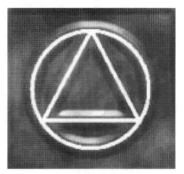

Addictions and Life Page.
http://www.addictions.org/

Jewish Grapezine
http://www.jacsweb.org/

Subtitled: Jews in Recovery from Alcoholism and Drugs.

National Families in Action Online
http://www.emory.edu/NFIA/

This group considers the cultural and ethnic connections of drug abuse, and provides helpful information on drugs and drug abuse. Site has an "Ask the Experts" question submission capability, a catalog of publications, and additional resources.

National Institute on Alcohol Abuse and Alcoholism

http://www.niaaa.nih.gov/

Offers publications and databases, news and events about alcohol abuse and addiction. Site includes the bulletin *Alcohol Alert*, a scientific journal entitled *Alcohol Health and Research World*, pamphlets, reports, research monographs and databases, as well as grant information and links.

Prevention Online (NCADI)

http://www.health.org/

National Clearinghouse for Alcohol and Drug Information.

Secular Organization for Sobriety (SOS) Home Page

http://www.codesh.org/sos/

An alternative to the 12-step program that separates sobriety from religion or spirituality. This site describes SOS and its history, provides contact information and links to the *SOS International Newsletter*.

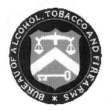

Sober Space

http://www.aa-erie-pa.com/

Sobriety and Recovery Resources

http://www.winternet.com/~terrym/sobriety.html

The Bureau of Alcohol, Tobacco and Firearms.
http://www.atf.treas.gov/

Substance Abuse Information for Parents

http://www.commnet.edu/QVCTC/student/ GaryOKeefe/drugfacts.html

U.S. Recovery, Addiction and Abuse Resources

http://www.contact.org/usrecov.htm

Web of Addictions

http://www.well.com/user/woa/

Accurate information about alcoholism and other drug addictions. Contains fact sheets, resources and contacts both on and off-line, meeting information, and more.

Women for Sobriety

http://www.mediapulse.com/wfs/

Dedicated to helping women overcome alcoholism and other addictions.

Humor & Addiction

Humor and Addiction

http://www.users.cts.com/crash/e/elmo/funindex.htm

Internet Addiction

Internet Addiction Disorder

http://www.cmhc.com/guide/iad.htm

If you're reading this book, you may want to check this site out...

Net Overuse

http://www.addictions.org/netaddict.htm

Nicotine

Alt.Support.Stop-Smoking (AS3)

http://www.swen.uwaterloo.ca/~bpekilis/as3

The newsgroup's web site and archives.

American Cancer Society Pages on Tobacco Control

http://www.ca.cancer.org/services/tobacco/

ASH: Action on Smoking and Health

http://www.setinc.com/ash/

Blair's Quitting Smoking Resources Pages

http://www.chriscor.com/linkstoa.htm

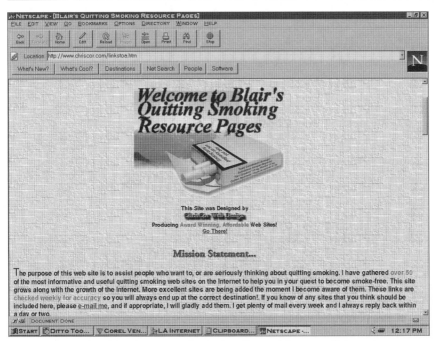

Blair's Quitting Smoking Resources Page. *http://www.chriscor.com/linkstoa.htm*

Cigarette Papers Online

http://galen.library.ucsf.edu/tobacco/cigpapers/

Master Anti-Smoking Page

http://www.autonomy.com/smoke.htm
Lots of links to anti-smoking and related web sites.

NicNet

http://ahsc.arizona.edu/nicnet/

Nicotine Anonymous

http://www.slip.net/~billh/nicahome.html
Enter both the official and unofficial Nicotine Anonymous web pages.

Nicotine Anonymous (Official)

http://rampages.onramp.net/~nica/

Nicotine Anonymous (Unofficial)

http://www.slip.net/~billh/nica/nic2home.html

Nicotine in Cigarettes and Smokeless Tobacco Products

http://www.fda.gov/tobacinfo/juristoc.html

Text of an FDA report from August, 1995.

NO SMOKE Software

http://www.autonomy.com/nosmoke.htm

Smoking, Tobacco and Cancer

http://www.oncolink.upenn.edu/causeprevent/smoking/

Tobacco Control Archives

http://galen.library.ucsf.edu/tobacco/

Recovery/Support

Challenges

http://www.well.com/user/woa/chall.htm

Monthly online publication.

Christian Recovery Site

http://www.tfs.net/~iugm/

DOC: Doctors Ought to Care

http://www.bcm.tmc.edu/doc/

The mission of this group is to fight tobacco and alcohol use among youths.

Guide to Clean and Sober Living: Steps for Recovery

http://www.pronex.com/80/steps/index.html

Online newspaper.

Join Together: Online

http://www.jointogether.org/jointogether.html

Self-described as a "resource center and meeting place for communities working to reduce harms [from] the use of illicit drugs,... alcohol and tobacco."

A Look at Relapse

http://www.recovery.org/aa/aa-related/relapse.txt

Mike and Terry's House
http://www.syix.com/mleahey/
> Narcotics Anonymous news, support, meeting information and more.

One Day at a Time
http://www.nmia.com/~khill/ODAAT.html

Prevention Primer
http://www.health.org/pubs/primer/index.htm

Recovery Anonymous
http://www.mlode.com/~ra/

Recovery Is Good for You
http://www.users.cts.com/crash/e/elmo/recovr.htm

Recovery Medicine Wheel (Native American)
http://www.recovery.org/aa/aa-related/medwheel.txt

Research

Addiction Research Foundation
http://www.arf.org/
> Combines research, information and community action.

Brown University Center for Alcohol and Addiction Studies
http://center.butler.brown.edu/

Center for Addiction and Alternative Medicine Research
http://www.winternet.com/~caamr/

Center for Substance Abuse Research
http://www.bsos.umd.edu/cesar/cesar.html

Research Institute on Addictions
http://www.ria.org/

AGING / GERONTOLOGY

Covered in this section: *Alzheimer's Disease; Caregivers; General Topics; Incontinence; Nutrition & Aging.*

Related sections: *Death & Dying; Hospice Care.*

Alzheimer's Disease/Dementia

Aging and Dementia Web Resources

http://www.biostat.wustl.edu/ ALZHEIMER/submit.html

Site provides resources for caregivers, offers clinical care guides, research about the aging process, products and services for the aging, links to personal home pages, information on "assisted living" and more.

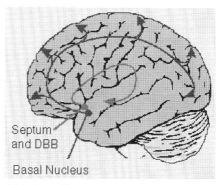

Alzheimer Web.
http://dsmallpc2.path.unimelb.edu.au/ad.html

Alzheimer Bookshelf

http://www.nbn.com/people/elder/alzheimer.html

Alzheimer Web

http://dsmallpc2.path.unimelb.edu.au/ad.html

Alzheimer's Association

http://www.alz.org/

Alzheimer's Disease Education and Referral Center

http://www.cais.com/adear/index.html

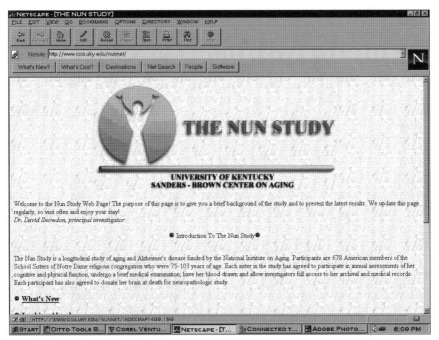

The Nun Study. *http://www.coa.uky.edu/nunnet/*

Alzheimer's Disease Fact Sheets

http://www.cais.com/adear/adfact.html

Symptoms of Alzheimer's; information on diagnosis, research and resources.

Alzheimer's Disease Resource Page

http://www.cwru.edu/orgs/adsc/intro.html

This page from Case Western Reserve University includes general information, research results, and resources for caregivers and for practitioners specializing in health care for the aging.

Alzheimer's Disease Web Page

http://med-amsa.bu.edu/Alzheimer/home.html

Alzheimer's Support Network

http://gator.naples.net/presents/Alzheimer/

Pages on Alzheimer's Disease and wandering; library, newsletter and links.

Early Alzheimer's Disease: Recognition and Assessment
http://www.ahcpr.gov/guide/alzover.htm

Overview of the AHCPR clinical practice guidelines for diagnosing early Alzheimer's Disease.

Final Report and Recommendations on Alzheimer's Disease and Other Dementias
http://www.health.state.ny.us/nysdoh/consumer/alzheimer/alzeihm.htm

These PDF files contain the contents of the *New York State Task Force on Alzheimer's Disease and Other Dementias, Final Report and Recommendations.*

The Nun Study
http://www.coa.uky.edu/nunnet/

This site describes the background and latest results of a longitudinal study of aging and Alzheimer's. The participants were 678 nuns ranging from 75-103 years of age.

Caregivers

Caregiving Online Newsletter
http://www.caregiving.com/

Elder Care Navigator
http://www.mindspring.com/~eldrcare/elderweb.htm

Subtitle to this site is "Helping People Navigate the Elder Care Maze."

Eldercare Locator: How to Find Community Assistance for Seniors
http://www2.ageinfo.org/naicweb/elderloc/elderloc.html

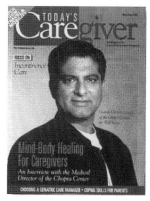

Today's Caregiver Magazine.
http://www.caregiver.com

Eldercare Site
http://pw2.netcom.com/~lehdoll/caretaker1.html

Support and understanding for people who provide care for the elderly.

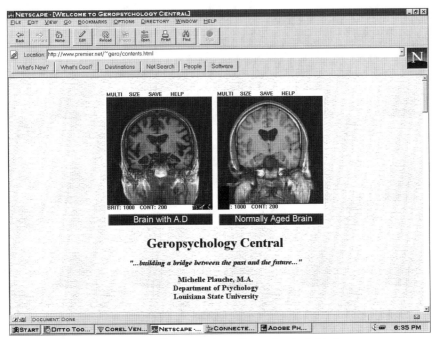

Geropsychology Central. http://www.premier.net/~gero/contents.html

Eldercare Web

http://www.elderweb.com/

Today's Caregiver Magazine

http://www.caregiver.com/
Bimonthly magazine.

General Topics

Administration on Aging

http://www.AoA.DHHS.GOV/aoa/pages/info.html
Information for older persons, their families, and people interested in aging. This site includes statistics, electronic booklets on health and living topics, women and aging, retirement, and Alzheimer's Disease.

AGE NET

http://elo.mediasrv.swt.edu/goldenage/script.htm

Aging Research Centre (ARC)
http://www.hookup.net/mall/aging/agesit59.html
> Services for researchers who are studying the aging process.

American Association of Retired Persons
http://www.aarp.org/

American Physical Therapy Association: Geriatrics Section
http://geriatricspt.org/
> Intended for physical therapists, geriatric clients and their families, students and anyone interested in healthcare issues relating to older people.

Andrus Gerontology Library
http://www.usc.edu/Library/Gero/
> The Andrus Library contains 11,000 book titles, 110 journals, 300 newsletters, videos and other media.

Center for Aging
http://garnet.berkeley.edu/~aging/
> All about the Center and its programs, publications and resources.

Directory of Web and Gopher Sites on Aging
http://www.AoA.DHHS.GOV/aoa/webres/craig.htm

Dr. Frank On-Line!
http://www.drfrank.com/
> Advice for seniors from Dr. Frank, a syndicated newspaper columnist.

ElderPage
http://www.aoa.dhhs.gov/elderpage.html

Geropsychology Central
http://www.premier.net/~gero/geropsyc.html
> Site describes itself as an "online resource devoted to the study of the neurological, psychological and sociological aspects of the aging process." It includes resources and services for seniors, as well as information about and links to geropsychology and gerontology sites.

GeroWeb

http://www.iog.wayne.edu/IOGlinks.html

Useful site includes the GeroWeb Virtual Library on Aging.

Hardin Meta Directory: Geriatrics

http://www.arcade.uiowa.edu/hardin-www/md-ger.html

Health/Prolongevity/Anti-Aging Resources

http://www.aeiveos.com/resource/index.html

Healthtouch: Older Americans

http://www.healthtouch.com/level1/leaflets/102179/1021/102179.html

Information on aging and the body, mental health, retirement, pain treatment, home care and more.

Internet and E-Mail Resources on Aging

http://www.aoa.dhhs.gov/aoa/pages/jpostlst.html

Longevity Game

http://www.northwesternmutual.com/games/longevity/longevity-main.html

Input personal information to receive an estimate on how long you will live, based on research done by the life insurance industry.

Medication Information Line for the Elderly (MILE)

http://www.mbnet.mb.ca/crm/health/mile.html

MedWeb: Geriatrics

http://www.gen.emory.edu/medweb/medweb.geriatrics.html

Provides a large number of website links.

National Aging Information Center

http://www.ageinfo.org/

This site collects policy-related materials, demographic and other statistical data on the health, economic and social status of older Americans. Links to many resources and bibliography of reading materials.

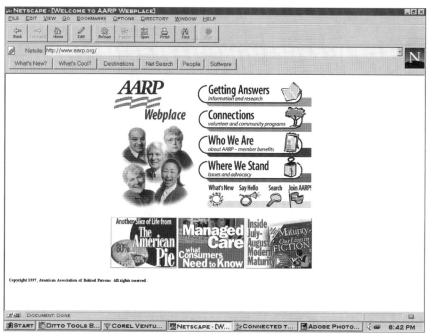

American Association of Retired Persons. http://www.aarp.org/

National Institute on Aging

http://www.nih.gov/nia/

This is a biomedical research agency that promotes healthy aging by supporting biomedical, social and behavioral research and public education. The site describes NIA's research, and offers publications on health and aging topics.

NetWatch TopTen - Senior Issues

http://www.pulver.com/netwatch/topten/tt21.htm

Older, Wiser and Wired: A Virtual Community for Netsurfers Over 50

http://www.oww.com/index.html

Links to associations; health, wellness and medical issues; news; recreation and additional resources for computer-savvy seniors.

Physical Activity and Health: Older Adults

http://www.cdc.gov/nccd/php/sgr/olderad.htm

Report from the U.S. Surgeon General.

Portals Aging
http://www.portals.pdx.edu/~isidore/aging.html
> Includes aging-related web sites, discussion groups, and databases.

Senior Access
http://www.hooked.net/users/sraccess/senior.html
> This site provides information to promote independent living for seniors.

SeniorNet
http://www.seniornet.com/

Seniors-Site
http://seniors-site.com/

SeniorSites
http://www.seniorsites.com/

Stroke and Aging Research Project
http://www.columbia.edu/~dwd2/
> Bibliography and links to related sites.

Incontinence

Incontinence Resources
http://ourworld.compuserve.com/homepages/ivy/incontin.htm

InContiNet Home Page
http://InContiNet.com/

Nutrition & Aging

Food Guide Pyramid for Older Adults
http://ianrwww.unl.edu/ianr/pubs/nebfacts/nf93-03.htm

National Policy and Resource Center on Nutrition and Aging
http://www.fiu.edu/~nutreldr/

ALLERGIES / IMMUNOLOGY

Covered in this section: *Allergies; General Topics; Organizations.*

Related sections: *HIV/AIDS; Lungs/Respiratory & Pulmonary.*

Allergies

Allergies and Asthma

http://www.best.com/~gazissax/chealth3.html

Site provides general information and links to newsgroups and other resources relating to allergies and asthma. It is part of the Children's Health Page web site.

Allergy, Asthma and Immunology Online

http://allergy.mcg.edu/

This web site is maintained by allergists and contains information and news for patients, their parents, physicians, and "individuals purchasing group health care programs." Information for patients includes an *Asthma Life Quality Test*, when to see and how to find an allergist, information on insect allergies, exercise and additional advice. Information for physicians includes practice parameters and clinical immunology. In addition, an Allergy-Immunology Glossary is offered, as well as helpful links to medical and general resources.

Allergy Discussion List

http://www.io.com/~kinnaman/
allergy/html

This site describes how to subscribe to the list server and how to read and/or search the Allergy Archives. To subscribe via e-mail, send a message to: LISTSERV@listserv.tamu.edu and in the body of the message, type: "Subscribe Allergy Yourfirstname Yourlastname."

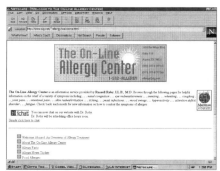

The On-Line Allergy Center.
http://www.sig.net/~allergy/welcome.html

Allergy Information Center

http://www.kww.com/allergy/

Includes information about allergies and about ALLERGY-LIST, a moderated newsgroup.

Allergy Internet Resources

http://www.Immune.Com/allergy/disclaim.html

This site offers a collection of information links on allergy topics, which include a long and well-organized list of text files. Main topics include: General Allergy texts, Asthma texts, Food Allergies, Kids' Allergies, Latex Allergies, and more.

Allergy Online

http://allergy.hno.akh-wien.ac.at/allergy/

The allergology server at Vienna Medical School offers patient and scientific information on allergies, pollen and related topics in English and German. Interesting historical trivia about allergies also provided.

National Allergy Bureau Report

http://execpc.com/~edi/nab/nab.html

Receive information on pollen and mold aeroallergen levels around the country. Reports are updated every Thursday, and particle counts and predominant allergen are provided.

On-Line Allergy Center

http://www.sig.net/~allergy/
welcome.html

Allergy facts, tips and feature articles as well as news updates are provided for allergy sufferers worldwide.

General Topics

Jeffrey Modell Foundation

http://www.mssm.edu/peds/modell/home-pag.html

Information on primary (or inherited) immune deficiency.

National Institute of Allergies and Infectious Diseases

http://www.niaid.nih.gov/

News, facts, publications and research updates; clinical research trial information, grant information and more.

National Jewish Center for Immunology and Respiratory Medicine

http://www.njc.org/

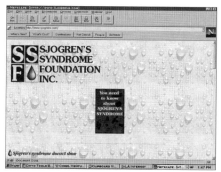

Sjogren's Syndrome Foundation.
http://www.sjogrens.com/

The National Jewish Center treats asthma, tuberculosis, emphysema and other respiratory and immune system diseases. This site offers information for health care consumers and professionals on topics such as asthma, chronic bronchitis, and sleep-related breathing disorders.

Sjogren's Syndrome Foundation

http://www.sjogrens.com/

This site acts as information clearinghouse for Sjogren's Syndrome, an incurable autoimmune disorder where the body attacks its own moisture-producing glands causing dry eye, mouth, and potentially worse effects.

Organizations

American Academy of Allergy, Asthma and Immunology

http://www.aaaai.org/

American Association of Immunology

http://www.scienceXchange.com/aai/

ALTERNATIVE MEDICINE

Acupuncture & Acupressure

Acupressure Point of the Day

http://www.inforamp.net/~holshe/acu.html

Acupuncture.com

http://www.acupuncture.com/

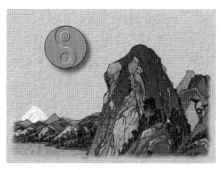

The traditional Oriental therapies of acupuncture, herbology, qi gong, Chinese nutrition and massage are addressed. Also find marketplace and resources for consumers, students and practitioners, as well as links to related sites.

Acupuncture.Com.
http://www.acupuncture.com/

Acupuncture Home Page

http://www.rscom.com/tcm/index.html

Acupuncture Resource Pages

http://homepages.enterprise.net/joo/

Acupuncture Therapy and Research Clinic

http://www.wt.net.acupudoc/

American Academy of Medical Acupuncture

http://www.medicalacupuncture.org/

Introduction to Acupuncture

http://198.150.8.9/acupuncture.html

James Roy Holliday III Guide to Acupressure

http://falcon.cc.ukans.edu/~moriarty/acupressure/acuguide.html

Medical Acupuncture Web Page

http://www.med.auth.gr/~karanik/

Aromatherapy

Aromatherapy Internet Resources

http://www.tiac.net:80/users/mgold/www/aromatherapy.html

Aromatherapy Links

http://galen.med.virginia.edu/pjb35/Aromatherapy.html
    Virtual doorway to hundreds of sites.

Ayurveda

Ayurvedic Foundations

http://www.ayur.com/
    Workshops, tapes and counseling about the Ayurvedic lifestyle.

Ayurvedic Health Center Online

http://www.ayurvedic.com/

Ayurvedic Resource List

http://www.ayur.com/practitioner/index.html

Good Care Inc.

http://www.technimed.com/GoodEarth/
    Herbs, massage oils, teas, and other products for the Ayurvedic market.

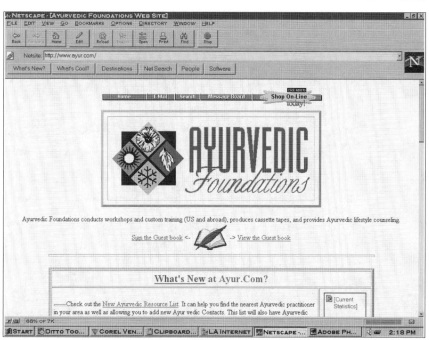

Ayurvedic Foundations. *http://www.ayur.com/*

Complementary Medicine

Complementary Medicine Directory

http://www.peinet.pe.ca/homepage/Health/vhccomp.html

A major key in complementary medicine is a good patient/provider relationship. This site describes some of the most popular alternative therapies, from acupuncture to yoga.

General Complementary Medicine References

http://www.forthrt.com/~chronicl/archiv.htm

Links to many complementary medicine resources. Includes general and specific physical/body and mind/spirit focused medicine resources, e-zines, journals, newsletters, newsgroups, discussion groups, mailing lists, organizations and related links.

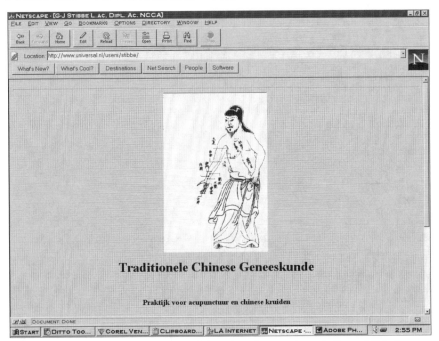

Dutch Site on Traditional Chinese Medicine. *http://www.universal.nl/users/stibbe/*

Eastern Medicine

ChinaMed: The Scientific Information Centre on Traditional Chinese Medicine

http://ourworld.compuserve.com/homepages/chinamed/

Abstracts of laboratory, clinical and scientific research on general traditional Chinese medicine, herbal medicine, dietetics and many specialties.

Chinese Herb and Health Discussion Forum

http://geog.hkbu.edu.hk/health/listinfo.txt

To subscribe, send e-mail to: majordomo@geog.hkbu.edu.hk and write: "subscribe herb yourname" in the body of the note.

Chinese Medical News

http://www.dmu.ac.uk/ln/cmn/

Free, bi-monthly publication.

Chinese Medicine

http://hanwei.com/culture/medic.htm

East Meets West International

http://www.eastmeetswest.com/

European University of Chinese Medicine

http://www.eucm.org/sinobiology/

Foundation for Traditional Chinese Medicine

http://www.rscom.com/tcm/ftcm.htm

Or Med Mailing List WWW Page

ftp://ftp.cts.com/pub/nkraft/ormed.html
> Information on the mailing list, as well as FAQs, archive and articles.

Tibetan Studies WWW Virtual Library

http://coombs.anv.edu.au/WWWVL-TibetanStudies.html

Traditional Chinese Acupuncture Information (Dutch)

http://www.universal.nl/users/stibbe/

General Topics

Alive and Well Institute of Conscious Body Work

http://iplex.com/adler/aliveandwell/

Alternative Medicine Digest

http://alternativemedicine.com/
> Online journal.

Alternative Medicine Homepage

http://www.pitt.edu/~cbw/altm.html

Ask NOAH About: Alternative (Integrative) Medicine

http://www.noah.cuny.edu/alternative/alternative.html

Many links to alternative medicine internet sites. Gathered by NOAH, the New York Online Access to Health.

Auto Urine Therapy

http://www.samart.co.th/hps/hurine.htm

Conscious Choice

http://www.consciouschoice.com/

Bi-monthly magazine that reports on environmental issues and natural alternatives in health care, food, and nutrition.

Directory of Healing Arts and Sciences

http://www.bbc.org/~rcarr/Organizer/learn.html

Dr. Bower's Complementary and Alternative Medicine Home Page

http://galen.med.virginia.edu/~pjb35/complementaryHomePage.html

Exploratory Centers for Alternative Medicine Research

gopher://gopher.nih.gov:70/00/res/nigh-guide/rfa-files/RFA-OD-94-004/

Guide from the National Institutes of Health.

Feldenkrais Method Web Pages

http://www.feldenkrais.com/

Gerson Therapy

http://www.gerson.org/

This site provides information about Gerson therapy, which is a nutrition-based and detoxifying medical treatment for cancer care, heart disease, diabetes and other degenerative diseases.

Health Source

http://www.healthsource.com/

Natural health care products, information, and internet services.

Natural Health and Longevity. *http://www.all-natural.com/*

Hemi-Sync

http://www.monroe-inst.com/programs/hemi-sync.html

According to this site, "Hemi-Sync effectively concentrates the inherent resources of your mind, brain and body" for an enormous number of uses, from greater emotional well-being, sleeping better, deeper transcendent experiences, better mental performance, and easier pregnancy. It claims to work by adjusting vibration frequencies that affect human brain wave patterns.

Horizon Quest Pure Pollen Extract

http://floralsnw.ark.com/health.html

Hypnosis.com

http://www.hypnosis.com/

Jim Sease's Kombucha Home Page

http://www.sease.com/kombucha/index.html

Kombucha tea is considered a health elixir.

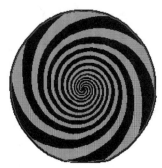

Hypnosis.Com.
http://www.hypnosis.com/

Living Soils Northeast, Inc.
http://www.livingsoilsne.com/
This company sells and discusses the healthful uses of wheatgrass.

Medical Astrology Catalog of Books
http://www.astroamerica.com/medical.html

Meditopia!
http://www.meditopia.com/

Mind-Body Medicine
http://www.fis.utoronto.ca/~mckenzie/documents/mind-body.html

Natural Health and Longevity
http://www.all-natural.com/
Information on natural health, complementary medicine, healing methods, and holistic health.

Natural Health and Nutrition Shop
http://www.pixi.com/~gedwards/health/
welcome.html

Natural Medicine, Complementary Health Care and Alternative Therapies
http://www.teleport.com/~amrta/

Natural Remedies and Products
http://nrd.com/maindir.html#sect4

New Age
http://www.newage.com/
Holistic health resources. Includes journal and marketplace.

Noah's Natural Foods Home Page
http://www.interlog.com/~noah/
Supplies herbs and herbal products.

Oxygen and Ozone Therapies

http://www.oxytherapy.com/

Shamanism

http://deoxy.org/shaman.htm

Shiatsu: Therapeutic Art of Japan

http://www.doubleclickd.com/shiatsu.html

Skeptics Sanctuary

http://user.itl.net/~brian/scepfr.htm

>Site expresses doubts about alternative medical practices..

Yahoo's Alternative Medicine

http://www.yahoo.com/Health/Alternative_Medicine/

>Covers everything from acupuncture, to music therapy to... urine therapy(?).

Herbal Medicine

Algy's Herb Page

http://www.algy.com/herb/index.html

Common Kitchen Herbal Remedies

http://watarts.uwaterloo.ca/~ijrosens/kitchenherbs.html

Essential Garden

http://essentialgarden.com/

Garden Forum: Herbs

http://www.gardenweb.com/forums/herbs/

Henriette's Herbal Homepage

http://sunsite.unc.edu/herbmed/

HerbNET

http://www.HerbNET.com/

>Information about herbs, herbal products, remedies, and more.

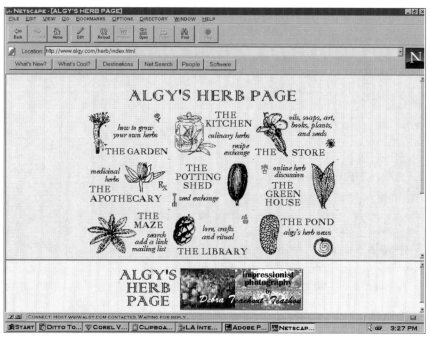

Algy's Herb Page. *http://www.algy.com/herb/index.html*

Herbs for Healing

http://watarts.uwaterloo.ca/~ijrosens/herbs.html

HerbWeb

http://www.herbweb.com/

Reference Guide for Herbs

http://www.realtime.net/anr/herbs.html

Southwest School of Botanical Medicine

http://chili.rt66.com/hrbmoore/HOMEPAGE/HomePage.html

Images, folios, manuals, journals, and pharmacology resources on the medicinal uses of plants.

Well Being Journal

http://essentialgarden.com/wbj/

A bi-monthly journal on herbal health.

World of Herbs
http://pages.prodigy.com/FL/Tampa/lemon/hercoi.htm
> Great list of internet links with descriptions.

Holistic Medicine

Aesclepian Chronicles
http://www.forthrt.com/~chronicl/homepage.html
> Synergistic Health Center.

American Holistic Medical Association
http://www.doubleclickd.com/about_ahma.html

Hidden Spirit Holistic Health Center
http://acxes.com/hiddenspirit.hhc.html

Holistic Dental Association
http://simwell.com/hda/

Holistic Healing Web Page
http://www.tiac.net/users/mgold/health.html
> Articles, weblinks, mailing lists, conferences and more about holistic health.

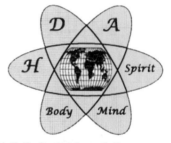

Holistic Dental Association.
http://simwell.com/hda/

Holistic Health Care Books
http://www.allcreaturesonline.com/booklist.htm

Holistic Internet Community
http://www.holistic.com/~holistic/

Holistic M.D.
http://www.consciouschoice.com/holisticmd/index.html

WorldWide Wellness: Internet Resources for Wholeliving
http://www.wholesliving.com/

Homeopathy

Homeopaths Without Frontiers
http://antenna.nl/homeoweb/noborder.html
Organization of volunteers that provide international homeopathic medical services.

Homeopathy
http://www.healthy.net/clinic/therapy/homeopat/index.html
Introduction to homeopathy, homeopathic remedies and treatment, and homeopathic research and resources.

Homeopathy Articles
http://lifematters.com/homeointro.html
A series of articles on homeopathy.

Homeopathy Homepage
http://www.dungeon.com/~cam/homeo.html
Resources and frequently asked questions (FAQs), references, mailing lists, and newsgroups regarding complementary medicine and homeopathy, in languages ranging from Czech and Polish to English.

Homeopathy Mailing List
http://www.dungeon.com/~cam/homlist.html
Information about the mailing list and archive as well as FAQs, etc.

Homeopathy Mailing List Archives
ftp://ftp.lyghtforce.com/pub/homeo/archives/by_subject/
To subscribe, send an e-mail to: Homeopathy-request@dungeon.com and type "subscribe" in the subject line.

Homeopathy Online
http://www.lyghtforce.com/homeopathyonline/
A journal of homeopathic medicine.

Homeoweb Home Page
http://antenna.nl/homeoweb/index.html

National Center for Homeopathy
http://www.healthy.net/pan/pa/homeopathic/natcenhom/index.html

Leeches

Bloodletting
*http://www.library.ucla.edu/libraries
/biomed/his/blood/blood1.htm*

FAQ about Leeches and Anticlotting Agents
*http://outcast.gene.com/ae/TSN/SS/
leeches_questions.html*

Leech Neurobiology Newsletter
*http://leechnews.bio.purdue.edu/
leechnews/leech.html*

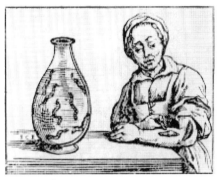

Bloodletting.
http://www.library.ucla.edu/libraries/biomed/

Massage Therapy

Art of Good Massage
http://www.maui.net/~gwr/spa/massage.html

Chinese Remedial Massage
http://ourworld.compuserve.com/homepages/CalmSpirit/tuina.html

Illustrated Guide to Muscles and Medical Massage Therapy
http://www.concentric.net/%7EOrthodoc/

International Massage Association
http://www.nationweb.com/business.ima/ima.html

Massage Therapy Homepage
http://www.lightlink.com/massage/
    Articles, links to education resources, products, and massage therapists.

Massage Therapy Web Central
http://www.qwl.com/mts.html

MassageTherapy.com
http://www.massagetherapy.com/

Therapeutic Message for Health and Fitness
http://www.doubleclickd.com/theramassage.html

Meditation

Foundation for International Spiritual Unfoldment
http://www.cityscape.co.uk/users/ea80/fisu.htm

How to Meditate
http://janus.saturn.net/~entropy/meditation.html

Maharishi University of Management
http://www.miu.edu/
This school studies transcendental medicine, yogic flying, and other holistic practices.

Meditation Mount
http://www.meditation.com/
Group meditation as a service to humanity.

Networks, Sites and Mailing Lists on Meditation
http:/zeta.cs.adfa.oz.au/Spirit/networks.meditation.html

Practicing the Presence: A Course in Meditation
http://netnow.micron.net/~meditate/

Shambhala: Worldwide Network of Meditation Centers
http://www.shambhala.org/

Stress Space
http://www.foobar.co.uk/users/umba/stress/

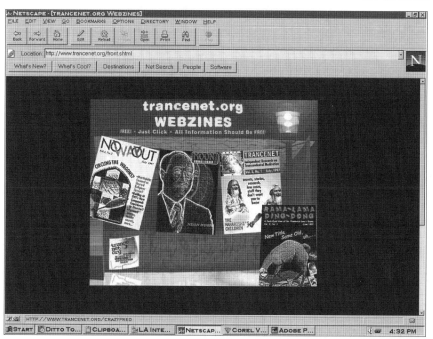

Trance Net. *http://www.trancenet.org/front.shtml*

Technique of Meditation

http://www.hookup.net/~greenr/files/meditate.html

Trance Net

http://www.trancenet.org/front.shtml
Publications and webzines.

Transcendental Meditation and TM-Sidhis Program

http://www.lmiu.edu/TM_public/TM_Home.html

What Is Zen Buddhism? A Dhyarma Discourse

http://www.inter-link.com/Dharma/nanhua/whatzen.htm
Information from the Nan Hua Zen Buddhist Society.

Naturopathy

American Association of Naturopathic Physicians
http://www.infinite.org/Naturopathic.Physician/Welcome.html

National College of Naturopathic Medicine
http://www.ncnm.edu/

Natural Resource Directory
http://www.itlnet.com/natural/nrd/

NaturMedia
http://www.geocities.com/WallStreet/1133/

Naturopathic Medicine in the UK
http://www.compulink.co.uk/~naturopathy/welcome.htm

Naturopathic Medicine Internet Resources
http://www.tiac.net/users/mgold/www/naturopath.html

Naturopathic Medicine Network
http://www.pandamedicine.com

Definition of naturopathy, directory of resources, discussion groups and newsletter, education links, and classified ads.

Reiki

Angels, Guides and Helpers
http://home.earthlink.net/%7ELightWrk11/guides.html

Center for Reiki Training
http://www.reiki.org/

Reiki Healing Energy
http://www.whidbey.com/turtle/reiki/

Reiki Threshold

http:/mypage.direct.ca/r/reiki/

Traditional Japanese Reiki

http://www.geocities.com/HotSprings/6542/

Welcome to REIKI

http://www.cyb1.com/reiki/default.htm

Welcome to Reiki.
http://www.cyb1.com/

Schools

Alternative Medical Schools

http://www.antioch.edu/~peace/studes/kcomerford.html

BIOMEDICAL ETHICS

Covered in this section: *Advance Directives/Euthanasia; Bioethics; Cloning; Medical Ethics.*

Related sections: *Death & Dying; Pain & Pain Management; Transplantation.*

Advance Directives/Euthanasia

See also: Death & Dying; Pain & Pain Management.

Advance Directives International

http://www.adiwills.com/

Choice in Dying

http://www.choices.org/
> Living will database for the United States.

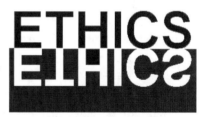

Do Not Resuscitate Orders: A Guide for Patients and Families

http://wings.buffalo.edu/faculty/research/ bioethics/dnr-p.html

Online Science Ethics Resources.
http://www.chem.vt.edu/ethics/vinny/ ethxonline.html

Euthanasia and Assisted Suicide

http://www.religioustolerance.org/euthanas.htm

Living Wills Registry (Canada)

http://www.sentex.net/~lwr/

When Death Is Sought

gopher://gopher.health.state.ny.us:70/1/.providers/.ethics/.death/
> Gopher menu containing the text of New York State Task Force on Life and the Law report entitled, *When Death Is Sought: Assisted Suicide and Euthanasia in the Medical Context.*

Bioethics for Beginners. *http://www.med.upenn.edu/~bioethic/outreach/bioforbegin/*

Bioethics

American Society of Law, Medicine & Ethics
http://www.aslme.org/

Basic Resources in Bioethics
http://guweb.georgetown.edu/nrcbl/sn15.htm

Bioethics Discussion Pages
http://www-hsc.usc.edu/~mbernste/index.html

Recent discussion-topics include cloning, physician-assisted suicide, and the definition of death.

Bioethics for Beginners
http://www.med.upenn.edu/~bioethic/outreach/bioforbegin/

Well-written and well-constructed site, offering many links.

Bioethics Online Service
http://www.mcw.edu/bioethics/

Center for Bioethics at the University of Pennsylvania
http://www.med.upenn.edu/~bioethic/

Center for Medical Ethics and Mediation
http://www.wh.com/cmem/

Conduct in Science
http://sci.aaas.org/aas-bin/wioma/scicond/

DIANA: International Human Rights Database
http://www.law.uc.edu:81/Diana/

Ethics in Biomedicine
http://www.mic.ki.se/Diseases/k1.316.html
> Lots of good information to be found at this site.

Eubios Journal of Asian and International Bioethics
http://www.biol.tsukuba.ac.up/~macer/EJAIB.html

Human Subjects/Participants and Research Ethics
http://www.psych.bangor.ac.uk/deptpsych/Ethics/HumanResearch.html

International Calendar of Bioethics Events
gopher:/rwja.umdnj.edu/ethicweb/upcome.htm

MedWeb's Search Engine - Bioethics
http://www.gen.emory.edu/MEDWEB/keyword/bioethics/bioethics.html
> Links to bioethics sites on the internet.

On-line Science Ethics Resources
http://www.chem.vt.edu/ethics/vinny/ethxonline.html

Research Involving Human Subjects
http://www.gdb.org/HTB/htb.html
> A database of research involving human subjects as collected by the Department of Energy.

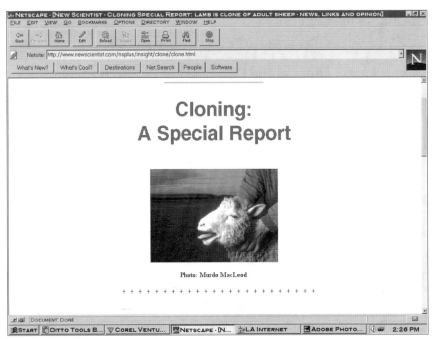

Cloning: A Special Report. *http://www.newscientist.com/nsplus/insight/clone/clone.html*

Sheffield Institute of Biotechnological Law and Ethics

http://www.shef.ac.uk/uni/projects/sible/sible.html

This site was created in response to the legal and ethical problems generated by developments in biotechnology.

Cloning

Cloning: A Special Report

http://www.newscientist.com/nsplus/insight/clone/clone.html

NPR Talk of the Nation: Cloning

http://www.realaudio.com/contentp/npr/ne7f24.html

Audio file of National Public Radio news program and interview on cloning.

Penn Cloning Site

http://www.med.upenn.edu/~bioethic/Cloning/

What's New in Nature: A Flock of Clones

*http://www.nature.com/Nature2/serv?SID=17204120&CAT=NatGen&PG
=sheep/sheep4.html*

Original research article, commentary, news items, and letters to the editor regarding the cloning of a sheep.

Medical Ethics

American Counseling Associations Code of Ethics and Standards of Practice

http://www.counseling.org/ethics.htm

Biomedical Ethics and Legal Issues

gopher://gopher.health.state.ny.us:70/11/.providers/.ethics/

Center for Medical Ethics and Health Policy

http://www.bcm.tmc.edu/ethics/ethics-newsletter.html

Library of Bioethics and Medical Humanities Texts and Documents

http://wings.buffalo.edu/faculty/research/bioethics/texts.html

MacLean Center for Clinical Medical Ethics

http://ccme-mac4.bsd.uchicago.edu/CCME.html

Medical Decision Making

http://www.uic.cdu/orgs/mdm/

Physician Codes and Oaths

http://ccme-mac4.bsd.uchicago.edu/CCMEPolicies/MedCodes/Hippo/

Role of Bioethics in Health Care Policy - Conference

http://ccme-mac4.bsd.uchicago.edu/CCMEDocs/Confs/Greenwall94/

BIOMEDICINE

Covered in this section: *Anatomy; Biochemistry; Biotechnology; General Topics; Genetics; Medical Informatics.*

Related sections: *Medical Equipment; Medical Imaging/Telemedicine; Virtual Medicine and Multimedia.*

Anatomy

Human Anatomy Resources
http://www.sunshine.net/folkstone/anatomist/anatomy/

Links to anatomy projects, products, academic resources, image collections, publications, and medical and legal resources.

Neuroanatomy Study Slides
http://www.mcl.tulane.edu/student/1997/Kenb/neuroanatomy/
readme_neuro.html

University of Washington Anatomy Teaching Modules
http://www.rad.washington.edu/AnatomyModuleList.html

Biochemistry

NetBiochem
http://ubu.hahnemann.edu/Heme-Iron/NetWelco.htm

This is a multimedia hypertext environment intended to be a complete medical biochemistry center. Tutorials consist of linked text documents with graphics, animations and sounds.

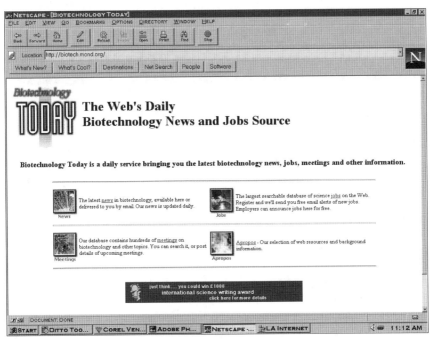

Biotechnology Today. http://biotech.mond.org/

Biotechnology

Bio Online
http://cns.bio.com/bio.html

Information and services related to biotechnology and pharmaceutical research.

Biological Data Transport: Biological Science and Product Information
http://www.data-transport.com/

BioTech
http://biotech.chem.indiana.edu/

An interactive educational resource and biotechnology reference tool.

BioTechNet WWW
http://www.biotechniques.com/

Biotechnology

http://www.cato.com/interweb/cato/biotech/

Biotechnology Information Center

http://www.nal.usda.gov/bic/

Biotechnology Information Sources

http://www.webpress.net/interweb/cato/biotech/

Extensive listing from the World Wide Web Virtual Library.

Biotechnology Links

http://schmidel.com/bionet/biotech.htm

Biotechnology Today

http://biotech.mond.org/

News, jobs, meetings and resources about biotechnology.

E-Forum of Medical Laboratory Technology

http://ourworld.compuserve.com/ho mepages/Eric_Masseus_eforum/

Health Services Technology Assessment Texts

http://text.nlm.nih.gov/

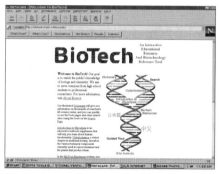

BioTech. *http://biotech.chem.indiana.edu/*

From the U.S. National Library of Medicine. Search AHCPR Guidelines, Technology Assessments, ATIS (HIV/AIDS Treatment Information Service) publications, NIH Clinical Studies, NIH Consensus Development Programs and other databases.

National Center for Biotechnology Information

http://www.ncbi.nlm.nih.gov/

Physiology and Biophysics - World Wide Web Virtual Library

http://physiology.med.cornell.edu/WWWVL/PhysioWeb.html

Includes biomedical and physical science links.

World Wide Biotech Information

http://www.aba.asn.au/links.html

General Topics

Biomedical Information Resources and Services

http://www.mic.ki.se/Other.html

Biomedical information resources and services by subject. Includes sites on specific diseases and disorders, as well as sites related to molecular biology, ethics, history and occupation.

BioSites

http://galen.library.ucsf.edu/biosites/

HistoWeb

http://www.kumc.edu/instruction/medicine/anatomy/histoweb/

Cellular images.

HyperCLDB

http://www.biotech.ist.unige.it/cldb/indexes.html

Hypertext access to Interlab Project's Cell Line Data Base which shows the cell culture availability of over 3,300 human and animal cell lines.

Journal of Molecular Biology

http://www.hbuk.co.uk/jmb/

Med Nexus Med Illustrator Home Page

http://www.med.nexus.com/mi/

National Institute of General Medical Sciences

http://www.nih.gov/nigms/

This Institute of the NIH supports biomedical research that is not targeted to specific diseases, but focused on understanding life processes and advancing disease diagnoses, treatment and prevention efforts.

National Institute of General Medical Sciences. *http://www.nih.gov/nigms/*

NRL 3D Database

http://www.gdb.org/Dan/proteins/nrl3d.html

Database of 3-dimensional structure of proteins.

OWL Database

http://www.gdb.org/Dan/proteins/owl.html

A non-redundant protein sequence database.

Genetics

Cooperative Human Linkage Center

http://www.chlc.org/

GeneNet: The Worldwide Resource for Genetics

http://www.genenet.com/

Genome Database
http://gdbwww.gdb.org/

Hereditary Disease Foundation
http://www.hdfoundation.org/
    Nonprofit, basic science organization dedicated to the cure of genetic diseases.

Human Genome Project
http://www.nhgri.nih.gov/HGP
    This is an international research program whose goal is to map the human genome and to locate the estimated 50,000 to 100,000 different genes within it. The site describes the project goals, summarizes the progress done thus far, and provides historical and bibliographical information.

Human Genome Research Centre
http://www.genethon.fr/genethon_en.html

International Centre for Genetic Engineering and Biotechnology Home Page
http://base.icgeb.trieste.it/

Master Index of Images for On-Line Mendelian Inheritance in Man
http://www.csmc.edu/genetics/omimpix/index.html

Primer on Molecular Genetics
http://www.gdb.org/Dan/DOE/intro.html
    From the Department of Energy. Also available in PDF (Adobe Acrobat) file format.

Medical Informatics

American Medical Informatics Association
http://amia2.amia.org/
    Answers questions about AMIA operations, meetings, membership, publications.

The Cooperative Human Linkage Center. http://www.chlc.org/

Department of Medical Informatics

http://www.imbi.uni-freiburg.de/medinf/mi_list.htm

Sites listed alphabetically by country. This page is maintained by the University of Freiburg in Germany.

Internet Links to Medical Informatics Sites

http://brasil.emb.newdc.us/NIB/links.htm

Journal of Informatics in Primary Care

http://www.ncl.ac.uk/~nphcare/PHCSG/Journal/index.htm

Medical Informatics and Medicine: Some Useful Links

http://www.cs.man.ac.uk/mig/people/medicine/medicine.html

Medical informatics involves the storage, retrieval and use of biomedical data and computer technology to solve problems and create models of biomedical systems.

Medical Informatics FAQ and Newsgroup Information
http://www.cis.ohio-state.edu:80/hypertext/faq/usenet/
medical-informatics-faq/faq.html

NIB News: An Electronic Newsletter on Medical Informatics
http://brasil.embnw.dc.us./NIB/nibnews/welcome.htm

BLOOD / HEMATOLOGY

Covered in this section: *Anemias; Blood Donation; General Topics; Hemophilia; Lymphedema; Pathology; Publications; Sickle Cell Disease.*

Related sections: *Cancer/Oncology; Pathology.*

Anemias

Anemia: An Approach to Diagnosis

http://www.ohsu.edu/cliniweb/handouts/anemia.html
> Outline for clinicians.

Anemias - Hypertext

http://weber.u.washington.edu/~conj/anemias/intro.htm

Aplastic Anemia

http://dpalm2.med.uth.tmc.edu/edprog/00000146.htm
> Etiology, incidence, diagnosis, pathophysiology and treatment of aplastic anemias.

Aplastic Anemia Answer Book

http://medic.med.uth.tmc.edu/ptnt/00001038.htm

Iron Deficiency in Adults

http://www.ironpanel.org.au/Acontents.html

Blood Donation

American Association of Blood Banks

http://www.aabb.org/
> Facts about blood, donations, transfusions, education, training, and AABB information.

Blood and Its Components. *http://www.jsc.nasa.gov/sa/sd/intro/blood.html*

America's Blood Centers

http://www.americasblood.org/

General Topics

Atlas of Hematology

http://www.med.nagoya-u.ac.jp/pathy/Pictures/atlas.html

View thumbnail images of a variety of blood stains, which may be enlarged to screen size. Images show healthy blood, as well as samples of iron deficiency anemia, leukemia, lymphoma, and about a dozen other kinds of blood disorders.

Blood and Its Components

http://www.jsc.nasa.gov/sa/sd/intro/blood.html

Blood basics for the public and beginning medical students.

Bloodline: The Online Hematology Resource

http://cjp.com/blood/

Contains Bayer's *International Atlas of Hematology* as wekk as a case-of-the-month, interviews and meeting updates, a professional directory, forums, bookstore of hematology and related resources, and a quarterly newsletter.

Cells of the Blood

http://www-micro.msb.le.ac.uk/imagemap/Bloodmap/Blood.html

Identify the basic blood cells such as neutrophils, eosinophils, monocytes, lymphocytes, basophils, and erythrocytes, and learn more about their activity.

Hematology/Oncology and Bone Marrow Transplantation

http://www.cc.emory.edu/PEDS/HEMONC/

Links to hematology, oncology and BMT sites.

Hemic and Lymphatic Diseases

http://www.mic.ki.se/Diseases/c15.html

Section on hematological diseases includes many links to sites on anemias, neutropenia, Job's syndrome, blood coagulation disorders and purpura. Also includes general hemic disease links.

Index of Hematology Cases

http://www.uchsc.edu/sm/pmb/medrounds/hemeindex.html

Hemophilia

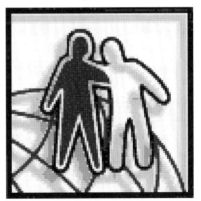

Haemophilia Forum

http://www.hemophilia-forum.org/

Haemophilia: Some Basic Facts

http://www.medicine.ox.ac.uk/ohc/Basics.htm

World Federation of Hemophilia.
http://www.wfh.org/

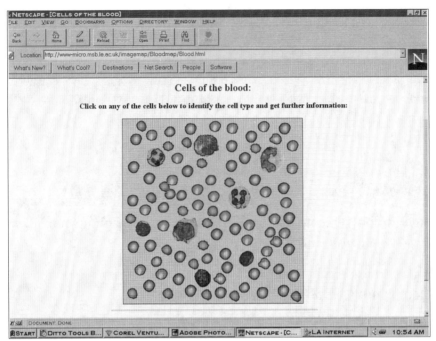

Cells of the Blood. *http://www-micro.msb.le.ac.uk/imagemap/Bloodmap/Blood.html/*

Hemophilia

http://www.geocities.com/WallStreet/1450/

Links and information about the HEMO Fact Mailing List.

Hemophilia: A Genetic Disease

http://chs-web.neb.net/usr/graham/hemophilia/index.html

The origin, etiology and progression of hemophilia, written for laymen.

Hemophilia Home Page

http://www.web-depot.com/hemophilia/AutoSite/AutoSite.cgi/

Good information on hemophilia, its relationship to AIDS, organizations, mailing lists, newsletters, legislative information, gene therapy and other treatments. Includes a section on women with bleeding disorders.

NIH Hemophilia Research Abstracts

gopher://gopher.nih.gov/77/gopherlib/indices/crisp/index?hemophilia

World Federation of Hemophilia

http://www.wfh.org/

Information and resources on hemophilia. Includes library and links, news updates, articles and press releases, frequently asked questions (FAQs) and an "Ask the Expert" department.

Lymphedema

National Lymphedema Network

http://www.wenet.net/users/lymphnet/

The Network is a nonprofit organization to educate and advise lymphedema patients, health care professionals and the general public. Lymphedema is chronic edema of the extremities due to lymph node disorders or lymph vessel blockage.

Pathology

American Journal of Pathology

http://www.at-home.com/PATHOLOGY/

From the American Society for Investigative Pathology.

Histology Lessons: An Outline of Blood

http://www.mc.vanderbilt.edu/histo/blood/

Publications

Blood: Journal of the American Society of Hematology

http://www.edoc.com/blood/

Site contains article abstracts, table of contents, and subscription information.

Blood Weekly

http://www.newsfile.com/1b.htm

Weekly newsletter with news reports, research, journal articles and summaries available online. Sample issue is available. Subscription information provided.

Sickle Cell Disease

Newborn Screening for Sickle Cell Disease and Other Hemoglobinopathies

http://text.nlm.nih.gov/nih/cec/www/61.html

Text of a National Institute of Health (NIH) Consensus Development Conference Statement.

Sickle Cell Disease: A Guide for Parents

http://text.nlm.nih.gov/ahcpr/sickle/www/scdptxt.html

An on-line booklet with valuable information and a glossary.

Sickle Cell Disease: Beyond the Pain

http://uhs.bsd.uchicago.edu/uhs/topics/sickle.cell.html

A comprehensive approach to care for people with sickle cell disease.

Sickle Cell Foundation of Georgia, Inc.

http://www.mindspring.com/~sicklefg/

Describes the disease and its prevalence in laymen's language. Describes the Foundation's education, screening and counseling programs.

BONES / ORTHOPEDICS

General Topics

Belgian Orthoweb
http://www.belgianorthoweb.be/index_uk.htm

Biomechanics World Wide
http://www.per.ualberta.ca/biomechanics/

This site covers the huge field of biomechanics and offers a large section of orthopedics links from around the world. Research, institute and laboratory sites, as well as associations are provided.

Bone and Joint Resources
http://www.orthop.washington.edu/bonejoint/zzzzzzzz1_1.html

Bonehome
http://www.bonehome.com/

Internet Journal of Orthopedic Surgery and Related Topics
http://www.rz.uni-duesseldorf.de/WWW/MedFak/Orthopaedie/journal/

La Pagina de Traumatologia & Cirugia Ortopedica
http://www.jet.es/~quique/

Spanish-language orthopedics links.

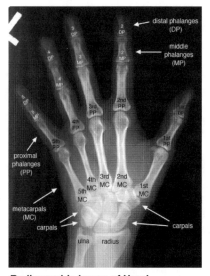

Radiographic Image of Hand.
http://www.scar.rad.washington.edu/
RadAnatomy/Hand/HandPALabelled.html

Link: Orthopaedics

http://www.dundee.ac.uk/orthopaedics/l
ink/welcome.html

"The scope of Orthopaedics is interpreted in the broadest sense and so links are included to sites covering such diverse topics as biomaterials, biomechanics, biomedical engineering, ergonomics, fracture fixation, functional anatomy, joint replacement, kinesiology, occupational therapy, orthotics, physiotherapy, prosthetics, rehabilitation, sports science and wheelchairs." Sites are listed by country and name, as well as by category.

MedWeb's Orthopedics

http://www.gen.emory.edu/medweb.orthopedics.html

Great set of links to organizations, diseases, and orthopedic-related sites.

Orthopaedic Links Page

http://virtualkamloops.com/cloughs/
orthlink.html

Aimed primarily at orthopedic surgeons and other health professionals, this site also offers information for the general public.

Orthopaedic Resident's Home Page

http://www.callisto.si/usherb.ca/~93110958/ortho.html

Orthopedic Resources

http://www.slackinc.com/bone/bone.htm

Osteovision

http://www.osteovision.ch/

Interactive information center in the bone field.

Radiographic Anatomy of a Skeleton
http://www.scar.rad.washington.edu/RadAnatomy/

Wheeless' Textbook of Orthopaedics
http://www.medmedia.com/

Features an image of a skeleton. When you click on a part of the skeleton, you get information about that bone, injuries to it and how to manage them. In addition, site offers research abstracts, radiographics and more.

WorldOrtho
http://www.worldortho.com/

Orthopedics and sports medicine sites on the web.

Organizations

Academic Orthopaedic Society
http://ortho1.uth.tmc.edu.

American Academy of Orthopaedic Surgeons
http://www.aaos.org/

Orthopedic Surgery

Anesthesia for Orthopedic Surgery
http://www.anes.ccf.org:8080/pilot/ortho/orthintr.htm

Orthopaedic Surgery on the Web
http://www.swmed.edu:80/home_pages/OrthoSurg/OrthoSites.html

Colleges, universities, societies, news and discussion groups, educational resources, clinics and institutes related to orthopedics.

Orthopedic Surgery Mailing List
http://www.sechrest.com/ortho/index.html

Site provides information on the orthopedic mailing list, but also membership directory, newsgroups, orthopedic surgery grand rounds, FTP site, and numerous

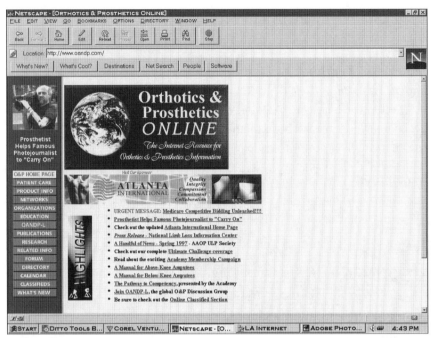

Orthotics and Prosthetics Online. *http://www.oandp.com/*

related links. To subscribe, send e-mail to: orthopedic-request@weston.com with the following message: "SUBSCRIBE Yourfirstname Yourlastname."

Orthotics

Orthotics and Prosthetics Online

http://www.oandp.com/

Osteoporosis

See also: Women's Health - Osteoporosis.

National Osteoporosis Foundation

http://www.nof.org/

    The causes of osteoporosis, as well as prevention, detection, and treatment.

Resource Center

http://www.osteo.org/

Site is presented in large type for easy reading.

Osteoporosis Information and Resources

http://www.pslgroup.com/OSTEOPOROSIS.HTM

Medical news, osteoporosis links, and related sites.

Osteoporosis Links

http://www.epibiostat.ucsf.edu/osteoweb/links.html

Osteoporosis Online

http://ntserver.ih2000.net/osteoporosis/

BRAIN & SPINE / NEUROLOGY

Acquired Brain Injuries

Acquired Brain Injury Forum

http://aztec.asu.edu/abi/welcome.html

This site serves the Arizona area, but includes a number of national resources as well.

Perspectives Network

http://www.tbi.org/

For survivors of acquired brain injury, their families, caregivers, friends and health professionals. Information, resources and support.

Anatomy

Layman's View on Brain Chemistry

http://www.maui.net/~jms/brainuse.html

This site discusses neurotransmitters, the parts of the brain that process perception and emotions, and effect personality. Information about brain size, brain tumors, and more. Written for laymen, in large type.

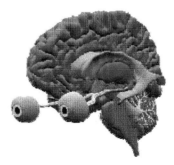

Layman's View on Brain Chemistry.
http://www.maui.net/~jms/brainuse.html

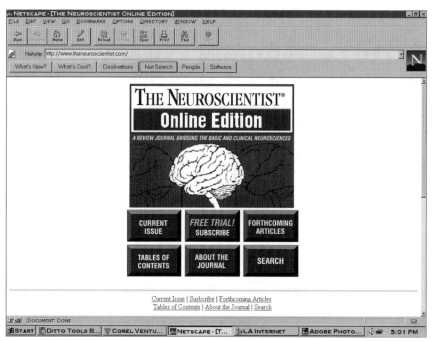

The Neuroscientist. *http://www.theneuroscientist.com*

Whole Brain Atlas Navigator

http://www.med.harvard.edu/AANLIB/cases/java/case.html

An amazing site for those with the ability to read Java.

Encephalocele

Encephalocele

http://www.icondata.com/health/pedbase/files/ENCEPHAL.HTML

Encephalocele is a congenital anomaly of the nervous system.

Encephalocele Disease Information

http://www.stepstn.com/nord/rdb_sum/867.htm

General Topics

Doug's Brain Storm
http://www.maui.net/~guestint/brainus2.htm

When a brain tumor was discovered in a man named Doug in March of 1997, he set up this page to keep others updated on his progress and to provide general information on brain tumors.

Gateway to Neurology at Massachusetts General Hospital
http://132.183.145.103

Neurological Information and Publications
http://www.ninds.nih.gov/healinfo/nindspub.html

From the NINDS Office of Scientific and Health Reports. Has much information about neurological disorders and stroke.

Neurological Services
http://neurosurgery.mgh.harvard.edu/

Clinical and educational information about neurovascular surgery, brain tumors, neurosurgical oncology, cranial injuries, spine surgery and epilepsy.

NeuroNet
http://www.neuronet.org/

Neurology online resource center for neurology professionals. To register, send an e-mail to the following address: synapse.info@ medlib.com. Sample pages are available for browsing.

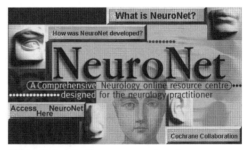

NeuroNet. *http://www.neuronet.org/*

Neuropsychology Central
http://www.premier.net/~cogito/neuropsy.html

This site describes the field of neuropsychology, which is the investigation of the brain and behavior.

Neuroscience Web Search. *http://www.acsiom.org/nsr/neuro.html*

Neuroscience Web Search

http://www.acsiom.org/nsr/neuro.html

Neurosciences on the Internet

http://www.neuroguide.com/

Neuroscientist

http://www.theneuroscientist.com/

Browse through a review copy of the online edition of this journal. Free subscription is available with registration.

NeuroSource

http://www.neurosource.com/

"The Global Directory of Neuromedicine" includes news, a library with access to neurological-related issues and links to disease information.

RebPage: The Brain in Health and Disease
http://www.uni-hohenheim.de/~rebhan/links.html

Information about the understanding, treatment and diagnosis of brain disorders.

Shuffle Brain
http://www.indiana.edu/~pietsch/home.html

Popular science articles on brain and brain transplanting; photographs of brains of humans and other animals; scientific articles, books and miscellaneous items experimenting and contemplating the activity and function of the brain.

Surgery

Brain Surgery Information Center
http://www.brain-surgery.com/

Center for Minimally Invasive Brain Surgery
http://nsi.tjh.tju.edu/MIBS/mibs.html

Gamma Knife
http://www.elekta.com/gkintro.html

Information about this non-invasive instrument for the treatment of brain tumors, vascular malformations and functional disorders. Information about the technology and procedures for use, indications treated, patient support, and bibliographical references.

Neurological Surgery: The Center for Spine Surgery at NYU
http://mcns10.med.nyu.edu/spine/spine_main.html

Includes information about some spinal disorders and their treatment.

Topics in Neurosurgery
http://neurosurgeon.com/

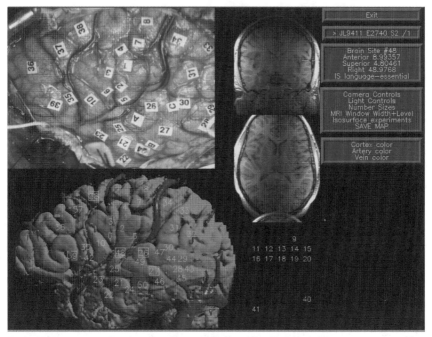

Brain Mapping. *http://www1.biostr.washington.edu/BrainProject.html*

Tumors

ABTA Dictionary for Brain Tumor Patients
http://neurosurgery.mgh.harvard.edu/abta/diction.htm

Al Musella's List of Clinical Trials and Noteworthy Treatments for Brain Tumors
http://www.virtualtrials.com/

Brain Tumor Society
http://www.tbts.org/

Primer of Brain Tumors
http://neurosurgery.mgh.harvard.edu/abta/abta/primer.htm

Virtual Medicine

Human Brain Project

http://WWW-HBP.scripps.edu/Home.html

Structural Information Framework for Brain Mapping

http://www1.biostr.washington.edu/BrainProject.html

Describes itself as a prototypical Human Brain Project application, the goal of which is to develop a system to organize, visualize, integrate and share information about human language function, and to generate the 3-D location and extent of cortical language sites with respect to a uniform, 3-D patient coordinate system.

Whole Brain Atlas

http://www.med.harvard.edu:80/AANLIB/home.html

CANCER / ONCOLOGY

Bone Marrow Transplantation

See also: Transplantation - Bone Marrow Transplantation.

BMT (Bone Marrow Transplant) Newsletter
http://nyernet.org/bcic/bmt/bmt.news.html

Bone Marrow Transplants: A Book of Basics for Patients
http://nysernet.org/bcic/bmt/bmt.book/toc.html

Lifeline Online: The Bone Marrow Foundation
http://www.bonemarrow.org/

National Marrow Donor Program
http://www.marrow.org/

For many people diagnosed with leukemia, aplastic anemia and other life-threatening diseases, their only hope for survival is a bone marrow transplant. Chances for a match are very small. To make it easier, this organization maintains a computerized registry of volunteer donors. Visit this site to find out how you can be a donor, or how to get help.

Colon Cancer

Colon Cancer
http://cancernet.nci.nih.gov/clinpdq/pif/Colon_cancer_Patient.html

Description, stages and treatment information on colon cancer. From the National Cancer Institute.

Colon Cancer Information Page
http://www.acor.org/colon_cancer/

Most of the information here relates to Stage IV colon cancer, where the cancer has metastasized to the liver or another distant organ. This site describes treatment and remission, colon/liver cancer stories, information on how to participate in a research study and how to obtain more information.

Colon Polyps and Colon Cancer
http://www.maxinet.com/mansell/polyp.htm

Common questions and answers, and information about the diagnosis, prognosis and treatment of colon polyps and colon cancer.

Esophageal Cancer

Cathy's Esophageal Cancer Café
http://www.missouri.edu/~cccathy/ec/index.html

Basic information on the causes of esophageal cancer, as well as treatment options (including alternative therapy, experimental therapy and surgery). Recommendations for special foods and nutrition for esophageal cancer patients.

Esophageal Cancer Mailing List
http://www.missouri.edu/~cccathy/ec/subscribe.html

To subscribe to this mailing list, send e-mail to: listserv@MAELSTROM. STJOHNS.EDU and in the message, write: "Subscribe EC-Group Firstname Lastname."

Seattle Barrett's Esophagus Program
http://www.fhcrc.org/~barretts/

Information and research, publications, articles and links.

General Topics

ATSDR Cancer Policy Framework
http://atsdr1.atsdr.cdc.gov:8080/cancer.html

Addresses public health concerns relating to carcinogens, from the Agency for Toxic Substances and Disease Registry.

Cancer Guide: Steve Dunn's Cancer Information Page
http://cancerguide.org/

Great place to start if you are investigating a certain type of cancer. Information on rare as well as more common cancers; bone marrow transplantation, treatment and alternative therapies; where to go for more information; and a "How to research medical literature" section.

Cancer Help
http://members.aol.com/abiaca/cancer.htm

Provides links to cancer resources located on the internet.

Cancer News on the Net
http://www.cancernews.com/quickload.htm

Includes sites of general interest, news and links to information on specific cancer types such as breast cancer, colon cancer, prostate cancer, etc. Also includes information on prevention, clinical trials, cancer support groups and research efforts. In addition, site features a Cancer News e-mail registry, where users can be electronically informed about new cancer developments.

Cancer Overview
http://www.mskcc.org/document/Cancer_Overview.htm

Cancer Patient Resources Available via WWW
http://www.charm.net/~kkdk/

Information for cancer patients, assembled by a cancer survivor.

Cancerhelp UK
http://medweb.bham.ac.uk/cancerhelp/index.html

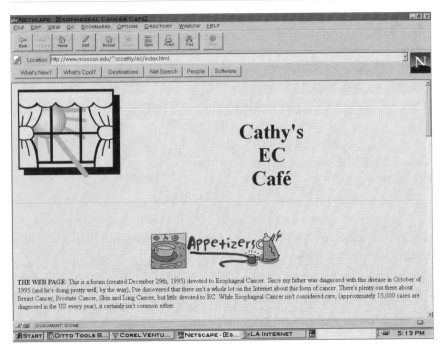

Cathy's Esophageal Cancer Café. http://www.missouri.edu/~cccathy/ec/index.html

CancerNet

http://wwwicic.nci.nih.gov/

This is the National Cancer Institute's cancer information source for patients and the public, health professionals, and basic researchers. The site offers fact sheets, treatment information, support, clinical trial updates, literature search capability, database access, and a page for children.

CancerNet Database Gopher Index

gopher://gopher.nih.gov:70/11/clin/cancernet

CancerTrack

http://www.nova.edu/~appu/cancertrack.htm

This site is a good starting place for cancer research, for it offers links to some of the bigger cancer information resources, including scientific literature, biotechnology sites, and pharmacology sites.

CancerWEB

http://www.graylab.ac.uk/cancerweb.html

A great source of information for cancer patients and their families and friends, clinicians and other health care professionals. Discusses cancer treatment, research, prevention, screening and support. Search the resources on CancerWEB, link to other indexes, or link to resources found on other servers.

CANSEARCH

http://www.access.digex.net/ ~mkragen/cansearch.html

Cancer resources from the National Coalition for Cancer Survivorship. Another great pointer to information about cancer and cancer issues.

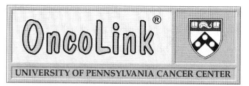

OncoLink. *http://www.oncolink.upenn.edu/*

Comprehensive Cancer Centers

http://www.cancernews.com/cancercenters.htm

Links to a dozen comprehensive cancer centers with a brief description of each center.

Guide to Internet Resources for Cancer

http://www.ncl.ac.uk/~nchwww/guides/clinks1.htm

Many pages of links to cancer-related information for the public and health care professionals.

MedWeb's Oncology

http://www.gen.emory.edu/medweb/medweb.oncology.html

A huge number of resources, broken down by topic, including kinds of cancer, treatment, institutions and research.

OncoLink

http://www.oncolink.upenn.edu/

One of the best, most highly touted information sources covering cancer on the net, maintained by the University of Pennsylvania's Cancer Center. Search research literature, link to journals and get the latest on cancer news.

OncoLink's "Editors' Choice" Awards
http://www.oncolink.upenn.edu/ed_choice

Oncology: From Web Doctor
http://www.gretmar.com/webdoctor/oncology.html

Index of links organized by type of cancer. Also includes caregiver resources, CancerLit link, and journals.

PDQ: NCI's Comprehensive Cancer Database
http://wwwicic.nci.nih.gov/pdq.htm

PDQ = Physician's Data Query. Use this tool to access peer-reviewed statements on treatment, supportive care, prevention and screening, as well as anti-cancer drugs. These statements are updated monthly. In addition, find a registry of open and closed clinical trials, directories of physicians, organizations and facilities that provide cancer care or cancer screening.

Powerlines and Cancer FAQ
ftp://rtfm.mit.edu/pub/usenet/news.answers/medicine/
powerlines-cancer-faq/

Recipes for Healthier Eating
http://www.aicr.org:80/recipe2.htm

This site is maintained by the American Institute for Cancer Research, and it provides tasty, nutritious, simple, low fat recipes.

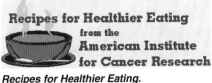

Recipes for Healthier Eating.
http://www.aicr.org:80/recipe2.htm

Kidney Cancer

Renal Cell Cancer
http://imsdd.meb.uni-bonn.de/cancernet/101070.html

Information for clinicians from MedNews.

Leukemia

GrannyBarb and Art's Leukemia Links

http://www.acor.org/diseases/hematology/Leukemia/leukemia.html

A great deal of information on leukemia, bone marrow transplant, support and resources for leukemia patients, leukemia survivor stories, and more.

Leukeamia Research Fund: Patient Information Booklets and Leaflets

http://www.leukaemia.demon.co.uk/patinfo.htm

Leukemia Information Center

http://www.meds.com/mol/leukemia/index.html

Leukemia Society of America

http://www.leukemia.org/

Leukemia, lymphoma, myeloma and Hodgkin's information and statistics, educational pamphlets and booklets; chapter finder, society and member information and events; research, patient services, links, and news and media briefs.

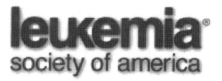

Leukemia Society of America.
http://www.leukemia.org/

OncoLink's Adult Leukemias

http://www.oncolink.upenn.edu/disease/leukemia1/

"Bone Marrow Transplant" newsletter and CancerNet updates on acute lymphoblastic leukemia, acute myeloid leukemia, hairy cell leukemia, and much more. Information for physicians and patients.

OncoLink's Pediatric Leukemias

http://www.oncolink.upenn.edu/disease/leukemia

CancerNet update and research on Hodgkin's disease, non-Hodgkin's disease, chronic myelogenous leukemia, cutaneous T-cell lymphoma, and more. Physician and patient information.

Yahoo's Diseases and Conditions: Leukemia

http://www.yahoo.com/Health/Diseases_and_Conditions/Cancer/Leukemia

Lung Cancer

American Cancer Society Lung Cancer Page

http://www.cancer.org/lung.html

The American Cancer Society describes incidence, morbidity, signs and symptoms, risk, treatment and chances of survival of lung cancer.

Lung Cancer: Understanding the Issues

http://meds.com/mol/u_lung.html

Medicine On Line offers a fact sheet on lung cancer, its causes, prevalence, diagnosis, types and treatment.

OncoLink's Lung Cancer

http://www.oncolink.com/disease/lung1/

This OncoLink web site addresses lung cancer, offering general information about the disease, as well as more specific articles on related topics.

Lymphoma

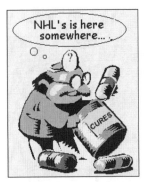

**Non-Hodgkin's
Lymphoma Web Site.**
*http://www.Westvirginia.net/
~sigley/NHL_Web_Site.htm*

AIDS-Related Lymphoma

*http://wwwicic.nci.nih.gov/clinpdq/pif/AIDS-related
_Lymphoma_Patient.html*

Information for patients suffering from AIDS-related lymphoma.

Cure for Lymphoma Foundation

http://www.clf.org/

This Foundation supports research and programs to find a cure for lymphoma.

Glossary of Lymphoma Terms
http://www.alumni.caltech.edu/~mike/lymphoma/glossary.html

Lymphoma Research Foundation of America
http://www.lymphoma.org/

Mike's Lymphoma Resource Pages
http://www.alumni.caltech.edu/~mike/lymphoma.html
   Information on Hodgkin's Disease and on non-Hodgkin's lymphomas.

Non-Hodgkin's Lymphoma Web Site
http://www.Westvirginia.net/~sigley/
NHL_Web_Site.htm

Pathfinder: Lymphatic Cancer Information
http://pathfinder.com@@0qNaTQQA@r7sM9*z/thrive/health/Library/CAD/
chronic/lymp.html
   Basic information, including off-line resources, relating to Hodgkin's disease and non-Hodgkin's lymphoma.

Melanoma

Malignant Melanoma Research Page
http://users.aol.com/zlphus/private/mel.html

Melanoma Information
http://www.arc.com/cgi-bin/Cancernet.
sh?english/patient=Melanoma
   Information on melanoma from the National Cancer Institute.

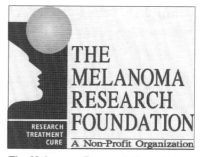

Melanoma List
http://www.geocities.com/HotSprings/
1704/marksmel.htm

The Melanoma Research Foundation.
http://www.acor.org/Melanoma/MRF/

Melanoma Patients' Information Page

http://www.sonic-net/~jpat/getwell/getwell.html

Introductory information, research, FAQs, clinical trials, articles and links.

Melanoma Research Foundation

http://www.acor.org/Melanoma/MRF/

Myeloma

Hem-Onc: Hematologic Malignancies ListServ/Support for Leukemia, Lymphoma and Multiple Myeloma

http://walden.MO.NET/~lackritz/hemonc.html

Information on and links to sites related to leukemia, as well as instructions on how to subscribe to the Hem-Onc List group, an unmoderated discussion list that primarily covers patient experiences, psychosocial issues, new research, clinical trials, and discussions of current treatment practices and alternatives. To subscribe, send e-mail to: listserv@maelstrom.stjohns.edu and in the message, type: "subscribe Hem-Onc yourfirstname yourlastname."

International Myeloma Foundation

http://myeloma.org/

Multiple myeloma is cancer of the bone marrow that results in the uncontrolled growth of plasma cells. This site provides good, basic information on this disease. Information provided in Spanish, as well.

Multiple Myeloma Research Web Server

http://myeloma.med.cornell.edu/

A multitude of information and links.

Myeloma Information Resources

http://myeloma.org/imf_ocir.html

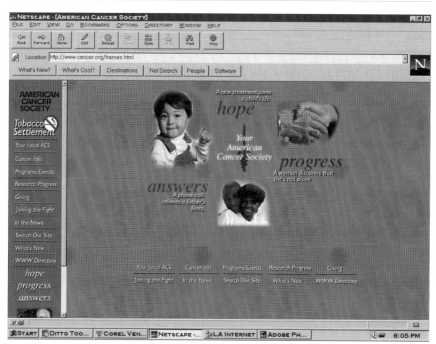

The American Cancer Society. *http://www.cancer.org/frames/*

Organizations

American Cancer Society

http://www.cancer.org/

Information on ACS programs, which include the Great American Smokeout, Relay for Life, and the Breast Cancer Network. General and specific cancer information (breast, prostate, colorectal and lung) is available, as well as cancer statistics addressing racial and ethnic patterns, nutrition and diet, environmental risks, etc. Also includes publications, meeting announcements, and links.

National Cancer Institute

http://www.nci.nih.gov/

The NCI is the federal government's principal agency for cancer research and training. It coordinates the National Cancer Program and the research efforts of various universities, hospitals and businesses, and it conducts research in its own laboratories and clinics. It also supports education and training, and collects and shares information on cancer. Links can be found at this site to CancerNet and other databases.

Pain Management

American Academy of Pain Management
http://www.aapainmanage.org/index.html

Cancer Pain Education for Patients and Families
http://www.nursing.uiowa.edu/www/nursing/apn/cncrpain/toc.htm
    Articles addressing a number of pain-related cancer issues.

Cancer Pain: Let's Talk About It
http://www.cancercareinc.org:80/clinical/page.htm
    This site is for health care professionals, and it discusses the causes, assessment, treatment and side-effects of treatment of cancer pain.

Cancer Pain Page
http://www.mdacc.tmc.edu/~acc/
    Home page for the University of Texas M.D. Anderson Cancer Center's Anesthesiology and Critical Care Department's Pain Program.

Home Care Guide for Advanced Cancer
http://www.acponline.org/public/homecare/
    From the American College of Physicians, this electronic pamphlet is for family, friends and hospice workers caring for individuals with advanced cancer who are living at home, when the quality of life is the primary goal.

Management of Cancer Pain
http://gopher.nlm.nih.gov:70/1/hstat/ahcpr/cancer/
    Advice for clinicians and patients, including a guide for patients in Spanish.

Managing Cancer Pain: A Consumer's Guide
http://text.nlm.nih.gov/ftrs/pick?collect=ahcpr&dbName=capp&t=853344865/

Pain and Symptom Management
http://www.mdacc.tmc.edu/~neuro/neuroweb/pain.html
    The AHCPR Cancer Pain Management Guidelines and other resources.

Talaria

http://www.stat.washington.edu/TALARIA/TALARIA.html

Subtitled "The Hypermedia Assistant for Cancer Pain Management," this site for health care professionals addresses issues relating to the management of pain in cancer patients. It includes guidelines, a calculator for drug conversions, links and movie clips on pain management.

Pancreatic Cancer

Pancreatic Cancer

http://imsdd.meb.uni-bonn.de/cancernet/100046.html

Pathology

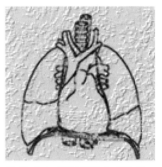

Pathology Simplified

http://www.erinet.com/fnadoc/path.htm

Good information for patients about lung cancer, breast cancer, and Pap smear tests. Includes photo archives, and hotlinks.

Pathology Simplified. *http:// www.erinet.com/fnadoc/path.htm*

Publications

CA: A Cancer Journal for Clinicians

http://www.lrpub.com/ca/

This is a peer-reviewed online journal from the American Cancer Society. View full text of articles from current and past issues. Searchable.

The Cancer Bulletin

http://www.mdacc.tmc.edu/~edpub/

Cancer Detection and Prevention

http://www.cancerprev.org/

Bimonthly cancer journal of the International Society for Preventive Oncology. Search through abstracts of current and previous issues.

Cancer Online

http://journals.wiley.com/cancer/

Search articles from current and previous issues of this interdisciplinary international journal published by the American Cancer Society. Subscription information and free sample available.

Journal of Clinical Oncology

http://www.jcojournal.org/

The official journal of the American Society of Clinical Oncology.

Journal of the National Cancer Institute

http://www.icic.nci.nih.gov/jnci/jnci_issues.html

Published twice a month. Abstracts and news summaries are available online.

Reviews on Cancer Online (ROCO)

http://www1.elsevier.nl/journals/roco/Menu.html

This journal deals with the new developments in cancer investigation at the molecular level. Both subscription and general cancer information can be obtained at this site.

Research

American Institute for Cancer Research Online

http://www.aicr.org:80/

This page discusses the relation of nutrition abd diet to cancer. According to this site, researchers estimate that 35% or more of cancer deaths are linked to our dietary choices. Find consumer information and information on AICR grants, as well as links and research news.

International Cancer Alliance for Research and Education
http://icare.ari.net/icare

Site serves as a cancer information network and includes access to cancer registry, *Cancer Therapy Review* and to research updates. Also includes a cancer newsletter, an area where patients are able to describe their own experiences, a library of cancer and related information, and areas entitled "think tanks" —where small groups of physicians, researchers and patients address therapy issues relating to specific forms of cancer.

Sarcoma

Kaposi Sarcoma Skin Cancer
http://www.lbcommunity.com/brochure/kaposi.html

Kaposi's Sarcoma
http://www.graylab.ac.uk/cancernet/201271.html

A lot of information on Kaposi's sarcoma.

Sarcoma Central
http://www.charm.net/~kkdk/sarcoma_html

General information, medical literature searches, treatment options, articles, case studies, and visual images of sarcoma.

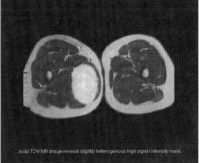

Soft-Tissue Sarcoma of the Extremities and Its Mimic
http://rpisun1.mda.uth.tmc.edu/se/sts/index2.html

Magnetic resonance images of sarcoma.

Surviving Sarcomas
http://www.geocities.com/HotSprings/4667/

Soft Tissue Sarcoma. *http://rpisun1.mda.uth.tmc.edu/se/sts/post_chemo/patient01/*

News, information, profiles, support groups and links relating to sarcomas.

Skin Cancer

Introduction to Skin Cancer

http://www.maui.net/~southsky/introto.html

Site provides a general introduction to skin cancer and offers links to specific information sources on the net. The cause for, description of and risk for skin cancer are addressed, as are diagnosis and treatment information. There is also a daily UV index forecast for 30 cities in the United States.

OncoLink's Skin Cancer

http://cancer.med.upenn.edu/diseases/skin1/

The University of Pennsylvania's OncoLink has assembled information on melanoma, Kaposi's sarcoma and other skin cancers. Online brochures and articles.

Skin and Cancer Foundation Australia

http://www.scfa.edu.au/

This site provides basic information and advice on skin cancer and its prevention. News and information for specialists are also provided.

Skin Cancer

http://www.medinfo.org/nci/cancernet/2/201228.html

The National Cancer Institute offers basic text and information on skin cancer. Includes descriptions of skin cancer, its stages, and treatment options.

Skin Cancer - An Undeclared Epidemic

http://www.derm-infonet.com/SkinCa.html

The American Academy of Dermatology text file on skin cancer types, treatment, and self-examination.

Tumors of the Skin and Integument

http://www.bioscience.org/bioscience/atlases/turnpath/skin/resource.htm

Information and resources for both clinicians and patients suffering from tumors of the skin and integument.

Support for Cancer Patients

Cancer Forum Chat
http://vitamins.net/forums/cancer/chat.html
Internet relay channel (IRC) group information for cancer survivors and their families.

Can.Survive
http://www.avonlink.co.uk/amanda/
There is an emphasis on Hodgkin's and non-Hodgkin's lymphoma, but information and resources on all kinds of cancers are available. Includes treatment and support.

Gilda's Club Home Page
http://www.jocularity.com/gilda1.html
This is a cancer support community formed in honor of Gilda Radner, the comedian who died of ovarian cancer. The mission is to serve as a place where cancer patients and their family members can share in building social and emotional support. It offers groups, lectures, workshops and social events.

OncoChat
http://www.oncochat.org/
Internet relay channel/peer support group. Also has a good list of internet cancer-related resources, sites and information to be found on the internet.

OncoLink Automated E-mail Discussion Group Subscriber
http://oncolink.upenn.edu/forms/listserv.html
Subscribe to more than 30 different listservers covering various cancers.

Treatment/Recovery
See also: Clinical Trials - Cancer.

Cancer Treatment Centers of America
http://www.cancercenter.com/
Maps the network of fully accredited cancer care centers. Provides some cancer basics, a risk profile, a glossary of cancer terms and related sites.

Complementary and Alternative Medicine Resources for Cancer

http://cpmcnet.columbia.edu/dept/rosenthal/Guide6.html

Inner Mountain Wilderness Education Center

http://kcd.com/innermtnindex2.htm

Site says that the Center "encourages adult cancer survivors to immerse themselves in the natural world, renew their trust in their bodies, rebuild confidence and vigor, and explore new personal boundaries."

National Comprehensive Cancer Network

http://www.cancer.med.umich.edu/NCCN/NCCN.html

This network is made up of 15 leading cancer centers across the U.S.

Oncology Drug Reviews

http://pharminfo.com:80/pubs/msb/msbonc.html

Updates on drug therapy for cancer treatment.

Rational Approach to the Use of Alternative Medicine in Cancer Therapy

http://www.teleport.com/~ormed/article1.htm

Text of an essay on alternative treatments for cancer.

CHILDREN'S HEALTH / PEDIATRICS

Adolescents

ADOL: Adolescence Directory On Line
http://education.indiana.edu/cas/adol/adol.html

Information on adolescent issues. Includes conflict and violence; mental health; physical health; counselor resources; and a section entitled "For Teens Only."

Adolescent Health Articles
http://www.ama-assn.org/insight/h_focus/adl_hlth/teen/teen.htm

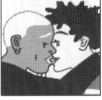

Positive Sexuality.
http://www.webcom.com/~cps/

AIDS Now! For Teens
http://www.itec.sfsu.edu/aids/aids.html

AIDS information for teenagers.

CAPS Hot Topic: Adolescents & AIDS Prevention
http://www.epibiostat.ucsf.edu/capsweb/hotteens.html

Chat-line and youth programs, descriptions, fact sheets and opinions, articles and research.

Asthma. *http://galen.med.virginia.edu/~smb4v/tutorials/asthma/asthma1.html*

Coalition for Positive Sexuality

http://www.webcom.com/~cps/

Information about sexuality for teenagers.

Asthma

Asthma

http://galen.med.virginia.edu/~smb4v/tutorials/asthma/asthma1.html

Multimedia asthma tutorial for kids and their parents. Audio and images discuss what is asthma, why it occurs, what are the symptoms of asthma, and how it is treated.

Wee Willie Wheezie Asthma Education Web Site

http://www.newcomm.net/ies/

This web site describes an educational interactive computer game created for asthma sufferers ages 5 through 12. Information on ordering the game is provided, as are related asthma information links.

Cancer

Candlelighters Childhood Cancer Foundation
http://www.candlelighters.org/

Childhood Brain Tumor
http://cure.medinfo.org/nci/cancernet/2/200047.html
> Good information about childhood tumors.

Emory University Pediatric Oncology Resources
http://www.emory.edu/PEDS/onc.htm
> Lots of links to online resources about pediatric cancer.

Guide to Internet Resources for Childhood Cancer
http://www.ncl.ac.uk/~nchwww/guides/guide2.htm
> Many links to online resources about pediatric cancer.

Jule's Home Page for CancerKids
http://www.geocities.com/Broadway/2616/

Kid's Home at NCI
*http://wwwicic.nci.nih.gov/
occdocs/KidsHome.html*

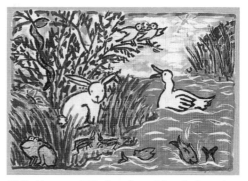

This site of the National Cancer Institute is for children's interest. It provides pictures and stories by and for kids who are receiving treatment for their cancer. It also offers information for parents.

*Kid's Home at NCI. http://wwwicic.nci.nih.gov/
occdocs/KidsHome.html*

Melinda's Page for Cancer Kids
http://www.monkey-boy.com/melinda/
> This site was created by a 15-year-old and contains lots of information, contacts, games and other fun sites for children.

National Childhood Cancer Foundation/Children's Cancer Group

http://www.nccf.org/

The NCCF is a non-profit organization that supports pediatric cancer and treatment projects. The Children's Cancer Group is a network of 2800 cancer specialists. This site includes fact sheets, information, news, resources, personal stories, and NCCF and CCG background.

National Children's Cancer Society, Inc.

http://zeus.anet-stl.com/~nccs/

This society offers financial assistance for bone marrow transplantation, donor harvest, donor search, donor recruitment and tissue typing, as well as emergency expenses and other program services to children with cancer.

NCI Childhood Brain Tumor

http://cancernet.nci.nih.gov/clinpdq/pif/Childhood-brain-tumor_Patient.html

OncoLink's Pediatric Cancers

http://oncolink.upenn.edu/disease/pediatric.html

Pediatric Oncology Group Web Site

http://www.pog.ufl.edu/

Research and clinical trials to fight childhood and adolescent cancers.

Pediatrics Childhood Brain Tumor Foundation

http://www.mnsinc.com/cbtf/

Articles, links, and Foundation news.

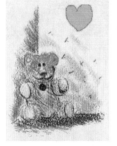

Ronald McDonald House.
http://www.multiactive.com/
McDonald/story.html

Ronald McDonald House

http://www.multiactive.com/McDonald/story.htm

The Ronald McDonald Houses are temporary lodging facilities where families of children being treated for cancer or other serious illnesses may stay while the child receives medical care at a nearby hospital. This site describes the program's start, its philosophy, and the facilities in the U.S. and Canada.

University of Chicago Pediatric Hematology/Oncology
http://rmoldwin.bsd.uchicago.edu/

This site offers great link to pediatric cancer resources..

Child Development

American Academy of Child and Adolescent Psychiatry Homepage
http://www.aacap.org/web/aacap/

This is a public service site that offers *Facts for Families*, a series of pamphlets for parents on issues that affect children. Issues covered include depression, parental divorce, abuse, violence, etc. Related topics regarding clinical practice, public health and managed care are also discussed. Find journals, publications and research papers, meetings and legislation updates here.

Behavior Online
http://www.behavior.net/index.html

Child Health and Development Information
http://www.public.health.wa.gov.au/CatChil.htm

National Institute of Child Health and Human Development
http://www.nih.gov:80/nichd/

Child Safety

Child Secure
http://www.childsecure.com/

Children's health and safety advice; "Ask the Doctor" e-mail action; pediatric news, consumer alerts, book reviews, parent's page and links to interesting sites.

International Society for Child and Adolescent Injury Prevention
http://weber.u.washington.edu:80/~hiprc/iscaip.html

National SAFE KIDS Campaign

http://www.safekids.org/

This organization is devoted solely to the prevention of unintentional childhood injuries. It includes helpful fact sheets, frequently asked questions, a check list of family safety, and an online quiz.

Protect Your Children on the Internet

http://www.med.jhu.edu/peds/neonatology/protect.htmlprotect

U.S. Consumer Product Safety Commission

http://www.cpsc.gov/

Includes a number of pamphlets related to child safety; for example, children's furniture and toy safety, child drowning prevention, poison prevention, and more. Also includes an area where consumer advertisements and items that have been recalled are announced.

Dental Health

American Academy of Pediatric Dentistry

http://www.aapd.org/

Diabetes

Children with Diabetes

http://www.castleweb.com/diabetes/

Diabetes basics and diabetes product information. Includes diabetic nutrition and a diabetes dictionary, as well as "Ask the Diabetes Team." Communicate with the diabetes community. For parents, kids and friends. Includes chat rooms and surveys, news and links, and a search engine.

Juvenile Diabetes Foundation

http://www.jdfcure.com/

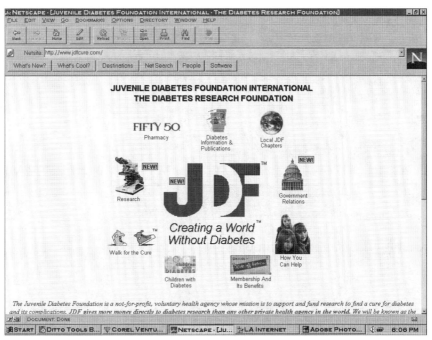

Juvenile Diabetes Foundation International. *http://www.jdfcure.com/*

Diet and Nutrition

Children's Nutrition Research Center

http://www.bcm.tmc.edu/cnrc/

Includes "Nutrition and Your Child," a newsletter, as well as research overviews, news items and links to related sites.

Disabled Children

Our Kids

http://rdz.stjohns.edu/library/support/our-kids/

Archive for the Our Kids mailing list, which is devoted to raising children with special needs. It offers information about the mailing list, as well as a reading list, nutrition list, newsgroup and network resources, adaptive technology, toy sites, and organization links.

Our-Kids List Welcome Message

http://wonder.mit.edu/ok/list-welcome.html

Archives and information about this mailing list. To subscribe, send e-mail to: listserv@maelstrom.stjohns.edu and in the body, type: "subscribe our-kids Firstname Lastname."

General Topics

Achoo! Pediatrics Links

http://www.achoo.com/achoo/practice/medicine/fields/pediatri.htm

Common Childhood Ailments

http://www.msn.com:80/MSHealth/Library/Child_Health/Common_Childhood _Ailments/

Articles about the symptoms, treatments, outlook, possible causes and prevention of dozens of early childhood illnesses.

Facts for Families

http://www.aacap.org/factsfam/index.htm

Family Web Home Page

http://www.familyweb.com/

Johns Hopkins Hospital Virtual Children's Center

http://www.med.jhu.edu/peds/pedspage.html

Kids Doctor

http://www.kidsdoctor.com/

MedWeb's Pediatrics

http://www.gen.emory.edu/medweb/medweb.pediatrics.html

Offers great links, organized by topic.

Mount Sinai Department of Pediatrics

http://www.mssm.edu/peds/www_peds.html

Features children's health internet site links.

National Parent Information Network

http://ericps.ed.uiuc.edu/npin/npinhome.html

Clearinghouse on elementary and early childhood education, including the special challenges for urban education. This site provides news and resources for parents and those who work with parents. Materials include a question-answer service available through "Parents Ask ERIC" and PARENTING-L, an electronic e-mail discussion group.

Paediapedia: An Imaging Encyclopedia of Pediatric Diseases

http://vh.radiology.uiowa.edu/Providers/TeachingFiles/PAP/PAPHome.html

PEDBASE: Pediatric Database Homepage

http://www.icondata.com/health/pedbase/index.html

Great starting point to search for pediatric health topics.

Pediatric News at Your Desktop

http://www.medconnect.com/finalhtm/pedjc/pedclbhm.htm

News summaries and abstracts. Requires registration, but it's free.

Pediatric Points of Interest

http://www.med.jhu.edu/peds/neonatology/poi.html

PEDINFO: A Pediatrics Web Server

http://www.uab.edu/pedinfo/index.html

Information for pediatricians and others interested in children's health issues. Site offers a great deal of material on disease-specific conditions, health education, subspecialties and related issues. A convenient subject search engine is also provided.

Rare Genetic Diseases in Children

http://mcrcr4.med.nyu.edu/~murphp01/support.htm

This support resources directory for parents whose children suffer from rare genetic disorders, and it offers links to hospice groups, death and dying support sites, parent-to-parent groups, respite care information, mailing lists, newsgroups and bulletin boards. Both disease-specific and more general support links may be found.

Vanderbilt Pediatric Interactive Digital Library
http://www.mc.vancderbilt.edu/peds/pidl/index.html

Virtual Hospital: Pediatrics
http://vh.radiology.uiowa.edu/Providers/ProviderDept/InfoByDept.Peds.html

Special Hearts Online.
http://www.sentex.net/~s_hearts/

Heart (Cardiology)

Special Hearts Online
http://www.sentex.net/~s_hearts/

Support and information for families of children with heart problems, cardio/apnea monitors, and pacers. Features general information, e-mail contacts and support.

HIV/AIDS

Adolescent AIDS Prevention and Treatment
http://www.mssm.edu/peds/aids.html

AIDS Information for Young People
http://www.oneworld.org/avertyoung.htm

CAPS Hot Topic: Adolescents & AIDS Prevention
http://www.epibiostat.ucsf.edu/capsweb/hotteens.html

Chat-line and youth programs, descriptions, fact sheets and opinions, articles and research.

Children with AIDS Project
http://www.aidskids.org/

Children's AIDS Network
http://www.itribe.net/candii/

Current Pediatric AIDS Protocols

http://wwwicic.nci.nih.gov/proto/pedaids.html

From the National Institutes of Health, provides the current treatment protocols for children with AIDS.

Mothers' Voices United to End AIDS

http://www.mvoices.org/

Pediatric AIDS

http://www.medaccess.com/h_child/aids/p_toc.htm#toc

Overview of research involving infants with HIV infection. Also has information on pediatric symptoms, diagnosis and prevention; AIDS in adolescents; and international pediatric AIDS research.

Pediatric AIDS Foundation

http://www.pedaids.org/

Immunizations

Ask NOAH About: Childhood Immunization

http://noah.cuny.edu/wellness/healthyliving/ushc/childimmuniz.html

Information and immunization schedule.

Childhood Immunization

http://www.os.dhhs.gov/hrsa/mchb/immun.htm

Describes the Maternal and Child Health Bureau's involvement in immunization programs.

Childhood Immunization Schedule for the United States

http://www.dynares.com/nip/child.htm

This site provides a link to the Adult Immunization Schedule.

Hot News in Immunization

http://www.kidscampaigns.org/Hot/immunenews.html

Latest national news on vaccines and immunization campaigns.

Parent's Guide to Childhood Immunization
http://www.hoptechno.com/book42.htm

Recommended Childhood Immunization Schedule
http://www.aafp.org/family/pracguid/rep-520.html
From the American Academy of Family Physicians.

VaCCINe: The Virginia Computerized Children's Immunization Network
http://galen.med.virginia.edu/~smb4v/immune.html

Infant Care

Baby Booklet
http://members.aol.com/allianceMD/booklet.html
Online information for parents of newborns.

Baby Web
http://www.netaxs.com/~iris/infoweb/baby.html

Babyhood
http://www.babyhood.com/
Information for parents on infant care (from birth to 24 months).

Neonatology on the Web Teaching Files, Outlines and Guidelines
http://www.csmc.edu/neonatology/syllabus/syllabus.html

Neurosurgery

Pediatric (Developmental) Neurosurgery Unit
http://neurosurgery.mgh.harvard.edu:80/pedi-hp.htm

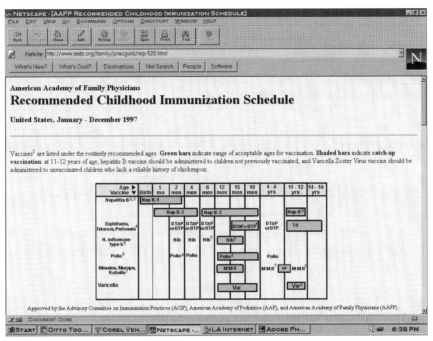

AAFP Recommended Childhood Immunization Schedule.
http://www.aafp.org/family/pracguid/rep-520.htm

Pediatric Neurosurgery

http://cait.cpmc.columbia.edu/dept/rsg/PNS/

This page from Columbia-Presbyterian Medical Center was written for parents and friends looking for answers to common pediatric neurosurgical questions. It is organized in text files on the most common conditions, from hydrocephalus to vascular aneurysms. Links to resources and support groups are also provided.

Organizations

American Academy of Pediatrics

http://www.aap.org/

Membership information, publications, family and professional resources, advocacy and research.

Institute for Child Health Policy

http://mchnet.ichp.ufl.edu/

Maternal and Child Health Bureau
http://www.os.dhhs.gov/hrsa/mchb/

Part of the Health Resources and Services Administration, this site offers Bureau information, newsletters and publications, an online forum, Federal Register notices and related internet sites.

Orthopedics

Dupont Hospital Department of Pediatric Orthopaedics
http://gait.aidi.udel.edu/

Three interactive learning modules ranging in level; for general physicians and specialists. Includes clinical services and clinical case presentations, along with pediatric orthopedic radiology lessons.

Pain Management

Pediatric Pain: Science Helping Children
http://is.dal.ca/%7Epedpain/pedpain.html

Parenting

Parent News
http://parent.net/

Parenting Questions and Answers
http://www.parenting-qa.com/

Parents at Home Newsletter
http://iquest.com/~jsm/moms/newsletter.shtml

Parent's Place
http://www.parentsplace.com/

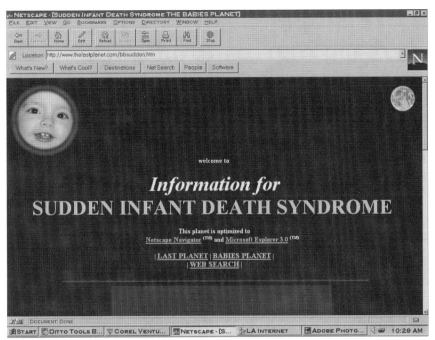

Information for Sudden Infant Death Syndrome.
http://www.thelastplanet.com/bbsudden.htm

Positive Parenting On-line
http://www.positiveparenting.com/

Tracy Mahan's Parenting Page
http://www.healthtrek.com/tracyhm.htm

Publications

Pediatric Pathology and Laboratory Medicine
http://path.upmc.edu/spp/pubs/pplm.htm

Sudden Infant Death Syndrome

American Sudden Infant Death Syndrome Institute
http://www.sids.org/

Back to Sleep Campaign

http://www.nih.gov/nichd/news/SIDS_HP_2/home1B.html

A campaign to reduce the risk of SIDS. Their major mantra is that infants should always sleep on their backs.

Information for Sudden Infant Death Syndrome

http://www.thelastplanet.com/bbsudden.htm

SIDS FAQ Archive

http://www.cis.ohio-state.edu/hypertext/faq/usenet/misc-kids/sids/faq.html

SIDS Network

http://www.sids-network.org/

Includes resources and advice for parents and siblings, and frequently asked questions about SIDS. A large amount of information.

SIDS: What You Can Do to Reduce the Risk

http://161.119.100.19/sids.html

Surgery

Common Ear, Nose and Throat Surgeries

http://kidshealth.org/parent/healthy/ent/tonsil.html

Questions and answers on tonsillitis, adenoids, ear infections and other topics for children and their parents.

Pediatric ER Cases

http://www.rad.washington.edu/PedERCaseList.html

Pediatric Surgery Web Site

http://pedsurg.surgery.uab.edu/

For pediatric surgeons and other health care professionals with an interest in the surgical care of children. This site provides access to news and editorials, CME programs, meeting information, case studies and surveys, as well as links to related listservers and web sites.

CHIROPRACTICS

Covered in this section: Discussion Groups; General Topics; Organizations; Publications; Schools.

Related sections: Bones/Orthopedics; Muscles & Musculoskeletal Disorders.

Discussion Groups

Chiro-List

http://www.chiro.org/chat/chiro-list.html

Parcelus

http://www.mbnet.mb.ca/~jwiens/paracel.txt

Mailing list for "eclectic" health care professionals, including chiropractors.

General Topics

Chiro-Web

http://pages.prodigy.com/CT/doc/doc.html

Chiropractic resources on the internet, including chiropractic research, education, networking, licensure, associations, products and services.

Chirogenesis

http://www.chirogenesis.com

For the general public and physicians. Includes information, referrals, links, and a publication.

ChiroNet: Managed Chiropractic Care

http://www.chiro-net.com/~chironet/

A PPO that contracts with insurance carriers and managed health care organizations to provide chiropractic benefits.

ChiroNet. www.chiro-net.com/~chironet/

ChiroPages

http://www.creativeye.com/icreate/chiro/

Chiropractic Glossary

http://www.bworks.com/chiro/gloss.htm

Chiropractic Page

http://www.mbnet.mb.ca/~jwiens/chiro.html

Information for students and patients, including links to colleges, organizations, research sites, mailing lists, and bulletin boards.

Chiropractic Radiology WebPage

http://web.idirect.com/~xray/chiro.html

Chiroweb

http://www.chiroweb.com

Information on and for chiropractors.

Directory of Chiropractic and Bodyworker Suppliers
http://www.makura.com/dir1/dir_top.html

Rick's Chiropractic Page
http://www.geocities.com/HotSprings/7780/index.html

Organizations

American Chiropractic Association
http://www.amerchiro.org/

Publications

Chiropractic Online Today
http://www.panix.com/~tonto1/dc.html
> Includes discussion and chat group, links, advertising and referral pages.

Chiropractic Research Journal
http://lifenet.life.edu/newlife/crj/crj.html

Schools

Chiropractic Colleges
http://www.bworks.com/chiro/college.htm
> Mailing addresses, phone numbers and, where applicable, web site addresses.

Life University Home Page
http://chiropractic.life.edu/
> Four-year academic university that teaches chiropractics.

Clinical Trials

Covered in this section: Cancer; HIV/AIDS; General Topics.

Cancer

Clinical Trials: Cancer
http://cancer.med.upenn.edu/clinical_trials/

USC/Norris Comprehensive Cancer Center Clinical Trials
http://norm41.hsc.usc.edu/Norris/Departments/trials.html
> Covers radiation oncology, medical oncology and hematology.

What Are Clinical Trials All About?
http://cancernet.nci.nih.gov/clinical_trials/trialintro.html
> *A Guide for Patients with Cancer* from the National Cancer Institute.

HIV/AIDS

AIDS Clinical Trial Results Database
http://www.actis.org/database.html

AIDS Clinical Trials Center
http://www.mc.vanderbilt.edu/dl/aids_project/actu/actu.html

AIDS Clinical Trials Information Service
http://www.actis.org/
> Current information on federally and privately sponsored clinical trials for people with AIDS or HIV infection.

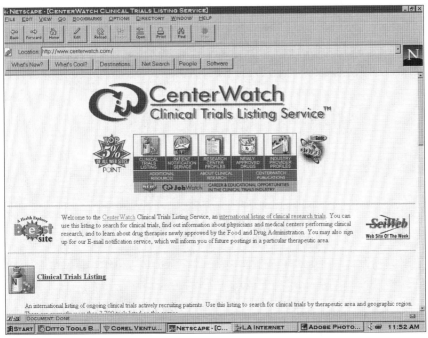

CenterWatch. http://centerwatch.com/

Canadian HIV Trials Network

http://www.hivnet.ubc.ca/ctn.html

Information on clinical trials for treatments, vaccines and cures for HIV/AIDS in Canada.

General Topics

CenterWatch Clinical Trials Listing Service

http://www.centerwatch.com/

Site describes clinical trials currently being undertaken and provides a patient notification service for when new clinical trials are begun. Also describes newly approved drug therapies, provides background information on clinical research, and offers links to industry providers.

Clinical Solutions

http://gamma132.s-online.com/sol/clsolutions

Opportunities for patients to be part of a clinical trial. Frequently asked questions, disease information, information for investigators, and a patient questionnaire.

Clinical Trials Advisor

http://www.medville.com/cta.html

A twice-monthly advisor on the practicalities of clinical trials. Offers free sample subscription, or you can read articles from a sample issue online.

Clinical-Trials Discussion Group

http://pharminfo.com/conference/cltrl.html

For professionals engaged in clinical trials, this site discusses techniques for performing, managing and analyzing them. To subscribe, send e-mail to: LISTSERV@shrsys.hslc.org and in the message, write "SUBSCRIBE CLINICAL-TRIALS firstname lastname."

ClinicalTrials.Com

http://www.clinicaltrials.com/

Attractive site offering support services, clinical trials posting, patient registry, frequently asked questions and newly approved drugs.

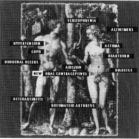

ClinicalTrials.Com.
http://www.clinicaltrials.com/

In Site Clinical Trials

http://www.insitenet.com/

Frequently asked questions about clinical trials and how to participate.

Medical Matrix: Clinical Trials

http://www.medmatrix.org/Spages/Clinical_Trials.stm

Online Journal of Current Clinical Trials

http://www.thomson.com/ojcct/default.html

Society for Clinical Trials Home Page

http://www.members.aol.com/sctbalt/index.htm

International professional organization to develop and disseminate information about clinical trials.

Trials Search: The On-line Guide to HIV Clinical Trials in California

http://sfghaids.ucsf.edu/researchlvel3search.html

DEATH & DYING

Covered in this section: Cryonics; "Dark" Humor; Euthanasia; General Topics; Grief & Bereavement; Living Wills; Organ Donation.

Related sections: Aging/Gerontology; Hospice Care.

Cryonics

Alcor Foundation and Cryonics

http://www.alcor.org/

According to this site, Alcor currently cares for 33 patients in cryonic suspension and has over 397 signed-up members.

American Cryonics Society, Inc.

http://www.jps.net/cryonics/

CryoCare: Human Cryopreservation Services

http://www.cryocare.org/

CryoNet Home Page

http://www11.pair.com/kqb/cryonet.html

Cryonics is defined as an experimental procedure for select patients who cannot be kept alive with today's medical abilities. They are are preserved at low temperatures with the hope that medical treatment will be available in the future. Site provides links to many online cryonics resources, including organizations and institutions that offer the service.

Cryonics Frequently Asked Questions List

http://www.cs.cmu.edu/afs/cs/user/tsf/Public-Mail/cryonics/html/overview.html

Life Extension Society

http://www.clark.net/pub/kfl/les/les.html

Prometheus Project

http://www.prometheus-project.org/prometheus/
> Suspended animation.

"Dark" Humor

City of the Silent

http://www.best.com/~gazissax/city/html
> Learn about cemeteries in culture, history, and art.

Los Angeles Grim Society

http://felix.scvnet.com/~highlites/grim/

You're Outta Here!!

http://www.cjnetworks.com/~roryb/outta.html
> Recent obituaries, including "Stoopid Death of the Month."

Euthanasia

See also: Biomedical Ethics - Advance Directives/Euthanasia.

Ethical Issue: Euthanasia

http://www-hsc.usc.edu/~mbernste/ethics.euthansia.html

Euthanasia World Directory

http://www.efn.org/~ergo/
> Includes a list of Right-to-Die societies, as well as a list of the patients Dr. Kevorkian has assisted. Also features news developments, statistics about euthanasia and suicide, book previews, frequently asked questions, bibliography and glossary, and other information.

The Hemlock Society

http://www.irsociety.com/hemlock.htm
> Information about the Society, which believes in the right to end one's life. Includes the organization's mission, principles, programs and services.

Index and Glossary of the Scottish Voluntary Euthanasia

http://www.netlink.co.uk/users/vess/a_z.html

Not Dead Yet!

http://acils.com/NotDeadYet/

This group fights euthanasia, especially when the disabled are involved.

Oregon Death with Dignity Act

http://www.islandnet.com/~deathnet/ergo_orlaw.html

Suicide Machine

http://www.freep.com/suicide/index.htm

Six-part article on Dr. Kevorkian; as published in the *Detroit Free Press*.

General Topics

Brain Injury and Brain Death Resources

http://www.changesurfer.com/BD/Brain.html

Death & Dying

http://www.newciv.org/worldtrans/BOV/death.html

Miscellany of news items on death and dying, as well as *The Natural Death Handbook.*

DeathNET: Advancing the Art and Science of Dying Well

http://www.islandnet.com/~deathnet/

Doctors Cry, Too

http://dr-boehm.com/ dr_cry.htm

A collection of essays on how death affects doctors.

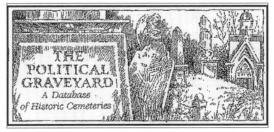

The Political Graveyard. *http://www.potifos.com/tpg/ index.html*

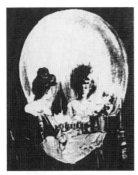

Tod (Death).
http://members.aol.com/
kmedeke/tod.htm

End of Life Resources

http://ccme-mac4.bsd.uchicago.edu/CCMEDocs/Death

Information on all perspectives regarding the end of life, including euthanasia, do-not-resuscitate (DNR) orders, advanced directives, body donation, life extension, religious beliefs, etc. Site has related essays and web links.

Essay on Dealing with Death

http://www.med.harvard.edu/publications/Focus/May12_1995/On_Becoming_A_Doctor.html

History of Cadaver Dissection

http://meded.com.uci.edu/~anatomy/willed_body/dissect.html

International Network for the Definition of Death

http://www.changesurfer.com/BD/Network.html

Medical, philosophical and psychological definitions of death.

Natural Death Handbook

http://198.68.36.114/GIB/natdeath/ndhbook.html

Political Graveyard: A Database of Historic Cemeteries

http://www.potifos.com/tpg/index.html

Sociology of Death and Dying

http://www.Trinity.Edu/~mkearl/death.html#di

Thanatolinks

http://www.lsds.com/death/

Tod (Death)

http://members.aol.com/kmedeke/tod.htm

Lots of links to all kinds of sites related to death; in English and German.

Transhumanist Resources

http://www.aleph.se/Trans/

Crisis, Grief & Healing. *http://www.webhealing.com/*

Widow Net

http://www.fortnet.org/widownet/

Information and self-help resources for widows and widowers.

Grief and Bereavement

See also: Mental Health - Grief and Bereavement; Pregnancy & Childbirth - Miscarriages.

Bereavement Education Center

http://www.bereavement.org/

Find brochure reprints, newspaper articles and web links to help deal with your own bereavement and grief, or the bereavement of children and friends. Includes information on outreach, funerals, palliative care, and suicide. Special section for helping men who have suffered a loss.

Crisis, Grief and Healing

http://www.webhealing.com/

Includes an honor page, where people write of their grief and healing process, as well as columns, discussion groups, links and a search engine.

Grief, Loss and Recovery

http://pages.prodigy.com/gifts/grief.htm

GriefNet

http://rivendell.org/

A collection of resources valuable to those who are experiencing loss and grief. Includes a list of usenet and mailing list support groups.

Pen-Parents, Inc.

http://pages.prodigy.com/NV/fgck08a/PenParents.html

Support group for grieving parents.

Willowgreen

http://www.opn.com/willowgreen/

Living Wills

See also: Biomedical Ethics - Advance Directives/Euthanasia.

Living Wills

http://www.mol.com.my/cancare/canwill.htm

Definition, description, and examples of living wills.

Organ Donation

UCI Willed Body Program

http://www.com.uci.edu/~anatomy/willed_body/index.html

Information about a program in which people can donate their body for medical science after death. Sponsored by the Department of Anatomy and Neurobiology in the College of Medicine at the University of California at Irvine.

DENTISTRY

Covered in this section: *General Topics; Implants; Organizations; Publications.*

Related sections: *Children's Health/Pediatrics; Surgery.*

General Topics

American Breath Specialists

http://www.breath-care.com/

How to treat bad breath, and/or hook up with a bad-breath treatment center.

Careers in Dentistry

http://www.dent.unc.edu/careers/cidtoc.htm

DDS-Online

http://www.dds-online.com/

Dental Consumer Advisor

http://www.toothinfo.com/

This site is intended for the public and includes advice on how to find a good dentist and what kind of dental benefits are practical. Also includes dental health basics, fact sheets, dental terminology, dental images and diagrams. Links to related internet sites.

Dental Cyberweb

http://www.vv.com/dental-web/

Worldwide exchange of dentistry-related information.

Dental Directory Service

http://www.teeth.com/

Find a dentist or a dental-related company online. Over 1,000 listings.

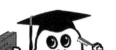

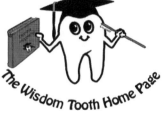

The Wisdom Tooth Home Page.
http://www.umanitoba.ca/outreach/wisdomtooth/

Dental Ethics

http://ourworld.compuserve.com/homepages/SEYMOUR_YALE/

Dental FAQ

http://www.dentistinfo.com/topics/faq.htm

Dental Globe

http://dentalglobe.com/public.html

Site advises on how to find a dentist and provides definitions of dental terminology and information about dental insurance. In addition, it offers opportunities for online chat time with a dentist and links to dental web sites written in Spanish.

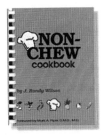

Non-Chew Cookbook.
http:// www.rof.net/yp/randyw/

Dental Icon

http://www.dentalicon.com/

Dental services, products and dealers, classified advertising, and an area devoted to professional education.

The Dental Information Home Page

http://129.146.79.87/

Dental Phobia and Anxiety

http://www.dentalfear.org/

Dental-Related Internet List of Links (DRILL)

http://www.citizen.infi.net/~dmtrop/dental/dental3.html

Dental Related Internet Resources

http://www.dental-resources.com/

Site claims to have links to over 1,000 dental resources. Topics include education, insurance, mail lists, and more.

Dental Site

http://www.dentalsite.com/

Provides links of interest to dental patients, dentists, dental assistants, dental hygienists, dental technicians, and vendors.

Dental Resources. http://www.dental-resources.com/

Dental Society Internet Sites and E-mail Addresses

http://www.ada.org/sites/ass-soc.html

State-specific dental society contact information.

Dental X Change

http://dentalxchange.com/

Information for the public and for dental professionals. Includes products and discussion forums, as well as a directory of dentists.

DENTalTRAUMA Server

http://www.unig.ch/smd/orthotr.html

Dentistry

http://www.mic.ki.se:80/Diseases/e6.html

Dentistry Homepage

http://www.pitt.edu/~cbw/dental.html

Dentistry On-Line

http://www.cityscape.co.uk/users/ad88/dentpunt.htm
   Information for dental patients.

Doctor B., Virtual Dentist

http://www.virtual-dentist.com/

Electronic Discussion Groups in Dentistry

http://www.vh.org/Beyond/Dentistry/Faculty/leslie.html

Galaxy's Dental Resources by Specialty

http://galaxy.einet.net/galaxy/Medicine/Dentistry.html

Gingivitis Disease

http://www.familyinternet.com/peds/top/001056.htm

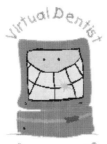

Dr. B. *http://www.
virtual-dentist.com/*

Internet Dentistry Resources

*http://galaxy.tradewave.com/galaxy/Medicine/
Health-Occupations/Dentistry.html*

Internet Dentistry Resources

http://indy.radiology.uiowa.edu/Beyond/Dentistry/sites.html
   Links to dental colleges, organizations and journals, as
well as dental education pages and commercial/dental vendor
home pages.

MedWeb's Dentistry

http://www.gen.emory.edu/medweb/medweb.dental.html
   Index containing many links on every facet of dental health.

Non-Chew Cook Book

http://www.rof.net/yp/randyw/
   Provides recipes for people suffering from chewing, swallowing and dry
mouth disorders.

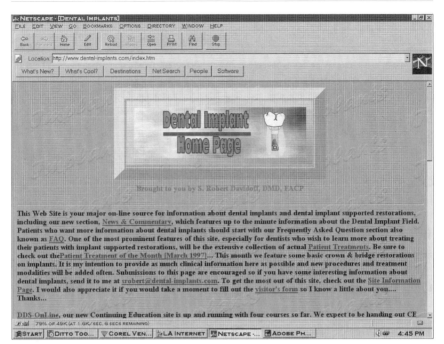

Implants. *http://www.dental-implants.com/index.htm*

Orthodontic Information Page

http://www.bracesinfo.com/

Information about braces for children and adults. Includes jokes, products, and links to other orthodontic sites.

Tooth Fairy Online

http://www.toothfairy.org/

University of Michigan Dentistry Library

http://www.lib.umich.edu/libhome/Dentistry.lib/index.html

"Virtual" Dental Center

http://www-sci.lib.uci.edu/HSG/Dental.html

This site includes numerous resources including medical and dental dictionaries and glossaries, a dental anatomy browser, teaching files and tutorials, and dental images.

WHO Oral Health Country Profile Programme

http://www.whocollab.odont.lu.se./index.html

Wisdom Tooth Home Page

http://www.umanitoba.ca/outreach/wisdomtooth/

A page primarily for children that includes frequently asked questions (FAQs) and tips on proper oral health care. Offers a special section for parents.

Implants

Dental Implant Home Page

http://www.dental-implants.com/

Implant Dentistry Information Services

http://www.implantdentistry.com/

Oral Implantology

http://www.personal.u-net.com/~implants/

Basic information about oral implants.

Organizations

American Association of Pediatric Dentistry Online

http://aapd.org/

This page provides parent, media and member information on pediatric dentistry, including internet links and publications, as well as links to kids' pages and to an online dental-themed coloring book.

American Dental Association Online

http://www.ada.org/

Find information for both consumers and professionals about dental care products and services, as well as news updates and links to related internet sites.

National Institute of Dental Research

http://www.nidr.nih.gov/

Research, news, publications, funding and health information relating to oral and dental health. Part of the National Institutes of Health.

Publications

Dental News Digest

http://www.ada.org/dnewdig/dnd-menu.htm

Dentalbytes Mag-E-Zine

http://www.dentalbyte.com/
  A bi-monthly online journal.

Dentistry Tomorrow

http://dentistry.mal.it/dentistry/index.html

  This international dental journal is available online in English and Italian. Read articles from the current issue or draw from the archives.

DIABETES

Blood Sugar

Goals for Blood Sugar Control
http://www.joslin.harvard.edu/wbggoal.html

Questions to ask Your Doctor about Blood Sugar Control
http://www.niddk.nih.gov/Questions/Questions.html

Diet

Diabetes and a Vegetarian Diet
http://www.envirolink.org/arrs/VRG/diabetes.html

Online article explaining the basics of diabetes. It covers general nutritional advice, including the goals of the diabetic diet, good sources for fiber and the effects of alcohol. The general idea is to limit (or eliminate) animal fat, to control blood lipid levels and weight, and to keep carbohydrate and fiber intake high.

Discussion Groups

Diabetic Mailing List Home Page
http://www.Lehigh.EDU/lists/diabetic/

Subscription information, frequently asked questions (FAQs), and archives. To subscribe, send e-mail to: listserv@lehigh.edu and in the message type: "SUBSCRIBE DIABETIC Yourname."

Diabetes and Hypoglycemia Forum on CompuServe

http://ourworld.compuserve.com:80/homepages/Curtise/

USENET FAQ's on Diabetes

http://www.cis.ohio-state.edu/hypertext/faq/usenet/diabetes/top.html

Eye Care

Diabetes and Your Eyes

http://www.jdfcure.com/brch14.htm

Don't Lose Sight of Diabetic Eye Disease

http://www.niddk.nih.gov/DiabeticEyeDisease/DiabeticEyeDisease.html
Important information for people with diabetes.

General Topics

AADEnet

http://www.addenet.org/
The American Association of Diabetes Educators home page.

Bob's Good Diabetes Stuff

http://www.orphanage.com/goodstuff/diabetes/diabetes.shtml

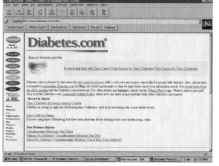

Diabetes.com. *http://www.diabetes.com/site/*

Diabetes.com

http://www.diabetes.com/site/

Diabetes Homepage

http://www.nd.edu/~hhowisen/diabetes.html
Over 70 diabetes-related links and 200 e-mail addresses of diabetics. Lots of information and chat rooms.

Living with Diabetes. *http://www.macatawa.org/~tdr/*

Diabetes Information

http://www.lilly.com/diabetes/

For health care professionals, patients and consumers.

Diabetes Information Page

http://www.geocities.com/Athens/
Forum/5769/diabete.html

Diabetes Insipidus and Related Disorders Network

http://members.aol.com/ruudh/dipage1.htm

Diabetes Mall

http://www.diabetesnet.com/

Diabetic products and publications, information and links.

Diabetes Mellitus: Links

http://www.pharmiq.com/pat/htmlpage/dm.htm

Links to diabetes-related materials, including background, diet, children, management, exercises and organizations.

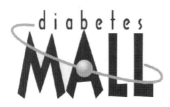

Diabetes Mall. *http://www.*
diabetesnet.com/

Diabetes Mellitus Tutorial
http://www-medlib.med.utah.edu/WebPath/
TUTORIAL/DIABETES/DIABETES.html

Diabetes Self-Management
http://www.enews.com/magazines/diabetes/
Online magazine.

Diabetic Data Centre
http://www.demon.co.uk/diabetic/index.html
   Good information, news, frequently asked questions (FAQs) and pages for children.

DM Survey
http://members.aol.com/DMSurvey/index.htm
   New online experiment to gather and share information about diabetes among "diabetic netizens."

Doctor's Guide: Diabetes Information and Resources
http://www.pslgroup.com/DIABETES.htm
   Lots of news and medical alerts. Information on diabetes for patient education and health care professionals.

Facts about Diabetes
http://www.novo.dk/backgrou/backgrou/badia1uk.htm

Family's Guide to Diabetes
http://www.geocities.com/HotSprings/1962/
   A guide for diabetic kids and their families, based on experience.

Joslin's Online Diabetes Library
http://www.joslin.harvard.edu/wlist.html

Living with Diabetes
http://www.macatawa.org/~tdr/
   Diabetes discussion, questions and answers, penpals, news, recipes and links.

National Diabetes Information Clearinghouse

http://www.niddk.nih.gov/Brochures/NDIC.htm

Includes "Diabetes Dateline" newsletter, *The Diabetes Dictionary*, bibliographies, and links to the Combined Health Information Database (CHID).

On-line Resources for Diabetics

http://www.cruzio.com/~mendosa/fq.htm

All about mailing lists, newsgroups and chat rooms for people interested in diabetes.

Patient Information on Diabetes

http://www.niddk.nih.gov/DiabetesDocs.html

Lots of information about diabetes, diabetes control, complications, kidney diseases, support and research information. Links to the National Diabetes Information Clearinghouse.

Reducing the Burden of Diabetes

http://www.cdc.gov/nccdphp/ddt/ddthome.htm

Diabetes basics and advice from the Centers for Disease Control.

Organizations

American Diabetes Foundation

http://www.diabetes.org/

The mission of the ADF is to prevent and cure diabetes and to improve the lives of all people affected by the disease. The site provides information for people with diabetes types I and II, as well as for their families, teachers, child-care providers and health professionals. "Living with Diabetes" addresses issues of sex, pregnancy, parenting, complications and nutrition. ADF research programs and grant support is also described. Legislation news and updates are offered in the form of a newsletter, "Diabetes Advocate." Another monthly publication, *Diabetes Forecast*, presents the latest diabetes research and treatment news as well as day-to-day coping issues. Browse current and past issues, or subscribe. Links to related sites.

International Diabetic Athletes Association
http://www.genet.com/~idea/

Having diabetes doesn't mean a person can't be physically active, as this association proves.

National Institute of Diabetes and Digestive and Kidney Diseases
http://www.niddk.nih.gov/

This site provides health information for the public about diabetes, digestive diseases, endocrine and metabolic diseases, hematological and kidney diseases, nutrition and obesity, and urologic diseases. In addition, it offers clinical information and databases, news, and funding resources for health professionals.

National Kidney Foundation
http://www.kidney.org/diab.html

Includes facts about diabetes and kidney disease.

Organizations Offering (Diabetes) Support
http://www.demon.co.uk/diabetic/orgs.html

Organizations are listed geographically.

Publications

Diabetes Interview World
http://www.diabetesworld.com

Publication comes out every two months. Subscription information and articles are available at this web site.

Diabetes Monitor
http://www.mdcc.com/

Diabetic Gourmet Magazine
http://gourmetconnection.com/ezine/diabetic

Good recipes for those on a restricted diet.

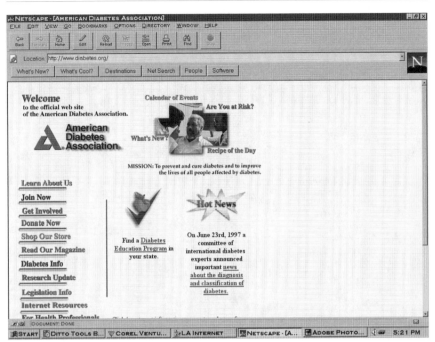

American Diabetes Association. *http://www.diabetes.org/*

Research

Academy for the Advancement of Diabetes Research and Treatment

http://drinet.med.miami.edu/

Diabetes Action Research and Education Foundation

http://www.daref.org/

Diabetes Education and Research Center

http://www.libertynet.org/~diabetes/

Includes frequently asked questions (FAQs), tips for individuals with the disease, and a diabetes chat area.

DIET & NUTRITION

Celiac Diet

See also: Digestive Disorders - Celiac Disease.

Celiac Support Page

http://www.celiac.com/

Celiac disease is gluten or wheat intolerance. This site provides frequently asked questions, overview of the disease, and support, as well as lists of similar diseases, recipes and cooking tips and doctors who specialize in its treatment.

Information for Gluten-free and Wheat-free Diets

http://www.wwwebguides.com/nutrition/diets/glutenfree/index.html

Fat Acceptance

Big Folks Health FAQ

http://www.cis.ohio-state.edu/hypertext/faq/usenet/fat-acceptance-faq/health/ faq.html

Brotherhood of Girth

http://home.sprynet.com/sprynet/imac/

Network of overweight men looking to experience life to its fullest.

Fat-Acceptance FAQs

http://www.cs.ruu.nl/wais/html/na-dir/fat-acceptance-faq/.html

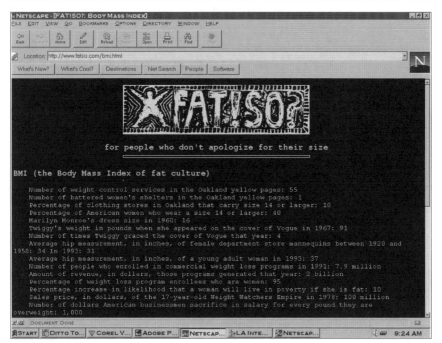

Fat! So? http://www.fatso.com

Fat Acceptance Stuff
http://www.wolfenet.com/~marymc/fatacc.htm

Fat Acceptance Support
http://www.comlab.ox.ac.uk/oucl/users/sharon.curtis/BF/SSFA/home.html

Fat Friendly Health Professionals List
http://www.bayarea.net/~stef/Fat/ffp.html

Alphabetical list (by country, state and city) of health professionals that some fat people have deemed fat friendly or who declared themselves fat friendly.

Fat Person's Home Page
http://www.io.com/~joeobrin/fat.html

Fat! So?
http://www.fatso.com/

Web-zine for individuals who are not ashamed of their weight.

Largesse: The Network for Size Esteem

http://www.fatso.com/fatgirl/largesse/

This site is described as a resource center and clearinghouse for "size diversity empowerment."

Lee Martindale's Rump Parliament

http://web2.airmail.net/lmartin/

Veteran size rights advocate.

National Association to Advance Fat Acceptance

http://www.naafa.org/

Radiance: The Magazine for Large Women

http://www.radiancemagazine.com/

Read back issues and get subscription information.

Food Allergies

See also: Allergies/Immunology.

Food Allergy and Intolerance

http://www.xs4all.nl/~maxdes/health/food-int/food-int.html

The Food Allergy Network

http://www.foodallergy.org/

Great Recipes for People with Food Allergies and Intolerances

http://www2.skyisland.com/skyisland/recipes/index.html

Mastering Food Allergies

http://www.nidlink.com/~mastent/

Food Safety

See also: Public Health.

Food Safety Consortium

http://www.uark.edu/depts/fsc/

The
**National Food
Safety Database**
World Wide Web Site

The National Food Safety Database.
http://www.foodsafety.org/

FoodLaw

*http://www.ift.org/divisions/foo
d_law/*

Food laws and regulations.

Institute of Food Technologists

http://www.ift.org/

The society for food science and technology has a web site that offers career information, publications and scientific communications, as well as meetings, membership and employment news.

National Center for Food Safety and Technology

http://www.iit.edu/~ncfs/

National Food Safety Database

http://www.foodsafety.org/

Food safety materials for consumers, the food industry, and educators, along with coverage of critical issues in food safety.

General Topics

Absolute Health Secrets

http://www.juiceguy.com/healthinfo/

American Society for Clinical Nutrition

http://www.faseb.org/ascn/

The goal of this organization is to promote nutritional education among medical and health care professionals. It presents several press releases and a position paper on trans fatty acids.

Arbor Nutrition Guide

http://netspace.net.au/%7Ehelmant/index.htm

Catalog of internet nutrition resources.

Ask the Dietician

http://www.dietician.com/

Nutritional advice.

Blonz Guide: Nutrition, Food and Health Resources

http://www.blonz.com/blonz/index.html

Site offers a large number of resources on varying subjects. Some topics include nutrition, food and fitness resources and associations; food resources, companies and associations; health and medical resources and associations; online newspapers, magazines and networks; government resources, U.S. and other; food and nutrition discussion groups; health, medical and wellness publications; nutrition resources; and agriculture and gardening resources.

CyberDiet

http://www.cyberdiet.com/

Nutritional profile, food court, and Fast Food Quest. Includes a device that tells nutritional content of popular fast-food items.

Dietetics Online

http://www.dietetics.com/

Information on nutrition and the dietetic profession.

Dole 5-a-Day Homepage

http://www.dole5aday. com/

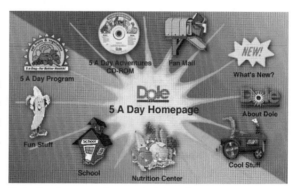

Dole 5-a-Day. *http://www.dole5aday.com/*

Dole sponsors this site for children, to remind them to eat five servings of fruit and vegetables every day. According to research, the health benefits of eating fruit and vegetables are indisputable, but Americans average only half of the recommended five servings. Along with some basic information, the site offers fun stuff for kids, using custom characters to tell details about asparagus, apples, bananas, blueberries, broccoli, cauliflower, carrots and other fruits and veggies.

Eating Plan for Healthy Americans

http://www.amhrt.org/pubs/ahadiet.html

The latest advice from the American Heart Association. Also find news and web resources, and the AHA's *Heart and Stroke A-Z Guide*.

Food Pyramid Guide

http://www.ganesa.com/food/index.html

Click on a food group to get a brief description of what is included as well as recommended serving suggestions.

Full USDA Nutrient Database Listings

http://www.fatfree.com/usda/all.shtml

Gourmet Connection Magazine

http://gourmetconnect.com/

Gourmet food and health news, advice, recipes, columns, articles and features.

Grand Style Spa

http://www.grandstyle.com/spa.htm

Promoting a healthy lifestyle, no matter what your weight.

International Food Information Council

http://ificinfo.health.org/

Food safety and nutritional information, including facts about food labeling, food allergies. The purpose of the IFCC is to provide sound and scientific information on food safety and nutrition for journalists, health professionals, educators, government officials and consumers.

Internet FDA

http://www.fda.gov/

Information about the U.S. Food and Drug Administration and product alerts.

Krispin Komments on Nutrition and Health

http://www.krispin.com/

This site provides information on potassium and protein and the sources from which they can be derived. Also find information on thyroid disease and an article linking abuse and nutrition.

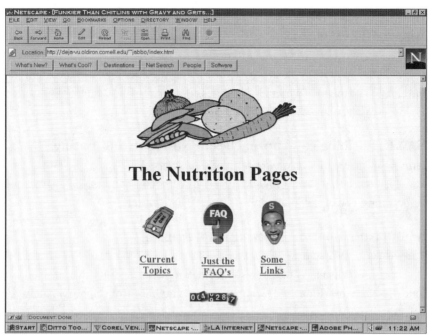

The Nutrition Pages. http://deja-vu.oldiron.cornell.edu/~jabbo/index.html

My Virtual Encyclopedia: Health and Nutrition
http://www.refdesk.com/health.html

Nutrition and Health
http://www.medlib.arizona.edu/educ/nutrition.html
A lot of information and links.

Nutrition Pages
http://deja-vu.oldiron.cornell.edu/~jabbo/index.html
Forum on nutrition articles of current interest, frequently asked questions and selected internet links.

Penn State Nutrition
http://nutrition.hhdev.psu.edu/
Graduate and undergraduate programs in nutrition.

People's Place
http://www.peopleplace.com/

Professor Geoff Skurray's Food, Nutrition and Health Information Page

http://www.hawkesbury.uws.edu.au/~geoffs/

Includes adult RDA dietary guidelines, a free dietetic simulation program and information on the food pyramid. Describes courses from the Centre for Advanced Food Research and provides exam questions.

SANE: Sociological Approaches to Nutrition and Eating

http://www.newcastle.edu.au/department/so/tasa/tasa16.htm

Discusses the social context of food with conferences, databases and associations, books and journal links.

Sound Nutrition: An International Appeal

http://www.fcs.uga.edu/~selbon/apple/guides/

Based on a display at the 1996 summer Olympics in Georgia, this site includes guidelines on nutrition and accompanying graphics from approximately 20 countries.

"Virtual" Nutrition Center

http://www-sci.lib.uci.edu/HSG/Nutrition.html

This site has a good section on nutritional calculations including body mass index, calories, heart rate and longevity. Also features courses and tutorials, links, news, journals and anatomy information.

Lactose Intolerance

Lactose Intolerance

http://www.niddk.nih.gov/LactoseIntolerance/LactoseIntolerance.html

No Milk Group

http://www.panix.com/~nomilk/

Lactose maldigestion, milk allergies, and casein intolerance: definitions, information and resources on the web.

Steve Carper's Lactose Intolerance Clearinghouse

http://ourworld.compuserve.com/homepages/stevecarper/welcome.htm

The Recipe Directory. *http://www.envirolink.org/orgs/vegweb/food/*

Macrobiotic Diet

Carbondale Center for Macrobiotic Studies
http://www.netoasis.com/health/macro/

Macrobiotics Online
http://www.macrobiotics.org/

The macrobiotic way of life is a holistic approach to health and diet. Site describes the macrobiotic diet, including its principles and philosophy, guidelines and recipes, recommendations, frequently asked questions and health information.

Macrons
http://www.macronews.com/

Phen/Fen

Note: In September, 1997, the Federal Drug Administration (FDA) removed fenfluramine and dexfenfluramine from the United States' market.

Appetite-Suppressant Drugs Can Cause Pulmonary Hypertension

http://www.bloodpressure.com/newsrsch/wrp.ulhyp.htm

Summary of article appearing in the New England Journal of Medicine.

Barbara's Phenfen Home Page

http://www.vais.net/~bhirsch/phenlink.htm

Phentermine and fenfluramine links. Includes frequently asked questions (FAQs), study reports, patient reports, information on phenfen and anesthesia, neurotransmitters and the neurotoxicity study.

Phen/Fen Pages

http://www.ulink.net/~dtison/

Information on phen/fen, Redux and other weight loss medications.

Phenfen Discussion

http://www.bolis.com/L/listinfo/phenfen/

To subscribe, send e-mail to: majordomo@bolis.com and in message, type either: "subscribe phenfen" or: "subscribe phenfen-digest" (for digest version).

PhenPhacts

http://members.aol.com/PhenFAQ/

For people using phen/fen or Redux to lose weight.

RxList: Fenfluramine

http://www.rxlist.com/cgi/generic/fenflur.htm

Description and additional information about fenfluramine, the weight loss drug used in combination with phentermine.

RxList: Phentermine

http://www.rxlist.com/cgi/generic/phenterm.htm

Weight-Loss or Health Loss?

http://www.familyville.com/bbj/phenfen/

Cautionary advice about the use of Phen/Fen.

Recipes

FATFREE: The Low-Fat Vegetarian Archive
http://www.fatfree.com/

HealthGate Healthy Eating
http://www.healthgate.com/healthy/eating/index.shtml

Mama's Pasta Glossary
http://www.eat.com:80/pasta-glossary/index.html
>From Angel Hair to Ziti. Also features links to recipes and to learning Italian.

Nutritiously Gourmet
http://www.aimnet.com/~gourmet/

The Recipe Directory
http://www.envirolink.org/orgs/vegweb/food/
>Healthy, vegetarian recipes arranged both alphabetically and by course.

Research

Purdue University Food Science
http://www.foodsci.purdue.edu/
>Describes faculty research, publications, outreach programs, and the graduate and undergraduate programs. Also provides web links.

Rutgers University Department of Food Science
http://foodsci.rutgers.edu/
>Food scientists study the physical, microbiological and chemical make-up of food, and develop ways to process, preserve, package and store food safely. This site describes Rutgers' program and the work of a food scientist. Fact sheets on safe food preparation, handling and storage, along with frequently asked questions and web links are provided.

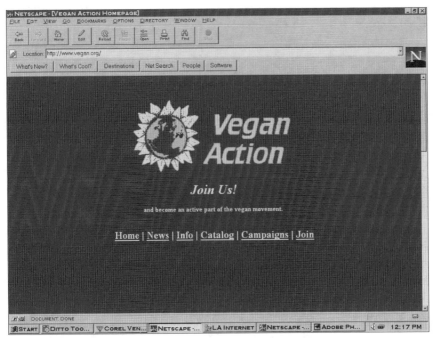

Vegan Action. *http://www.vegan.org/*

Vegan Diet

Vegan Action

http://www.vegan.org/

A non-profit organization formed to enhance public awareness of the benefits of a vegan lifestyle and to improve the availability of vegan food. Site provides information on veganism, a catalog of products and books, news alerts, campaign information and activist opportunities.

Vegan Awakening

http://www.vegan.org/awakening/

News, recipes, quotes, articles, information and a picture gallery of animals, all supporting a vegan lifestyle.

Vegan Biker's Domain

http://www.nildram.co.uk/veganmc/

Links to vegan and motorcyclist sites on the web.

Vegan News

http://www.vury-rd.demon.co.uk/

Newsletter for vegans.

Vegan Outreach Web Site

http://www.envirolink.org/arrs/vo/

Arguments for veganism, from health, ecological, theological and ethical perspectives. Newsletter and other resources.

Vegan-L's Most Frequently Asked Questions

http://www.envirolink.org/arrs/faqvegan.html

A vegan diet avoids all animal products, including dairy and egg. Living a cruelty-free lifestyle is the overall goal, and it includes avoiding clothing made from animal sources along with achieving greater personal and ecological health.

Vegetarian Diet

Mega Index to Vegetarian Information

http://www.veg.org/veg/Docs/vegindex.html

Tool for finding information on vegetarianism drawn from a variety of resources.

Vegetarian Pages

http://www.veg.org/veg/

Guide to the internet for vegetarians, vegans and others.

Vegetarian Resource Group

http://www.vrg.org/

Includes information on vegetarianism, lifestyle guides, nutrition and recipes, as well as a catalog of vegetarian products.

Vegetarian Resources

http://www.cyberspy.com/~webster/veg.html

Vegetarian Society of the United Kingdom

http://www.veg.org/veg/Orgs/VegSocUK/

Many links and good information.

The Net Loss Club. *http://www2.itw.com/~thinker/home.html*

Veggies Unite! Online Guide to Vegetarianism

http://www.envirolink.org/orgs/vegweb/

Very Vegetarian Sites

http://www.cyber-kitchen.com/pgvegtar.htm

Comprehensive list of web resources for vegetarians.

World Guide to Vegetarianism

http://www.veg.org/veg/Guide/index.html

Site lists vegetarian and vegetarian-friendly restaurants, stores, organization and services by country, state, county and city. In addition, it lists chain restaurants that offer vegetarian and vegetarian-friendly products.

Vitamins

Austin Nutritional Research Reference Guide for Vitamins

http://www.realtime.net/anr/vitamins.html

MN-NET Home Care

http://www.idrc.ca/mi/mnnet.htm

Micronutrient malnutrition information.

Prevention's Vitamin Dispenser

http://www.healthyideas.com/healing/vitamin/

Select from a number of health problems and receive information on vitamins recommended to help treat the condition.

Understanding Vitamins

http://www.critpath.org/aric/altern03.htm

This article reviews basic background information on vitamins and minerals and examines several individual vitamins that are frequently discussed in the context of HIV.

Vitamin Update

http://www.ozemail.com.au/~bookman/

Vitamins

http://www.doitnow.com/~gillick/ph05000.html

Vitamins Network UK

http://uk.vitamins.net/

Weight Loss

Burn Barometer

http://homearts.com/helpers/calculators/burnf1.htm

Circle of Hope

http://www.swlink.net/~colonel/coh.html

Open to anyone with a desire to lose weight and who is 100 or more pounds overweight. Costs $10 to subscribe indefinitely, with a free two-week trial period.

Diet and Weight Loss/Fitness Home Page

http://www1.mhv.net/~donn/diet.html

Diet and weight loss tips.

Dieter's Guide to Weight Loss During Sex

http://www.maui.net/~jms/weight.html

Have some fun!

Health Information About Fatness

http://www.comlab.ox.ac.uk/oucl/users/sharon.curtis/BF/Inf/main.html

Healthy Weight Loss

http://www.ComSource.net/~bwelch/healthy.html

Low-Fat Lifestyle Forum

http://www.wctravel.com/lowfat/

Tips, recommendations, recipes and links.

Magic of Believing

http://www.geocities.com/Athens/1953/

Weight loss support group. To subscribe, send e-mail to: majordomo@ angus.mystery.com and in the message, type: "subscribe mob."

Medical Information on Obesity and Weight Control

http://www.weight.com/

Net Loss Club

http://www2.itw.com/~thinker/home.html

E-mail support group for weight loss. Current membership is approximately 400 people. Be inspired, share stories, check out suggestions and recipes. Even if you don't wish to join this group, the site offers valuable diet advice and links.

Starting Your Weight-Loss Journal

http://homearts.com/gh/health/1196opb3.htm

Weight Watchers

http://www.weight-watchers.com/

Yeast

Candida Page

http://www.panix.com/~candida/

Links to *Candida albicans* and candidiasis web sites.

Yeast Connection

http//www.yeastconnection.com/

Information about yeast-connected (candida) disorders.

DIGESTIVE DISORDERS / GASTROENTEROLOGY

Covered in this section: *Celiac Disease; Colon; Esophagus; Gallstones; Gastritis; General Topics; Organizations.*

Related sections: *Diet & Nutrition; Eating Disorders.*

Celiac Disease

See also: Diet & Nutrition - Celiac Diet.

Celiac Disease

http://www.icondata.com/health/pedbase/files/CELIACDI.HTM
> Clinical information. on celiac disease, the inability to digest gluten or wheat.

Celiac Disease and Gluten Sensitivity

http://cpmcnet.cpmc.columbia.edu/dept/gi/celiac.html

Gluten-Free Page

http://www.panix.com/~donwiss/

What Is Celiac Disease and Dermatitis Herpetiformis?

http://www.wwwebguides.com/nutrition/diets/glutenfree/faq.html
> The Celiac Action Line fact sheet.

Colon

See also: Cancer/Oncology - Colon Cancer.

Crohn's and Colitis Foundation of America

http://www.ccfa.org/
> Information on inflammatory bowel disease.

Crohn's Disease Web Page

http://members.aol.com/bospol/
homepage/crohns.htm

General information, illustrations, articles, frequently asked questions and other resources.

Crohn's Disease/Ulcerative Colitis/Inflammatory Bowel Disease Pages

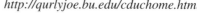

http://qurlyjoe.bu.edu/cduchome.html

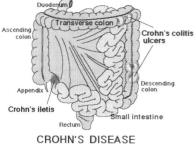

Culinary Couples Creative Colitis Cookbook

http://ourworld/compuserve.com/hom
epages/colitis_cookbook/

Disguises of Inflammatory Bowel Diseases

http://www.acg.gi.org/phyforum/gifoc
us/2eii.html

Crohn's Disease Web Page.
http://members.

Facts about Crohn's Disease and Ulcerative Colitis

http://www.ccfc.ca/facts.html

Information from the Crohn's and Colitis Foundation of Canada, presented in English and French.

IBS Page: Irritable Bowel Syndrome Web Sites

http://www.panix.com/~ibs/

Inflammatory Bowel Disease FAQ

http://www.ddc.org/pat/faqs/ibd_faq.html

International Foundation for Bowel Dysfunction

http://incontinet/adscopy/ads_nfpo/ifbd.htm

Support and education for patients and consumers.

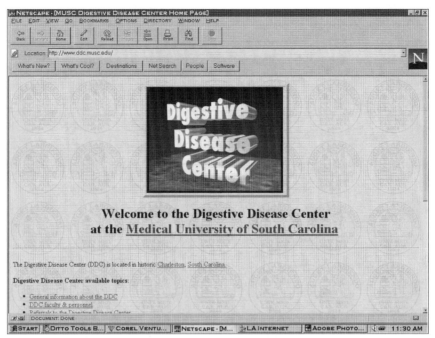

The Digestive Disease Center. *http://www.ddc.musc.edu/*

Irritable Bowel Syndrome Self Help Group

http://www.ibsgroup.org/

Scope

http://www.kitsap.net/health/ccl/scope.html

Newsletter by and for people with inflammatory bowel disease.

Esophagus

See also: Cancer (Oncology) - Esophageal Cancer.

Diseases of the Esophagus

http://edcenter.med.cornell.edu/CUMMC_PathNotes/Gastrointestinal/
Gastrointestinal.html

Dysphagia Resource Center

http://dysphagia.com/

Resources for swallowing and swallowing disorders.

Gastroesophageal Reflux Disease

http://www.niddk.nih.gov/Heartburn/Heartburn.html

The National Institute of Diabetes and Digestive and Kidney Diseases (NIDDK) information on hiatal hernia and heartburn.

GERD: Gastroesophageal Reflux Disease

http://www.pathcom.com/~minaise/gerd.html

GERD Information Resource Center

http://www.gerd.com/

Heartburn, Reflux and Esophagitis

http://www.cyberstreet.com/swfrmc/GI-HEART.HTM

Seattle Barrett's Esophagus Program

http://www.fhcrc.org/~barretts/

Gallstones

How Are Gallstones Treated?

http://www.healthtouch.com/level1/leaflets/nddic/nddic080.htm

Laparoscopic Cholecystectomy

http://www.anesthesia.org/public/guides/lap_chole.html

NIDDK Information on Gallstones

http://137.187.36.5/Gallstones/Gallstones.html

Power Points about Gallstone Disease

http://www.medicinenet.com/mainmenu/encyclop/ARTICLE/Art_G/gallston.htm

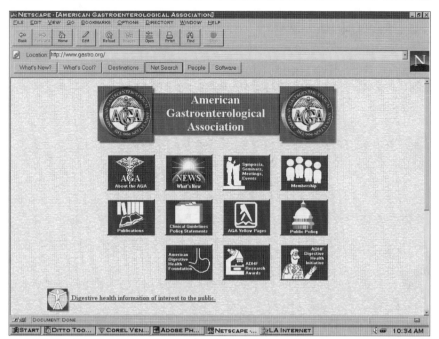

American Gastroenterological Association. http://www.gastro.org/

Gastritis

Helicobacter Foundation

http://www.helico.com/

All about *Helicobacter pylori*, its diagnosis, treatment and clinical correlations. Site includes frequently asked questions, discussion group, helicobacter movie, history and pathogenesis. *Helicobacter pylori* are the bacteria which cause gastritis, which may lead to ulcers and other digestive complaints.

Peptic Ulcer Disease: FAQ

http://www.ddc.org/pat/faqs/peptic_faq.html

Treatment for Helicobacter Pylori

http://www.vianet.net.au/~bjmrshll/table1.htm

General Topics

Atlas of Digestive Endoscopy
http://www.luz.ve/ICA/Atlas_med/i_index.html

English version of a site that includes a collection of endoscopic images.

Columbia University Gastroenterology Web
http://cpmcnet.columbia.edu/dept/gi/

Information about the faculty and department specialties, as well as information and links on specific digestive diseases. Includes links to academic gastroenterology sites, organizations, pathology, radiology, and endoscopy.

Constipation
http://niddk.nih.gov/Constipation/Constipation.html

Digestive Disease Center
http://www.ddc.musc.edu/

From the Medical University of South Carolina, information on endoscopy and endoscopic-related techniques, liver diseases, and digestive diseases.

Digestive Health and Disease: A Glossary
http://www.acg.gi.org/digest/gitrac/3ci.html

Digestive System Diseases
http://www.mic.ki.se/Diseases/c6.html

Articles about the digestive system, gastroenterology and specific digestive disorders. Sections on gastric, esophageal, biliary tract, pancreatic and liver disorders.

"Everything You Ever Wanted to Know about Gastroenterology" Page
http://www.cyberstreet.com/swfrmc/GI-PAGE.HTM

General information about gastroenterology and fact sheets on disorders of the digestive tract. From Barrett's Esophagus, Peptic Ulcer Disease, and swallowing disorders, to treatment and monitoring examinations such as colonoscopy, ambulatory 24-hour pH monitoring, and esophageal dilation.

Gastroenterology Consultants

http://www.gastro.com/

Gastroenterology Resources

http://cait.cpmc.columbia.edu/dept/gi/elsewhere.html

HealthWeb: Gastroenterology Disease Resources

http://www.medlib.iupui.edu/hw/gastro/

Disease and educational resources for health care professionals. Electronic publications and communications, academic and non-academic organizations and career opportunities.

Hemorrhoids

http://www.niddk.nih.gov/Hemmorhoids/Hemmorhoids.html

Information from the National Institute of Diabetes and Digestive and Kidney Diseases.

Patient Information Documents on Digestive Diseases

http://137.187.36.5/DigestiveDocs.html

Good information on digestive disorders including topics such as bleeding in the digestive tract, gallstones, pancreatitis and ulcerative colitis. Sstatistics, an overview of the digestive system and how it works, and professional organizations.

PharmInfoNet's Digestive Disease Center

http://pharminfo.com/disease/gastro.html

This site offers links to patient information and frequently asked questions (FAQs), sorted by organ and by disease.

Texas Virtual Clinic

http://websurg.uth.tmc.edu/digestive/index.shtml

UCLA Digestive Disease Center

http://www.ddc.org/

Non-profit site devoted to all aspects of digestive diseases. Addresses peptic ulcer disease, inflammatory bowel disease, ulcerative colitis, Crohn's disease, irritable bowel syndrome, gallstones, colon cancer and AIDS-related gastrointestinal problems. Information exchange for patients and consumers, as well as discussion area for doctors and other health care professionals.

UNC Division of Digestive Diseases and Nutrition
http://www.med.unc.edu/medicine/gi/

Organizations

American Gastroenterological Association
http://www.gastro.org/

American Gastroenterological Association news, meetings, clinical policy statements, publications and message board.

Directory of Digestive Diseases Organizations for Patients
http://www.niddk.nih.gov/DigDisOrgPat/DigDisOrgPat.html

Voluntary and private organizations offering educational materials and services about digestive diseases.

DISABILITIES

Adaptive Technology

Adaptive Computing Software Project

http://www.wildmantim.com/acsp/accuvoice.html

This site searches out shareware, freeware, and commercial vendors who offer products for disabled computer users working within an MS-DOS or Windows environment. Link to the Super Adaptoid column, which posts reviews of software.

Alliance for Technology Access

http://www.ataccess.org/

ATA is a network of resource centers dedicated to providing information and support services to the disabled, and increasing their use of standard assistive and information technologies. Provides list of vendors, frequently asked questions (FAQs), and links to other assistive technology resources.

Apple Computer Corporation's Disability Page

http://www2.apple.com/disability/welcome.html

Information on assistive technology and disability products.

AZtech, A to Z Assistive Technology

http://cosmos.ot.buffalo.edu/aztech.html

AZtech, Inc., is a nonprofit, community based enterprise that helps vendors and manufacturers develop assistive technology.

Designing an Accessible World

http://www.trace.wisc.edu/world/world.html

Discusses design principles and guidelines for making technology and structures more accessible to the disabled. Numerous web links are offered on subjects such as computers, telecommunications, ATMs, and recreation facilities.

Equal Access to Software and Information

http://www.isc.rit.edu/~easi/

Information and guidance in the area of access-to-information technologies for the disabled. Contains lists of adaptive technology resources and publications, including libraries without walls.

James Stanfield Publishing Company

http://www.stanfield.com/

Books, videos and other media programs for students with cognitive challenges and those who teach them. Includes programs on teaching assertiveness, sexuality, social and working skills.

Macintosh Disability Shareware and Freeware

http://www.ECNet.Net/users/gnorris/place.shtml

Survey of the shareware and freeware available for disabled Macintosh computer users. Site is maintained by Scott Norris, a disabled computer user.

Asperger Syndrome

Asperger's Syndrome

http://www.autism-society.org/packages/aspergers.html

Description of Asperger Syndrome and how it differs from autism; links.

O.A.S.I.S.: On-Line Asperger's Syndrome Information and Support

http://www.udel.edu/bkirby/asperger/

Asperger syndrome is a mild form of autism. This site describes research and educational projects; lists conferences, mailing lists and support groups. Included is a section of personal accounts and poetry written by individuals with AS.

OASIS. *http://www.udel.edu/bkirby/asperger/*

Ataxia

About Hereditary Ataxias and Euro-Ataxia

http://www.vsn.nl/euroatax/index.htm

Ataxia is a degenerative neurological disease that results in the loss of muscle coordination. This site describes and classifies the different kinds of ataxias, and tells about the activities of Euro-Ataxia and provides links to related sites.

International Ataxia Friends Mailing List

http://132.183.145.103/neurowebforum/ChildNeurologyArticles/
JoinourATAXIAmailinglist.html

To subscribe, send e-mail to: Majordomo@citi.doc.ca and in the body write: "Subscribe INTERNAF" or, to receive a digest version, in the body type: "Subscribe INTERNAF-DIGEST."

National Ataxia Foundation

http://www.nwwin.com/ATAXIA.htm

Basic information about NAF and its fight against the various kinds of ataxias.

Attention Deficit Disorder (ADD)

A.D.D. WareHouse
http://www.addwarehouse.com/

Site describes products for Attention Deficit/Hyperactivity Disorder (AD/HD) and related problems.

ADD Parents Mailing List
http://homepage.sease.upenn.edu/~mengwong/add/addparents.txt

To subscribe, send e-mail to: Majordomo@mv.mv.com with the following in the body of the message: "subscribe add-parents Yourfirstname Yourlastname."

Attention Deficit Disorder WWW Archive
http://www.seas.upenn.edu/~mengwong/add/

Lists interesting ADD information sites, with a brief description.

Attention Deficit Hyperactivity Disorder
http://www.healthguide.com/ADHD/biology.stm

Site addresses ADHD, its effects and treatment approaches. It describes symptoms and the biology of the brain. Written for non-professionals.

CH.A.D.D.: Children and Adults with Attention Deficit Disorders
http://www.chadd.org/

Non-profit, parent-based organization that offers family support and advocacy, public and professional education, and research support. Links to _Attention!_ a magazine for individuals dealing with ADHD, general information on ADD and how to treat or parent those individuals with ADHD.

Defined Diets and Childhood Hyperactivity
http://text.nlm.nih/cdc/www/32.html

One A.D.D. Place
http://www.iquest.net/greatconnect/oneaddplace/

Information and resources pertaining to Attention Deficit Disorder (ADD) and other learning disorders. Includes general information, products and services, articles, references, frequently asked questions (FAQs), calendar of events, and a general adult ADD symptom checklist.

Online Attention Deficit Disorder Test
http://www.med.nyu.edu/Psych/addc/addscr.htm

Autism

#Autism Channel
http://www.norwich.net/~kellysm/autism.html

All about proper procedure and etiquette for interacting with others through the Autism Channel, an internet relay channel (IRC) or real-time forum where parents and family, educators and health care professionals can talk about autism and other PDD-spectrum disorders, sharing personal stories and support, and discussing treatment options and other issues.

Autism Channel Link
http://www.telepath.com/canance/autism.html

This virtual newspaper was created to help parents and professionals learn more about autism. It includes links to the autism internet relay channel (IRC) and chat group, and provides a lot of information on news, treatment and therapies, legislation, organizations and personal pages.

Autism Frequently Asked Questions
http://web.syr.edu/~jmwobus/autism/autism.faq.html

In addition to answers to frequently asked questions, this site provides mailing list information, a glossary, information on coping with autism, educational methods and advice for parents, as well as a list of well-known individuals with autism or who have family members with autism. To subscribe to the AUTISM mailing list, send e-mail to: LISTSERV@MAELSTROM.STJOHNS.EDU with the message: "subscribe autism Firstname Lastname."

Autism Resources
http://web.syr.edu/~jmwobus/autism/

Links to web sites around the world having anything to do with autism. Broken down by topics, such as general information, online discussion, news, books, articles, treatment methods, academic and research programs, organizations and resources by language, and support for parents.

Autism Society of America

http://www.autism-society.org/asa_home.html

What is autism? This site has an autism checklist, and describes the activities and mission of the Autism Society of America.

Indiana Resource Center for Autism

http://www.isdd.indiana.edu/~irca/

The IRCA focuses on strategies to empower communities to support individuals with autism in typical work, school and community activities. Site describes IRCA programs and seminars. Bibliography also provided.

Cerebral Palsy

Cerebral Palsy

http://www.stayhealthy.com/hrd/dicopr_heneco_cepa.htm

Information, articles, contacts, chat groups and web links.

Cerebral Palsy: A Guide for Care

http://gait.aidi.udel.edu/res695/homepage/pd_ortho/clinics/c_palsy/cpweb.htm

Overview of a book by the same name.

Cerebral Palsy: A Multimedia Tutorial

http://galen.med.virginia.edu/~smb4v/tutorials/cp/cp.htm

For children and their parents.

Cerebral Palsy Fact Sheet

http://weber.u.washington.edu/~wscchap/NoMoreLabels/palsy.html

Basic information about cerebral palsy.

General Information about Cerebral Palsy

gopher://aed.aed.org:80/00/.disability/.nichcy/.online/.fact-general/.onlist/.cp/

List of United Cerebral Palsy Association National Affiliate Offices

http://web2.airmail.net/ucpdal/afflist1.htm

The Stuttering Homepage. *http://www.mankato.msus.edu/dept/comdis/kuster/stutter.html*

Susie's Cerebral Palsy Homepage

http://pw2.netcom.com/~wheels27/home.html

Personal account, and resources for those with cerebral palsy (CP), their parents, students and health care professionals.

United Cerebral Palsy Association

http://www.ucpa.org/

Communication/Speech Disorders

Aha! American Hyperlexia Association Home Page

http://www.hyperlexia.org/

Information about hyperlexia and related disorders, such as Semantic-Pragmatic disorder. Hyperlexia information, materials, conferences, and useful sites are found here, along with personal stories. Hyperlexia is a communication or language disorder where children have precocious reading abilities accompanied by significant problems in verbal, learning and social skills.

Net Connections for Communication Disorders and Sciences
http://www.mankato.msus.edu/dept/comdis/kuster2/welcome.html

Stuttering FAQ
http://www.casafuturatech.com/FAQ/faq.html

This text file is a shorter version of the book, *Stuttering, Science, Therapy and Practice* which is also available on the internet.

Stuttering Homepage
http://www.mankato.msus.edu/dept/comdis/kuster/stutter.html

Information about stuttering and other fluency disorders such as cluttering. Provides links to support groups, research and publications, case studies, news, personal accounts, therapy and discussion forums. Lists famous people who stutter.

Developmental Disorders

National Association of Developmental Councils Home Page
http://www.igc.apc.org/NADDC/

NADDC promotes a national policy which enables individuals with developmental and other disabilities to have the opportunity to make choices regarding the quality of their lives and to be included in the community.

Treatment of Destructive Behaviors in Persons with Developmental Disabilities
http://text.nlm.nih.gov/nih/cdc/www/75.html

This site contains text of a statement from the National Institutes of Health 1989 Consensus Development Conference.

Waisman Center's List of Web Sites
http://waisman.wisc.edu/www/mrsites.html

Lists dozens of web sites related to cognitive and developmental disabilities.

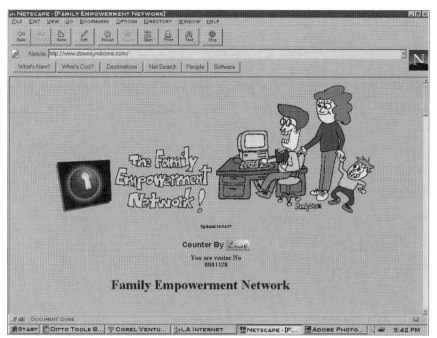

Family Empowerment Network. *http://www.downsyndrome.com/*

Down Syndrome

Down Syndrome Listserv
http://www.nas.com/downsyn/dslistserv.html

Down Syndrome WWW Page
http://www.nas.com/downsyn/

Articles, frequently asked questions, health care guidelines, organizations, resources, parent support groups, conferences, toy catalogs, and personal "Brag Pages" created about children with Down syndrome by their parents. Links to related sites include funding opportunities, educational and medical resources.

Hope for Parents of Children with Down Syndrome
http://www.efaxinc.com/~sgtms/downsyn.htm

Site created by the adoptive parent of a child with Down Syndrome. Addresses vitamins and supplements that can help children with Down Syndrome. Links.

Family Empowerment Network

http://www.downsyndrome.com/

UPSIDE!

http://www.telebyte.com/upside/upside.html

Self-described as an informal society of individuals, parents, and friends involved in the world of Down Syndrome. Includes child-of-the-month, newsletters, short articles, upcoming events, and lots of web links and USENET newsgroup addresses, listservers, as well as e-mail addresses, mailing addresses, and phone numbers for a number of Down Syndrome organizations.

World Wide Information Pages about Down Syndrome

http://alf.zfn.uni-bremen.de/~downsyn/down10e.html

Down Syndrome organizations from Europe, Asia, Australia, North America and South America.

Dyslexia

Dyslexia Archive

http://www.hensa.ac.uk/dyslexia.html

Contains information about dyslexia, including education, groups, events, articles and software. Also, human-interest information, such as a list of famous people with dyslexia and personal accounts.

Dyslexia Resources

http://www.phantom.com/~grow/dyslexia.html

Dyslexia resources on and off the web, including relevant newsgroups. Provides basic information on dyslexia, a bibliography, references, software, research, therapy, special needs resources and more.

Dyslexia 2000 Network

http://www.futurenet.co.uk/charity/ado/index.html

Information and advice about software, hardware and other tools for adult dyslexics. Link to the Adult Dyslexia Organization, which was founded by dyslexics to support others with dyslexia. Checklist on dyslexia provided, along with information on further resources.

Fragile X Syndrome

Fragile X Discussion List
http://www.counterpoint.com/fraxa/frx.html

Fragile X syndrome is the number-one cause of inherited mental retardation. List discusses fragile X, in particular its diagnosis and treatment stages. To subscribe, send e-mail to: majordomo@counterpoint.com and in the body type: "subscribe fragilex your_e-mail_address."

Fragile X Syndrome
http://www.kumc.edu/instruction/medicine/genetics/support/fragilex.html

Online resources and discussion group.

FRAXA Research Foundation
http://www.FRAXA.org/

Supports research in treating fragile X xyndrome. Describes symptoms, causes, diagnosis and treatment, and provides links to other web sites, medline associations and references. Newsletter available.

General Disability Resources

Ability OnLine Support Network
http://www.ablelink.org/

A penpal e-mail system that connects young people with disabilities or chronic illness with disabled and non-disabled peers and mentors. In addition, the site offers information to patients, their families and friends about medical treatments, educational strategies, and employment opportunities.

Access Media
http://www.human.com/mkt/access/index.html

Access Media is a non-profit organization that works to acquire important documents for individuals with disabilities, in forms that are usable to them (e.g., braille and audio tapes).

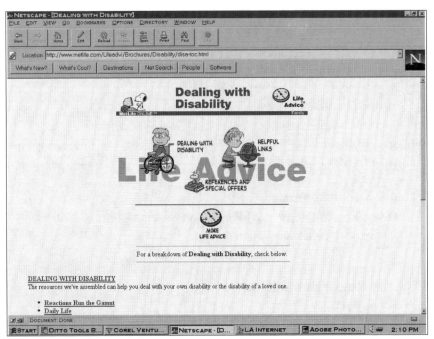

Dealing with Disability. *http://www.metlife.com/Lifeadvi/Brochures/Disability/disa-toc.html*

Boulevard

http://www.disprodpc.com/

Site provides information about products and services available to health care professionals and individuals with disabilities. Includes information on van conversions, elevators, wheelchairs and other assistive technology. Also offers dozens of links to sites of interest to the disabled and their families, including management services, medical links and publications.

Center for Independent Living

http://www.ci/berkeley.ca.us/agc-cil.html

The Center for Independent Living has a number of services that enable people with disabilities to live on their own. This site describes the Center's programs, which includes couseling for housing, personal assistant screening and referral, peer support, employment, and financial benefits.

Dealing with Disability: Life Advice

http://www.metlife.com/Lifeadvi/Brochures/Disability/disa-toc.html

Contains resources that help one cope with one's own disability or the disability of a loved one. Includes such topics as understanding reactions, adjusting to the disability in daily life, sources for financial support, medical assistance, and advice for interacting with people with disabilities. References and web links lead to additional resources.

Different Roads to Learning

http://www.difflearn.com/

Online catalog of learning materials and playthings for children with developmental delays and disabilities. Includes educational flash cards, manipulative toys and learning games. Describes each item and the skills it helps the child develop.

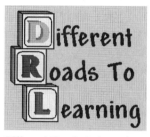

Different Roads to Learning.
http://www.difflearn.com/

Directory for the Disabled

http://www.wheeler.org/direct.html

The Metropolitan Society for Crippled Children and Adults has created a directory of resources for handicapped and disabled people around the country. Topics include but are not limited to home care, ramps and access, adaptive clothing, useful toll-free phone numbers, and veteran's assistance. Bulletin board and other online services are offered.

Disabilities by Category

http://www.seals.com/publish/category.html

From Alzheimer's to spinal cord, disabilities alphabetized by category.

Disabilities, Etc.

http://www-gse.berkeley.edu/program/SP/Disabilities/

Links to several disability compilations, as well as to individual sites for autism, Down syndrome, attention deficit disorder, dyslexia, epilepsy and fragile X syndrome.

Disability Information

http://galaxy.einet.net/GJ/disabilities.html

This is a condensed collection of web sites offering information on resources for the disabled. Many academic links and links to organizations based outside of North America.

Disability International Online

http://www.dpi.org/di.html

This is the magazine of the Disabled Peoples' International. It discusses the experiences of individuals with disabilities, the work of DPI, and provides information on products, technological advances and employment opportunities for individuals with disabilities, as well as news, commentaries and updates. Published quarterly; free sample issue is available; subscription information provided.

Disability Net

http://www.globalnet.co.uk/~pmatthews/DisabilityNet/

This is a service for the disabled and those with an interest in disability issues. Run by Muscle Power, a UK organization of people with neuromuscular impairmen, the site offers information on access, the arts, benefits, independent living, legislation, sex/relationships, sports, and much more. Penpals, classified advertisements and a search engine are also offered.

Disability Resources on the Internet

http://disability.com/links/cool.html

Huge listing of resources available on the internet for the disabled and their families and friends. This site covers disabilities due to aging, as well as physical, mental and sensory problems. Describes sites that provide emotional, legal, and medical support, technology and assistive products, along with information on rehabilitation programs, employment, governmental and educational resources, recreation and travel.

Disabled Peoples' International Home Page

http://www.dpi.org/

A grass-roots network that includes individuals from over 110 countries, devoted to promoting the human rights of people with disabilities.

DO-IT

http://weber.u.washington.edu/~doit/

DO-IT (Disabilities, Opportunities, Internetworking, and Technology) seeks to increase the participation of those with disabilities in science, engineering and mathematics academic programs and careers. The program serves high school students with disabilities who are interested in these fields and want to attend college. They are supported through mentoring and summer-study programs, as well as by being loaned computers and adaptive technologies for use in their homes. Newsletter, publications, video, and newsgroup information are provided as well.

DRM WebWatcher

http://www.geocities.com/CapitolHill/1703/DRMwww.html

The Disabilities Resources Monthly Guide provides an alphabetical list of online resources with links to specific disabilities, as well as to organizations whose scope is cross-disability. Includes a number of disorders and diseases not typically grouped in the disabled category, such as arthritis and chronic fatigue syndrome.

Evan Kemp Associates

http://disability.com

Evan Kemp Associates Home Page offers news and information about disability and disability resources, as well as products and services that help those who are disabled to live independently. The EKA Product Showcase boasts an online catalog of EKA and other company products, including mobility devices, clothing, and various aids to daily living. Medical, low-vision, mobility, and vision rehabilitation products are also presented.

The Hub

http://www.curbcut.com/

Information for people in wheelchairs, includes topics of sex, hope, law, therapy, sports, travel, and more. Lists related web sites with summaries of what you will find there.

Internet Resources for Special Children Home Page

http://www.irsc.org/

Large amount of information and web links for parents, educators, medical professionals and other people who interact with disabled children. Topics include specific disability information, support groups for parents and family members, special education and legal resources.

Invisible Disabilities Page
http://www1.shore.net/~dmoisan/invisible_disability.html

Job Accommodation Network
http://janweb.icdi.wvu.edu/

An international, toll-free consulting service that provides information about job accommodations and the employability of people with disabilities. Information on the Americans with Disabilities Act is also provided.

Lubin's disABILITY Information and Resources
http://www.eskimo.com/~jlubin/disabled.html

This site offers a collection of net and non-net resources for people with disabilities and those who work with them. It is maintained by Jim Lubin, a respirator-dependent quadriplegic who types 17 words per minute using a sip-and-puff switch.

Mainstream Online
http://www.mainstream-mag.com/

Self-described as "the leading news, advocacy, and lifestyle zine for people with disabilities." This site covers many facets of disability culture, including disability rights, news and current affairs, products, technology, personal profiles, education, employment, sexuality and relationships, housing, transportation, travel and recreation.

Monaco and Associates
http://zeus.kspress.com/monaco/

Products and services for individuals with disabilities such as computer software and video tapes.

National Sports Center for the Disabled
http://www.nscd.org/nscd/

Outdoor recreation for children and adults with disabilities.

NCSA Mosaic Access Page
http://bucky.aa.uic.edu/

The page provides information about how people with disabilities can use the internet and the World Wide Web.

Network Libraries for Blind and Physically Handicapped Individuals

http://lcweb.loc.gov/nls.libs.html

Alphabetical, by state.

New England INDEX

http://NE-INDEX.Shriver.Org/

Serving mostly the New England area, this INDEX (Information on Disabilities EXchange) invites users to call their specialists who can search a database for up-to-date information. Provides links to resources on the net, contains fact sheets and the "Exceptional Physician" newsletter.

New Mobility Magazine

http://www.newmobility.com/nmmag.htm

Recent issue and article archives available for this lifestyle magazine for the disabled. Includes personal interviews, columns, book reviews, articles on alternative medicine, cures, drugs, mobility, arts, sports, sex, travel, etc. Subscription information and links to related sites provided.

Northwestern University Rehabilitation Engineering and Prosthetics and Orthotics Center

http://pele.repoc.nwu.edu/repoc.html/

Research to improve prostheses and orthoses. Site describes programs and offers online movies demonstrating devices. Free, online "Capabilities" newsletter is also available, along with links to related sites.

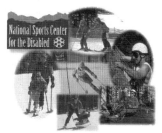

National Sports Center for the Disabled.
http://www.nscd.org/ nscd/

PeopleNet DisAbility DateNet Home Page

http://chelsea.ios.com/~mauro/

This page was created by a writer who has been disabled since the age of five as a result of polio . It contains articles, stories, poems and resources concerning love, dating, sex, intimacy and contraception as experienced by disabled individuals.

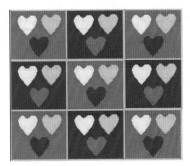

PeopleNet DisAbility DateNet.
http://chelsea.ios.com/~mauro/

Resources for Research on Disabilities

http://www.sped.ukans.edu/disabilities/

This University of Kansas site contains links to internet resources concerning people with disabilities, including academic and social programs, online texts and other references sources. Information on technology for people with disabilities, and links to disability-related gophers.

Rick and Joni's Home Page

http://www.access.digex.net/~vandyke/

Information about the Disabled-Able Travel Service; amputee resources with information about prosthetics; and links to social clubs and disability chatlines. Also has information about the annual Fascination Meeting, where interested abled individuals can meet disabled people.

Sibling Support Project

http://www.chmc.org/departmt/sibsupp/

National program dedicated to the brothers and sisters of people with special health and developmental needs. Site offers support and information to both child and adult siblings. Workshops, newsletters and listservers discuss the concerns and needs of these individuals. Directory offers listing of sibling programs and books about disabilities and illness for young readers.

Special Education Resources on the Internet

http://www.hood.edu/seri/serihome.htm

Large collection of internet-accessible resources for those involved in special education. This includes everything from physical disability and speech impairment, to learning disability, mental retardation and autism.

WebABLE!

http://www.yuri.org/webable/

News, articles and information on workshops and conferences to enhance web accessibility for the disabled.

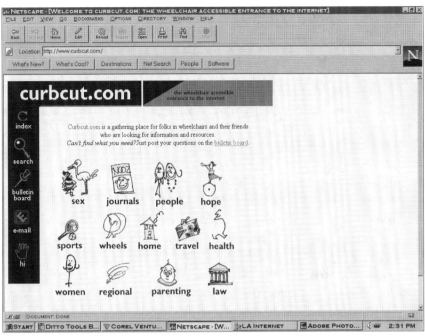

The Hub. *http://www.curbcut.com/*

W3C Disabilities Development

http://www.w3.org/pub/WWW/Disabilities/

This site is devoted to the developments and issues as they relate to implementing accessibility to the Web for people with disabilities. As such, it offers links to disabilities resources, guidelines and specifications, research projects and developments, utilities, tools, conferences, news and events information.

World Information on Disability

http://www.dais.is.tohoku.ac.jp/~iwan/
foreign_res.html

A long list of international weblinks, split into helpful sections including music, art and broadcasting; education; law; leisure and sports; products; publications; social support groups; technology, toys and travel; and work resources.

Hearing Impairment

See also: Ear, Nose & Throat/Otolaryngology.

AUDIES Net

http://www.tsi.it/contrib/audies/deafnet.html

Although this site is in Italian, many of the links are in English. Medical and technology links are listed, along with dozens of research projects, academic sites and institutes around the world.

Beyond-Hearing Mailing List

http://webcom.com/~houtx/b-h.html

To subscribe, send e-mail to: majordomo@acpub.duke.edu and leave the subject area blank. Type the following in the message: "subscribe beyond-hearing."

Center for Assistment and Demographic Studies

http://www.gallaudet.edu/~teallen/cards.html

CADS studies the deaf and hard-of-hearing population in the United States, and adapts tests to make them fair for those people.

Central Institute for the Deaf

http://cidmac.wustl.edu/

Information about the Institute's education department, outpatient clinic, research projects, and school which teaches deaf children to talk. Links to related internet sites are also offered.

Collection of Deaf Resources

http://darwin.clas.virginia.edu/~tms4s/deaf.html

Site provides a list of web sites about deaf culture, American Sign Language, deaf schools, and other resources for the deaf community.

Conditions of the Ear

http://www.bookmasters.com/marktplc/readroom/rr00055.htm

Check out this chapter of a book entitled, Deaf/Blindness: Essential Information for Families, Professionals, and Students. Written by Isabell Florence, who herself is deaf and blind.

Deaf/Hard of Hearing

http://www.familyvillage.wisc.edu/lib_deaf.htm

This site provides descriptions, names, mailing addresses, phone numbers and e-mail addresses for many organizations serving the deaf and hard-of-hearing community. It also directs browsers to e-mail lists, online magazines and other sites for the hearing impaired.

Deaf Magazine

http://WWW.Deaf-Magazine.Org/

News and communication with other deaf computer users. To subscribe, send e-mail to: listserv@listserv.deaf-magazine.org and leave subject area blank, but in body, type: "sub deaf-magazine firstname lastname."

Deaf Queer Resource Center

http://www.deafqueer.org/

This site is interested in promoting deaf lesbian, gay, bisexual and transgender visibility on the web. Library and information resources are provided, along with a bulletin board which includes announcements, a calendar, penpal matches, discussion groups, and the Point of View Café.

Deaf World Web

http://deafworldweb.org/

Provides information and social/cultural resources for the hearing-impaired. Includes news, chat and discussion groups, as well as the *On-line Deaf Encyclopedia*.

DeafWeb Washington

http://www.wolfenet.com/~hydronut/deafweb.htm

Articles, news, updates on assistive technology, book reviews, job information, educational, medical, governmental and kid's pages, and more resources for individuals who are hard of hearing.

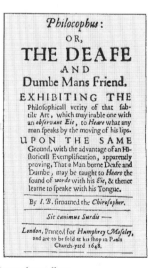

Speechreading.
http://mambo.ucsc.edu/psl/lipr.html

Early Identification of Hearing Impairment in Infants and Young Children

http://text.nlm.nih.gov/nih/cdc/www/92txt.html

Full text of a statement from the National Institutes of Health Consensus Development Conference, which states that approximately 1 of every 1,000 infants is born deaf. Present and future screening plans are discussed.

Gallaudet University

http://www.gallaudet.edu/

Admission and program information about the only four-year university for deaf and hard-of-hearing students.

Hearing Loss Resources

http://www.webcom.com/~houtx/

For those suffering from or interested in hearing loss. Primarily, this site is the vehicle of the SayWhatClub, an online group of late-deafened and hard-of-hearing individuals who support each other via e-mail. Includes essays and links to other hearing loss resources.

National Institute on Deafness and Other Communication Diseases

http://www.nih.gov/nidcd/

This NIH branch supports and conducts research on the normal and disordered processes of hearing, balance, smell, taste, voice, speech and language. This site describes current research and offers NIDCD publications and access to NIDCD Information Clearinghouse Database.

NIDCD Information Clearinghouse

http://www.aerie.com/chid/nidcd/dctest.html

This database provides titles, abstracts and availability information on articles related to deafness and other communication disorders. Includes a lot of material that is not classified elsewhere.

Speech on the Web

http://fonsg3.let.uva.nl/Other_pages.html

Links to sites related to phonetics and speech sciences.

Speechreading (Lipreading)

http://mambo.ucsc.edu/psl/lipr.html

This site offers a collection of essays and resources about speechreading. It begins with a 1648 essay entitled, "Philocophus: Or, the Deafe and Dumbe Mans Friend," an essay on lip-reading. Includes NATO studies and many more related web sites.

Travel Tips for Hearing Impaired People

http://www.netdoor.com/entinfo/herimaao.html

Advice on making travel arrangements. Provides useful phone numbers to services adapted for the deaf and hearing impaired.

Legal Issues

ADA and Disability Information

http://www.public.iastate.edu/~sbilling/ada.html

Long list of ADA resources on the web, including accessibility guidelines, reference books, compliance handbooks, and a newsgroup devoted to ADA issues. Other links to general and specific disability material are offered.

Americans with Disabilities Act Home Page

http://www.usdoj.gov/crt/ada/adahom1.com

The U.S. Department of Justice maintains this site. Information about the toll-free ADA phone line, ADA enforcement programs, ADA status reports, new or proposed regulations, and ADA Technical Assistance grants are provided.

Americans with Disabilities Act of 1990

gopher://wiretap.spies.com/00/Gov/disable.act/

Full text of the 1990 ADA passed by Congress to prohibit discrimination on the basis of disability.

Social Security Online

http://www.ssa.gov/SSA_Home.html

Information and publications on Social Security entitlement programs.

Mental Retardation

American Association on Mental Retardation

http://www.aamr.org/

The mission of the AAMR is to advance the knowledge and skills of those who work in the field of mental retardation by helping the exchange of information and ideas. The site contains membership information, abstracts, convention information, training and career opportunities, and a list of disability resources.

Arc of the United States Home Page

http://TheArc.org/welcome.html

The Arc is the nation's largest voluntary organization serving children and adults with mental retardation and their families. There are over 1,000 affiliated chapters of the Arc, and this site describes the organization's mission and activities, which include research, advocacy, education and training for the mentally handicapped. Fact sheets provide information on services, groups, Social Security benefits, the ADA and community living. Some pages are available in Spanish. Links to online chapter sites.

Disability-Related Sites on the World Wide Web

http://www.prostar.com/%7Ethe.arc/dislink.htm

The King County, Washington chapter of the Arc has assembled a thorough and helpful list of links to mental retardation and developmental disability resources available on the web.

Hydrocephalus Association Homepage

http://neurosurgery.mgh.harvard.edu/ha/

This site describes programs dealing with hydrocephalus, an abnormal accumulation of fluid in the brain. Includes articles and frequently asked questions.

Special Olympics International

http://www.specialolympics.org/

Special Olympics is a non-profit, international program of sports training and competition for individuals with mental retardation.More than one million athletes in nearly 150 countries participate in 22 sports. This official site describes the games, provides information on volunteering, coaching and competing, and offers information and links to U.S. chapters, and worldwide regional programs.

Paralysis

Cure Paralysis Now
http://cureparalysis.org/

This site is devoted to the advancement of a cure for spinal cord paralysis. Includes frequently asked questions, news, chat rooms, research and many related links.

Neuro-Implant Program
http://he1.uns.tju.edu:80/neuro/

Describes a program whose goal is to aid in the relief of head/spine injuries, multiple sclerosis, cerebral palsy, cancer and permanent pain injuries. The tactic is to surgically implant neuro-stimulation and neuro-chemical devices.

Spinal Cord Research Centre
http://www.scrc.umanitoba.ca/

Describes the Centre's activities and research to cure spinal cord injuries.

Spine and Peripheral Nerve Surgery
http://neurosurgery.mgh.harvard.edu/spine-hp.htm

The Neurological Service at Massachusetts General Hospital and Harvard Medical School provides information on spine evaluation and treatment, surgery, tumors, referrals, and links to related sites.

Polio

Polio E-mail Archives and Subscription Information
http://otpt.ups.edu/listservs/POLIO/

Site contains information on subscribing to the Polio e-mail list, as well as archives. To subscribe, send e-mail to: listserv@sjuvm.stjohns.edu and type in the body: "subscribe Yourfirstname Yourlastname."

Polio Survivors' Page

http://www.eskimo.com/~dempt/polio.html

This page provides links to polio and post-polio resources, and includes announcements, articles and research. A great deal of material may be found on Post Polio Syndrome (PPS), a muscle fatigue syndrome that occurs in patients who have suffered from polio years before.

Spina Bifida

Children with Spina Bifida

http://www.waisman.wisc.edu/%7Erowley/sb_kids.htmlx

This site serves as a resource page for parents of children with spina bifida. Includes mailing list information, words of encouragement, information resources, articles, research, photos and personal web page links, as well as links to related sites.

Spina Bifida Association of America

http://www.infohiway.com/spinabifida/

Facts about spina bifida, the SBAA, medical updates and related links.

Spina Bifida Information

http://www.bethisraelny.org/inn/myelo/mye_ind.html

Spina Bifida Occulta

http://www.icondata.com/health/pedbase/files/SPINABIF.HTM

Clinical information on this spinal defect.

Understanding Spina Bifida

http://seals.com/publish/understanding/usb.html

Spina bifida occurs when the spinal cord does not form properly during fetal development.

Visual Impairment

See also: Eye/Optometry & Ophthalmology.

American Council of the Blind

http://www.acb.org/

Provides general information about the ACB and recent issues of their monthly publication, *The Braille Forum*. Also offers updates from Washington, D.C. and ACB affiliates, as well as resources about blindness, Braille, product catalogs and financial help.

American Federation for the Blind Gopher Menu

gopher://gopher.afb.org:5005/1/

Includes Federation news and information, literacy program for the blind, research reports, policy papers, and fact sheets on aging, education and other issues related to blindness. Also contains the Computerized Braille Tutor User's Manual and software (requires a PC).

American Foundation for the Blind

http://www.igc.apc.org/afb/

Offers information on blindness, low vision and related issues, as well as access to AFB newsletters, the *Journal of Visual Impairment and Blindness*, and the AFB catalog of books. AFB activities fall within the non-medical aspects of blindness and vision impairment.

Associated Services for the Blind Information Page

http://www.libertynet.org/~asbinfo/

Speech-friendly option available at this site, which describes ASB activities and mission. Also offers recorded periodicals, including over 25 magazines on subjects ranging from archeology to home cooking and computers to science.

Blind Related Links

http://www.seidata.com/~marriage/rblind.html

Offers many links to resources of interest to the blind, including adaptive technology, training, publications, employment, commercial sites, medical sites and government sites.

Blindness-Related E-mailing Lists

http://www.hicom.net/~oedipus.blinst.html

There are over 60 e-mail listservers related to blindness, and subscriptions to them are offered at this site. Includes everything from access technology for the blind, to information about computer games accessible to the blind, everyday experiences, guide dog users chat list and legislation. Links that are not exclusively blindness-related are also available.

Blindness Resource Center

http://nyise.org/blind.htm

Collection of web sites related to assisting the blind and visually impaired. Provides a brief description of most of the sites, which include organizations, software and technology, schools and research sites, information on Braille, translators, deaf-blindness, eye diseases, libraries and vendors.

Cathy's Newstand

http://ww2.cdepot.net/~mist/

A long collection of online newspapers, magazines and web sites, many of which are identified as having been designed for the blind or visually impaired.

Dotmaker's Home Page

http://www.azstarnet.com/~dotmakr/index.html

Resources and information links for the blind, visually impaired, and deaf and blind. Offers sites of interest to Braille users, including the computerized Braille tutor, and a long list of home pages maintained by blind computer-users.

Guide Dog Laws

http://www.seeing.eye.org/laws.shtm

Type in the state or province (for Canada) abbreviation to receive a description of the regional laws relating to guide dogs.

Internet Phone Book of Blind Users and Services

http://www.crl.com/~phil/pmenu.html#

Site contains information on blind computer-users; organizations for the blind; web, ftp and gopher sites related to blindness issues; and blind ham radio operators.

Lions World Services for the Blind

http://www.rollanet.org/~rlions/web/

This site describes this organization's activities and mission, which is to help the visually impaired learn independent living and vocational skills.

Louis Braille

http://world.std.com/~duxbury/braille.html

Autobiographical information.

National Federation of the Blind

http://www.nfb.org/default.htm

This group was founded to help the blind help themselves and is the largest organization serving the blind in the U.S., according to this site. The NFB's activities and events are described, and information about *The Braille Monitor* magazine may be found. In addition, features information for children describing what it is like to be blind, as well as links to Braille resources, research, technological, legal and legislative information.

National Library Service for the Blind and Physically Handicapped

http://lcweb.loc.gov/nls/nls.html

A free library of Braille and recorded materials circulated through cooperating libraries. Search the online catalog at this site to see what is available. Book reviews, legal information, and a list of network libraries for blind and physically handicapped individuals may be found here.

On-line Books Page

http://www.cs.cmu.edu/books.html

Thousands of fiction and non-fiction books are available online, and are indexed at this site. Search by author, title, or subject, or browse through the new listings. Find links to other book repositories, in English and other languages.

Outpost

http://users.deltanet.com/~tdb/

A "speech-friendly" site created for the blind computer user as well as for those who seek information in accessible format. Contains links and material about adaptive technology companies, demos, guide dogs, automated online banking, shopping and products for the blind.

Recordings for the Blind and Dyslexic

http://www.rfbd.org/

National headquarters of this nonprofit organization that serves people who cannot read standard print because of a visual, perceptual or other physical disability. Site describes RFB&D's library, provides links and catolog of services.

Royal National Institute for the Blind, UK

http://www.trib.org.uk/

This site was designed not only to serve and provide information for blind and partially-sighted computer users, but also to demonstrate how an internet site can be designed to be usable by the visually impaired. The RNIB events, publications and products are described, and fact sheets on the eye and visual impairments are provided, along with an international guide to agencies and other links. There is a demonstration of a Braille translation software program, entitled "Braille It!"

Scotter's Low Vision Land

http://www.community.net/~byndsght/

Also known as Beyond Sight - Low Vision Resources. Scotter has assembled a list of resources for the blind and visually impaired, and offers computer assistance to any fellow vision-impaired individual. Internet resources listed include newsgroups, listservers, bulletin boards, online books and other sites. A brief summary of each site is provided.

Vision Impairments: A Guide for the Perplexed

http://vanbc.wimsey.com/~jlyon/index.html

Information and resources for people with vision impairments. Also provides a thorough, alphabetized index of recommended sites to visit on the internet.

DRUGS / PHARMACOLOGY

General Topics

American Society of Health-System Pharmacists
http://www.ashp.org/

Ask a Pharmacist
http://www.gis.net/~rogeryoung/
Medication counseling service. E-mail experts your questions.

Clinical Pharmacology Online
http://www.cponline.gsm.com/
Drug monographs.

Drug Database
http://pharminfo.com/drugdb/db_mnu.html

Drug Formulary
http://www.intmed.mcw.edu/drug.html

Drug Topics
http://www.drugtopics.com/
A twice-monthly news magazine for pharmacists and the pharmaceutical community. Includes continuing education articles, news flashes, new products and cover stories. Free to qualified recipients.

Edmund's Home Page/Pharmacy Sites
http://www.li.net/~edhayes/rx.html

FDA News
http://www.fda.gov/opacom/hpnews.html

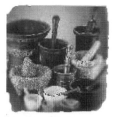

Grier's Pharmacy Page

http://members.aol.com/poison5249/GrierPharm/
ghpharm.html

Pharmacy and toxicology resources on the internet.

Hardin Meta Directory: Pharmacy and Pharmacology

http://www.arcade.uiowa.edu/hardin-www/md-pharm.
html

Links to lists of internet sites.

Healthtouch: Drug Information Search

http://www.healthtouch.com/level1/p_dri.htm

This site claims to have information on over 7,000 prescription and over-the-counter drugs.

Internet Mental Health: Medications

http://www.mentalhealth.com/p30.html

Monographs containing information on dozens of drugs, from Adapin (Cosepin), an antidepressant; to Zopiclone, a hypnotic. Information includes pharmacology, indications and contraindications, warnings, adverse effects, dosage and research.

Internet Self-Assessment in Pharmacology

http://www.cs.umn.edu/Research/GIMME/ISAP/intro.html

For health professionals, this self-study guide includes lecture outlines and pharmacological information on approximately 300 drugs, as well as exam questions and answers with explanations and clinical cases.

Merck Manual Online

http://www.merck.com/!!rfcLF3CgwrfcMm2tJj/pubs/mmanual/html/sectoc.htm

Mortar and Pestle Pharmacy Links

http://www.teleport.com/~keller/pharm.html

Attractive, informative site.

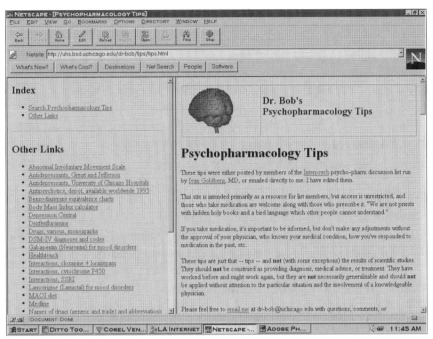

Dr. Bob's Psychopharmacology Tips. *http://uhs.bsd.uchicago.edu/dr-bob/tips/tips.html*

PDRnet.com

http://www.pdrnet.com/

Access to the PDR database, which includes a complete entry of each drug in the *Physicians' Desk Reference*, *PDR for Ophthalmology*, and *PDR for Nonprescription Drugs*, as well as MEDLINE, AIDSLINE, AIDSDRUGS, AIDSTRIALS and DIRLINE literature searches. Free to all MDs and DOs in full-time patient care.

Pharmacology Glossary

http://med-amsa.bu.edu/Pharmacology/Programmed/glossary.html

Includes symbols and terms, from "A:" to "Zero Order Kinetics." From Boston University Department of Pharmacology.

PharmInfoNet

http://pharminfo.com/

The Pharmaceutical Information Network contains a drug database, frequently asked questions (FAQs) and publications. Links to diseases and discussion groups, and related internet sites.

PharmWeb

http://www.pharmweb.net/

International pharmaceutical links and services. Lots of information.

Physicians GenRx: Mosby's Complete Drug Reference

http://www.mosby.com/Mosby/PhyGenRx/

Psychopharmacology Tips

http://uhs.bsd.uchicago.edu/dr-bob/tips/tips.html

U.S. Pharmacist

http://www.uspharmacist.com/

View the current issue of this magazine. Includes feature articles and departments, editorials, news, links and an index to earlier issues.

U.S. Pharmacopoeia Drug Information

http://www.usp.org/

Educational leaflets on prescription and non-prescription medications and their uses. USP is a private, nonprofit organization that seeks to disseminate unbiased information about drugs.

Virtual Library Pharmacy

http://www.cpb.uokhsc.edu/pharmacy/pharmint.html

Includes associations, schools, pharmaceutical companies, journals and books, databases, listservers and newsgroups on pharmacy-related topics.

"Virtual" Pharmacy Center

http://www-sci.lib.uci.edu:80/~martindale/Pharmacy.html

World Wide Drugs

http://community.net/~neils/new.html

World Wide Drugs Internet Links

http://community.net/~neils/news.html

Prozac

Fluoxetine Drug Monograph
http://www.mentalhealth.com/drug/p30-p05.html

Information on Prozac (Fluoxetine) which is classified as an antidepressant, antiobsessional and antibulemic.

Is Prozac for You?
http://www.adlist.com/psychiatry/prozac.html

Whether use of the antidepressant fluoxetine HCl (Prozac) is advisable.

Prozac Survivor's Support Group
http://syllabus.syr.edu/CHE/mlsage/CHE205/pro3.htm

Prozac Threads
http://pharminfo.com/drugdb/proz_arc.html

Includes basic information and "threads" from PharmInfo Net.

Yahoo's Prozac Links
http://www.yahoo.com/Health/Pharmacy/Drugs/Specific_Drugs/Prozac/

Ritalin

Factline on the Non-Medical Use of Ritalin
http://www.drugs.indiana.edu/pubs/factline/ritalin.html

Prescriptions for Ritalin have increased more than 600% in the last five years, and it is believed that this drug is often used inappropriately or recreationally. This site describes the "non-medical" abuse of this drug and its potentially dangerous health consequences.

Generic Name: Methylphenidate Hydrochloride
http://www.nmcp.med.navy.mil/neurolog/ritalin.htm

Basic information on Ritalin, prescribed for treating attention deficit/hyperactivity disorder, narcolepsy, and related medical conditions, from the Division of Neurology at the Naval Medical Center in Portsmouth, Virginia addresses indications, dosage, side effects, and precautions.

EAR, NOSE & THROAT / OTOLARYNGOLOGY

Acoustic Neuroma

Acoustic Neuroma Association Home Page

http://neurosurgery.mgh.harvard.edu/ana/

A patient-organized support and information group for people who have tumors affecting the cranial nerves, such as acoustic neuroma. Frequently asked questions, detection and treatment information provided.

Acoustic Neuroma Resources

http://www.netrail.net/~swiggins/neuroma.html

Ear Infections

Acute Otitis Media (Earache)

http://kidshealth.org/parent/common/otitis_media.html

Ear Infections

http://scendtek.com/darren/earhome.html

Answers to some frequently asked questions.

Ear Infections: What You Can Do

http://www.sig.net/~allergy/ear.html

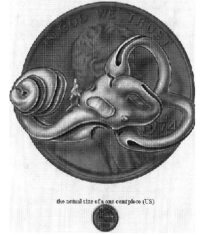

The world of Hearing and Balance
are the functions of these two important Ear parts
COCHLEA (left) controls hearing
SEMI-CIRCULAR CANALS (right) control Balance

the actual size of a one centpiece (US)

The Ear Surgery Information Center.
http://www.earsurgery.org/INDEX.html

General Topics

Cochlear Implants in Adults and Children
http://text.nlm.nih.gov/nih/cdc/www/
100.html

Text of the National Institutes of Health Consensus Development Conference statement. Addresses the issue of cochlear implants thoroughly and straight-forwardly.

Diseases of the Ear
http://www.hsc.wvu.edu/som/
otolaryngology/ears.htm

Dr. Edward Reiman's Chairside Consult on TMJ Disorders
http://www.saver.net/~enidrei/

Ear Surgery Information Center
http://www.earsurgery.org/

More than just ear surgery information, this site also describes how the ear functions, its anatomy, different ear diseases and injuries. Also includes glossary and research information.

Ideology Forum: Video Otoscopy
http://www.li.net/~sullivan/ears.htm

Noise and Hearing Loss
http://nlm.nih.gov/nih/cdc/www/76txt.html

Statement from the National Institutes of Health Consensus Development Congress regarding contribution to, susceptibility for, protection and prevention of hearing loss.

Otolaryngology Resources

http://www-tmc.edu/oto/others.html

From the Department of Otorhinolaryngology and Communicative Sciences at Baylor College of Medicine, this site provides links to discussion groups, education, publications, software, and organizations related to otolaryngology.

Otolaryngology Resources on the Internet

http://www.bcm.tmc.edu/oto/others.html

Provides links to discussion groups, academic programs, publications and research about otolaryngology and related studies.

Otology Online

http://www.ears.com/

Access to bulletins, discussion groups and medical library resources devoted to the diagnosis and management of diseases of the ears, hearing and balance. For physicians, patients and their families.

Ménière's Disease

Ménière's Disease

http://www.psych.ucsb.edu/~smits/meniere.htm

Ménière's is characterized by ear pressure, discomfort, and fullness; fluctuating hearing loss; fluctuating ringing in the ears; and episodic vertigo.

Symptoms and Incidence of Ménière's Disease

http://oto.wustl.edu/men/mn1.htm

Tinnitus

American Tinnitus Association

http://www.teleport.com/~ata/

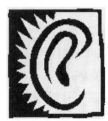

Hearnet

http://www.hearnet.com/

Information on how to prevent hearing loss and tinnitus, provided by Hearing Education and Awareness for Rockers (H.E.A.R.). Hearing evaluation referrals, hearing protection, hearing aids, music news and gossip are discussed.

American Tinnitus Association. http:// www.teleport.com/~ata/

Information about Tinnitus

http://users.bart.nl/~tomdeman/tinnitus.htm

Tinnitus FAQ

http://www.cis.ohio-state.edu/hypertext/faq/usenet/medicine/tinnitus-faq/faq.html

Questions about tinnitus (chronic "ringing" in the ears), including its diagnosis, treatment, complications, and further resources. The site also provides instructions to subscribe to a newsgroup about tinnitus.

Vestibular Disorders

In Balance: Vestibular Disorders Support Group

http://www.best.com/~lyceum/inbalance/

Support and help for individuals suffering from vestibular disorders such as dizziness, balance problems, hearing loss, ringing and/or pain in the ears.

Information about Dizziness, Ataxia and Hearing Disorders

http://hsinfo.ghsl.nwu.edu/neuro/programs/vestib/edu.html

Vestibular Disorders: An Overview

http://www.teleport.com/~veda/overview.html

Vestibular Disorders Association (VEDA)

http://www.teleport.com/~veda/

EATING DISORDERS

Anorexia and Bulimia

American Anorexia/Bulimia Association, Inc.
http://members.aol.com/amanbu/index.html

Anorexia
http://www.neca.com/~cwildes/
   A touching account of a woman with the disease; information and support.

Anorexia Nervosa and Bulimia Association (ANAB)
http://qlink.queensu.ca/~4map/anabhome.html

Anorexia Nervosa and Bulimia Nervosa: Basic Brain, Behavioral and Clinical Studies
http://charlotte.med.nyu.edu/woodr/nimh_anorexia.fund/

Coping with Bulimia
http://cybertowers.com/selfhelp/articles/health/bulimia.html/

Montreux Counseling Centre
http://www.riverhope.org/montrx/
   The Montreux Counseling Centre offers a program to treat emergency cases of eating disorder that is largely based on the creation of an unconditionally supportive environment.

Eating Disorder Recovery Online. *http://www.edrecovery.com/*

General Topics

Cath's Links to Eating Disorders Resources on the Internet

http://www.stud.unit.nostudorg/ikstrh/ed/ed.html

Eating Disorders Recovery Online

http://www.edrecovery.com/

Lucy Serpell's Eating Disorders Resources

http://www.iop.bpmf.ac.uk/home/depts/psychiat/edu/eat.htm

Myer's Information on Obesity, Weight Control, Eating Disorders, and Related Health Conditions

http://www.weight.com/

National Eating Disorders Alliance

http://www.kidsource.com/nedo/index.html

Something Fishy Website on Eating Disorders
http://www.something-fishy.com/ed.htm

Anorexia nervosa, bulimia nervosa, compulsive overeating and other eating disorders are discussed. Signs and symptoms, dangers, and resources are offered, along with articles on stress management and recovery.

Whitefuzz's Eating Disorder Web Site
http://www.fsci.umn.edu/~AAABL/default.htp

Obesity and Compulsive Eating

Binge Eating Disorder
http://www.medhelp.org/lib/binge.txt

Information from the National Institutes of Health.

Healing Hearts' Compulsive Eating Questionnaire
http://www.worldramp.net/~hearts/coesurvey.html

Health Implications of Obesity
http://text.nlm.nih.gov/nih/cdc/www/49txt.html

Overeaters Anonymous
http://www.overeatersanonymous.org/

Overeaters Recovery Group
http://www.HIWAAY.net/recovery/

Lists many different e-mail groups, as well as Overeaters Anonymous weekly meetings on the internet.

EMERGENCY MEDICINE & CRITICAL CARE

Covered in this section: *Critical Care; Disaster Relief; Emergency Home Safety; Emergency Preparedness; General Topics; Injury Control; Organizations; Trauma; Wilderness Medicine.*

Related sections: *Environmental Health; Public Health; Surgery.*

Critical Care

CCM-L
http://www.sfhs.edu/ccm-l/

Site provides archiving and subscription information for the International Critical Care Internet Discussion Group. To subscribe, send e-mail to: majordomo@list.pitt.edu and type in the body: "subscribe CCM-L."

Critical Care Forum
http://biomednet.com/forum/cc/

Critical Care Medicine Humorpage
http://www.ccm-l.med.edu/jokes/

International Critical Care Internet Discussion Group
http://ccm-l.med.edu

Disaster Relief

American Red Cross
http://www.redcross.org

Emergency-Related WHO Press Releases
http://www.who.ch/programmes/eha/press95.htm

Global Health Disaster Network

http://hypnos.m.ehime-u.ac.jp/GHDNet/index.html

Seeks to be an accurate information source about disasters in order to help coordinate efforts to quickly provide relief. Links to disaster-related networks, news sources, journals and conferences.

Internet Disaster Information Network

http://www.disaster.net/

Information on ongoing and historical disaster situations.

ReliefWeb

http://www.reliefweb.int/emergenc/index.html

WHO Division of Emergency and Humanitarian Action

http://www.who.ch.programmes/eha/eha_home.htm

World Association for Disaster and Emergency Medicine

http://www.pitt.edu/HOME/GHNet/wadem/wadem.html

Provides knowledge, techniques, education and policy information, and publications. Encourages the dissemination of information about disaster and emergency medicine.

Emergency Home Safety

Common Simple Emergencies

http://www.clark.net/pub/electra/cse0.html

CPR Instruction

http://www.heartinfo.org/cpr.html

CPR instruction in six simple steps.

Home Safety and Health Patient Education

http://www.vtmednet.org/diner/homeheal.htm

Emergency Preparedness

Earthquake Information

http://quake.wr.usgs.gov/

Earthquake Preparedness Handbook

http://www.ci.la.ca.us:80/dept/LAFD/
eqindex.html

Emergency Preparedness Information Exchange

http://hoshi.cic.sfu.ca/epix/

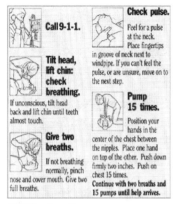

CPR Instruction.
http://www.heartinfo.org/pocket.html

General Topics

Department of Public Safety Online: Medic Alert Program

http://www.ou.edu/oupd/medalert.htm

The Medic Alert emblem is worn around the neck or wrist, and contains important information about the wearer's medical problem(s), name, and contact number to reach medical file information. On-call 24 hours a day.

Emergency Medical Humor

http://home.cwnet.com/catspaw/emshumor.htm

For the emergency room crowd.

Emergency Medicine and Primary Care Home Page

http://www.embbs.com/

Educational resources for emergency and primary care physicians and allied health care providers. Collections of relevant clinical photographs, radiographs, and EKGs; lectures, job opportunities and timely clinical information. Also includes patient care simulations and links to additional related web sites.

Emergency Medicine at the Crossroads

http://x-roads.com/directory.html

Includes journals, organizations, mailing list and a marketplace of emergency medical information resources.

Emergency Medicine Internetwork Gateway

http://oac.hsc.uth.tmc.edu/uth_orgs/emer_med/

Emergency Sciences WWW Site List

http://gilligan.uafadm.alaska.edu/www-911.htm

A list of known fire, rescue, EMS and emergency service sites that can be found on the internet.

EMT's World Wide Discussion Forum

http://monmouth-ocean.com/emt/

Global Emergency Medicine Archives

http://gema.library.ucsf.edu:8081/

World Wide Web of Emergency Services

http://dumbo.isc.rit.edu/ems/index.html

WWW Emergency Sites

http://www.desktop.com.au/~bolin/emlist.htm

Yahoo's Emergency Services

http://www.yahoo.com/Health/Emergency_Services/

Injury Control

Injury Control Resource Information Network

http://www.injurycontrol.com/icrin/

Internet-accessible resources related to the field of injury control and prevention. Injury specific resources include fire safety, burns, poisonings, firearms, violence, and occupational safety. Recent research and links to governmental, professional and commercial sites are provided, as well as many posting and discussion areas.

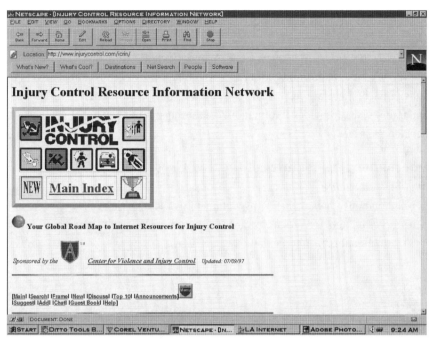

Injury Control Resource Information Network. http://www.injurycontrol.com/icrin/

Injury Prevention Resources on the Net

http://www.albany.edu/sph/injur_8a.html

Internet Resources for Injury Control

http://www.upmc.edu/icrin/

Organizations

American Association of Poison Control Centers

http://198.79.220.3/aapcc/aapcc.htm

American Trauma Society

http://www.amtrauma.org/index.htm

Site for this voluntary non-profit organization dedicated to the prevention of trauma and the improvement of trauma care.

Association of Emergency Physicians

http://www.aep.org/index.html

Federal Emergency Management Agency

http://www.fema.gov/

FEMA provides emergency relief to areas declared National Disasters. The site offers news about floods, tornadoes, and other disasters, and about efforts to aid victims of these events. It also sponsors programs in emergency preparedness and training, and provides information on assistance programs to help people get back on their feet.

International Committee of the Red Cross

http://www.icrc.ch/

International agency that helps victims of war and internal violence. Site has news, description of operations by country, discussion of special issues and topics, and international humanitarian law.

Trauma

American Association for the Surgery of Trauma Webnet

http://www.aast.org/

Site describes itself as providing "scientific information regarding the care of the trauma patient." Includes prevention, prehospital care, resuscitation, operative care, critical care, rehabilitation and trauma system design. Hyperlinks to other trauma resources and discussion groups on the internet.

American Trauma Society

http://www.amtrauma.org/index.htm

Site for this voluntary non-profit organization dedicated to the prevention of trauma and the improvement of trauma care.

Patient's Guide to Cumulative Trauma Disorder (CTD)

http://www.sechrest.com/mmg/ctd/stuff.html

Trauma and Injury Prevention WWW Servers

http://rmstewart.uthscsa.edu/traumasites.html

Links to trauma and injury prevention web sites, accompanied by a brief description. Includes professional organizations, research and academic centers.

TraumAID Project

http://www.cis.upenn.edu/~traumaid/

TraumAID is a program developed to assist physicians with the diagnosis and treatment of critical care and trauma patients. After the patient has been stabilized, the physician supplies some information and TraumAID proposes goals that need to be addressed; as well as produces a plan that will maximize the chance of meeting these goals.

Trauma.Org: Care of the Injured

http://www.trauma.org/

The main feature of this site is the Traumabank, which contains images, articles, case presentations and links divided by specific trauma area specialties, from neurotrauma, to trauma anesthesiology. Connections to Trauma Chat and archives are also offered.

UTHSCSA Trauma Home Page

http://rmstewart.uthscsa.edu/

The University of Texas Health Science Center at San Antonio focuses on issues dealing with injury, injury prevention and surgical critical care. Information for health care professionals, patients and the public is provided. Specifically, advice on pediatric emergency treatment, safety and injury prevention are offered, as well as links to web pages on critical care and emergency prevention.

Virtual ER

http://www.virtualer.com/

Includes tutorials, clinical and radiological images, a medical library, an emergency medicine professional network, residence and fellowship information, links.

Wilderness Medicine

AEE Wilderness Safety and Emergency Care Home Page

http://www.princeton.edu/~rcurtis/wildsafe.html

High Altitude Pathology Institute
http://www.geocities.com/CapeCanaveral/6280/

High altitude pulmonary edema, chronic mountain sickness and other illnesses related to altitude are addressed.

Medical Herpetology
http://www.xmission.com/~gastown/herpmed/med.htm

Medical herpetology (the study of reptiles and amphibians), emerging diseases, and wilderness medicine web sites.

Mountain Rescue Association
http://www.mra.org/

Outdoor Action Program
http://www.princeton.edu/~oa/oa.html

Wilderness first aid and safety for outdoor recreations, from rock climbing, biking and camping, to caving.

Snakebyte Emergency First-Aid Information
http://www.xmission.com/~gastown/herpmed/snbite.htm

ENDOCRINOLOGY

General Topics

Addison's Disease
http://www.niddkh.nih.gov/AD/AD.html

Addison's Disease is a rare endocrine disorder characterized by weight loss, muscle weakness, fatigue and darkening of the skin. Site describes AD symptoms, diagnosis and treatment, and offers suggested reading.

Center for the Study of Environmental Endocrine Effects
http://www.endocrine.org/

Database of material examining the potential effects that man-made or man-generated "endocrine disrupters" may have on the hormones of humans and other animals. Includes links to articles, abstracts, governmental information and an online discussion group.

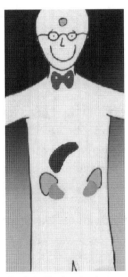

Craig's Endocrinology Project
http://users.iafrica.com/j/jr/jritchie/project/project.htm

Click on an endocrine gland to learn the basics of what it does and how it works. Links; glossary.

Craig's Endocrinology Project.
http://users.iafrica.com/j/jr/jritchie/project/project.htm

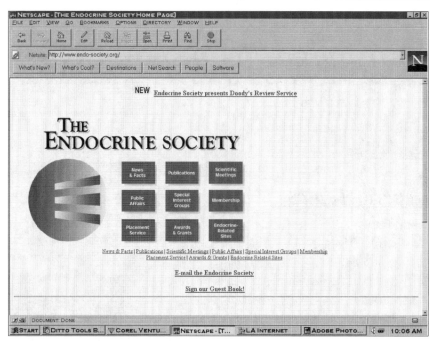

The Endocrine Society. http://www.endo-society.org/

Endocrine Diseases

http://coyote.einet.net:8000/galaxy/Medicine/Diseases-and-Disorders/
Endocrine-Diseases.html

Leads the web-browser to articles on different endocrine disorders, as well as to case studies, organizations, and databases relating to endocrinology.

Endocrine Diseases

http://www.mic.ki.se/Diseases/c19.html

The Swedish Karolinska Institute has assembled an extensive list of links to internet sites focusing on endocrinology in general, as well as to sites addressing specific diseases afflicting the organs of the endocrine system: e.g., diabetes mellitus, Addison Disease, Cushing Syndrome, breast diseases, pituitary diseases, parathyroid diseases, thyroid diseases, Kallmann Syndrome and endocrine gland neoplasms.

Endocrinology Databases

http://museum.state.il.us/isas/data2.html

The Illinois State Academy of Science maintains this site which provides tables showing the standard ranges of concentration of pituitary, steroid, thyroid and other hormones as well as levels of the insulin-like growth factors in humans (by age) and in other animals.

Endocrinology Home Page

http://www.endocrinology.com/

Links of Interest to Endocrinologists

http://www.geocities.com/HotSprings/1833/endolinks.htm

This site contains numerous references to endocrinology associations and journals, and points to sites providing patient information on endocrinology, and to guidelines and medical resources for physicians.

Medical Matrix Endocrinology Page

http://www1.slackinc.com/SPECIALT/ENDOCRIN.HTML

Thorough guide and index for endocrinology on the web. Includes news, abstracts, reviews, indices, guidelines, case studies, images, meetings, and concentration on specific endocrine disorders (e.g., adrenal diseases, diabetes, thyroid/parathyroid disease, chronic fatigue syndrome, and endocrine neoplasms).

MedWeb's Endocrinology

http://www.gen.emory.edu/medweb/medweb.endocrinology.html

Another choice starting-place for researching endocrinology topics. This site provides links to countless endocrine-related sites, including case studies, consumer health information, pediatric endocrinology and toxicology.

Patient Information Documents on Endocrine Disorders

http://www.niddk.nih.gov/EndocrineDocs.html

NIDDK information for patients and the general public offers information on acromegaly, Addison disease, Cushing syndrome, familial multiple endocrinoneoplasia, hyperparathyroidism and prolactinoma. Description of the disease, its cause, prevalence, symptoms, treatment and suggested readings are provided. Also offers a directory of organizations addressing endocrine and metabolic diseases.

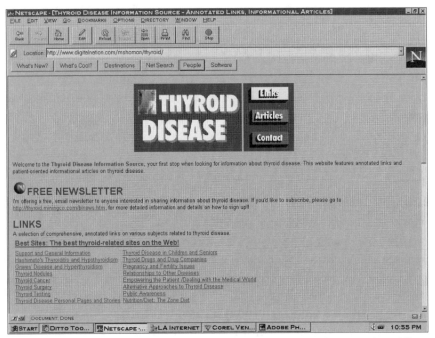

Thyroid Disease Information Source. *http://www.digitalnation.com/mshomon/thyroid/*

Reproductive Endocrinology and Infertility
http://www-leland.stanford.edu/dept/GYNOB/rei/

Site is maintained by the Division of Stanford Health Services, which helps those with fertility and reproductive problems, and addresses infertility as related to the endocrine system.

Organizations

American Association of Clinical Endocrinologists Home Page
http://www.aace.com/

This site offers information for AACE members and non-members about practice guidelines, continuing education opportunities, jobs, legislative updates, discussion groups and CPT coding issues as related to endocrinology. In addition, it offers access to the online edition of "The First Messenger," a bi-monthly newsletter.

228

Endocrine Society

http://www.endo-society.org/

Well-organized and well-written, this site offers many fact sheets on endocrine-related topics. In addition, *Endocrine News* may be received free to approved applicants, and it contains editorials, articles, and technical news.

Thyroid

Diagnosing Thyroid Disorders

http://www.hsc.missouri.edu/medicine/thyroid/thyindex.html

Describes the different thyroid disorders and various thyroid function tests. Presents case studies in the form of a "thyroid quiz," and offers links to other thyroid and endocrine sites.

Health Guides on Thyroid Disease

http://home.ican.net/~thyroid/English/Guides.html

Santa Monica Thyroid Diagnostic Center

http://www.thyroid.com/

As well as information specific to the Center, this site offers patient information on thyroid function and anatomy, hypothyroidism and hyperthyroidism. Describes the diseases and their symptoms, treatment, etc. Patient and physician links to articles, books, associations and online services are also provided. Thyroid-related questions may be e-mailed and will be answered by the Center's staff.

Thyroid Disease Information Source

http://www.digitalnation.com/mshomon/thyroid/

Site offers patient-oriented informative articles on thyroid disease, as well as links and a newsletter.

Thyroid Foundation of Canada

http://home.ican.net/~thyroid/Canada.html

Information in French and English for thyroid patients and their families. Includes educational materials, pamphlets, contacts, meetings, lectures and events, as well as links to an international directory of organizations devoted to the thyroid.

A quarterly publication entitled "Thyrobulletin Newsletter" is free with membership.

Thyroid Neck Check

http://www.aace.com/guidelines/card.html

All you need is a glass of water and a mirror to check out your thyroid gland.

ENVIRONMENTAL HEALTH

Covered in this section: _General Topics; Hazardous Substances/Toxicology;_
Multiple Chemical Sensitivity; Organizations.

Related sections: _Emergency Medicine & Critical Care; Public Health._

General Topics

Case Studies in Environmental Medicine

http://bios-3.bsd.uchicago.edu/Hhs/index.html

From the U.S. Department of Health and Human Services, Public Health Service, Agency for Toxic Substances and Disease Registry.

Environmental Health

http://chs-web.neb.net/usr/graham/ehealth/

Environmental Health and Safety Gopher

gopher://ehs.ucr.edu:70/00/welcome/

From the University of California at Riverside.

Environmental Health and Safety Resources

http://www.uwm.edu:80/People/rjg/ehslinks/ehslinks.html

Set of links gathered by the University of Wisconsin-Milwaukee.

Environmental Health Patient Education

http://www.vtmednet.org/diner/env.htm

Information on mercury, lead, radon, pesticides, air quality and other contaminants, for the general public.

History of Radiation Protection

http://www.sph.umich.edu/group/eih/UMSCHPS/hist.htm

National Institute of Environmental Health Sciences
http://www.niehs.nih.gov/

Research on environment-related diseases, including press releases, journal links, information clearinghouse, research and scientific programs.

News Page: Environmental Services
http://www.newspage.com/NEWSPAGE/cgi-bin/walk.cgi/NEWSPAGE/ infold14/d1/

The current day's hazardous waste contamination and clean-up efforts across the nation are summarized on this page. Access to complete reports requires registration, which is free.

Radiation and Health Physics Home Page
http://www.sph.umich.edu/group/eih/UMSCHPS/index.html

Right-To-Know Network (RTK Net)
http://www.rtk.net/

Access to government databases relating to environment and housing issues.

Hazardous Substances/Toxicology
See also: Emergency Medicine & Critical Care; Public Health.

Agency for Toxic Substances and Disease Registry
http://atsdr1.atsdr.cdc.gov:8080/

Chem-Tox.Com
http://www.chem-tox.com/

Subtitled "Chemical & Pesticide Health Effects Research."

Emergency Response Notification Center of the EPA
http://www.epa.gov/ERNS/

Find out the details about the top 10 oil and hazardous substance spills this past month, past year, and overall. Database.

Environmental Protection Agency. *http://www.epa.gov/*

ExToxNET: The Extension TOXicology NETwork

http://ace.orst.edu/info/extoxnet/

Provides a variety of information about pesticides. Includes fact sheets, news, technical information, newsletter, and additional resources.

Hazardous Substances and Public Health

http://atsdr1.cdc.gov:8080/HEC/hsphhome.html

Quarterly newsletter published by the Agency for Toxic Substances and Disease Registry.

Hazardous Substance Research Centers

http://www.gtri.gatec.edu/hsrc/

HazDat: Hazardous Substance Release/ Health Effects Database

http://atsdr1.atsdr.cdc.gov:8080/hazdat.html

Maintained by the Agency for Toxic Substances and Disease Registry.

Natural Hazards Center
http://www.Colorado.EDU/hazards/

Pesticide Information Profiles
http://ace.ace.orst.edu/info/extoxnet/pips/ghindex.html

Toxic Hot Spots
http://www.econet.apc.org/hotspots/

Chemicals Can Cripple

Multiple Chemical Sensitivity. *http://www.supernet.net/~jackibar/mcs.html*

Multiple Chemical Sensitivity

MC Survivors
http://www-rohan.sdsu.edu/staff/lhamilto/mcs/
Site for individuals suffering from multiple chemical sensitivity and environmental illness.

Multiple Chemical Sensitivity
http://www.supernet.net/~jackibar/mcs.html
Advice on living a non-toxic lifestyle.

Resources for the Chemically Sensitive or Enviromentally Ill
http://www.snowcrest.net/lassen/mcsei.html
Directory for individuals wishing to avoid excessive use of synthetic and chemical products.

Organizations

American Environmental Health Foundation
http://www.aehf.com/
AEHF is a non-profit organization seeks to further the practice of environmental medicine. Site offers educational materials and a product catalog.

U.S. Environmental Protection Agency
http://www.epa.gov/

EYES / OPTOMETRY & OPHTHALMOLOGY

Cataracts

American Society of Cataract and Refractive Surgery

http://www.ascrs.org/

This is the home page for member ophthalmologists specializing in cataract and refractive surgery. It offers: Society news as well as eye care information; *Eye World Magazine Online*; legislative and government updates; and a marketplace section which provides information on industry news, stocks, and a listing of eye care vendors. Links to other professional societies.

Cataract Image

http://www-medlib.med.utah.edu/WebPath/EYEHTML/EYE018.html

Eye Care Information

http://www.ascrs.org/patient.html

Patient information on refractive surgery and cataract surgery, and frequently asked questions (FAQs) about cataracts. Access to the American Society of Cataract and Refractive Surgery resources which includes publications, meetings information, search engine and additional web links.

General Topics

Conjunctivitis (Pink Eye) Patient Information

http://lib-sh.lsumc.edu/fammed/pted/pinkeye.html

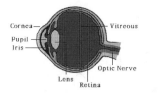

The Eye!
http://www.eyeinfo.com/wayworks.htm

The Eye!

http://www.eyeinfo.com/

All about the eye and eye care. Includes information about refractive surgery, cataracts, contact lenses, glaucoma, eye anatomy and physiology.

Eye Care FAQS

http://www.eyenet.org/public/faqs/faqs.html

Eye Care: Related Links

http://www.nerdworld.com/nw1041.html

Nerd World Media's long list of sites related to eye care, including acupressure, contact lenses, eye strain, questions and answers about glaucoma, eye diseases, eye surgery and eye-robics.

Eye Information

http://www.noah.cuny.edu/eye/eye.html

Information on anatomy, function, diseases and eye care.

Eye Page

http://haas.berkeley.edu/~dowis/eye/eye.html

Eyenet

http://www.eyenet.org/

Information from the American Academy of Ophthalmology.

Eyeville

http://www.eyeville.com/

Resources and information on eye care.

Information about Eye Conditions and Diseases

http://www.web-xpress.com/vhsc/iaecad.html

Information on astigmatism, cataracts, crossed eyes, dry eyes, glaucoma, eyelid surgery and more.

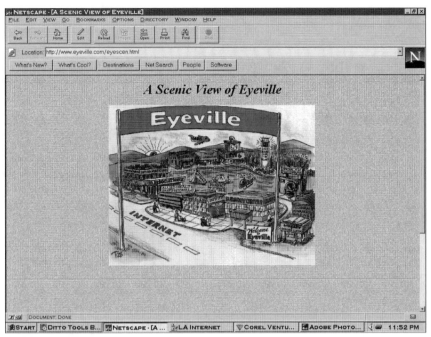

Eyesville. *http://www.eyeville.com/eyescen.html*

National Eye Institute

http://www.nei.nih.gov/

Information for researchers, health care professionals, the general public and patients, educators and the media on the research and activities being carried out or supported by the NEI.

Glaucoma

Glaucoma FAQ

http://www.iglou.com/KEC_eyedocs/glaucoma.htm

What glaucoma is, what causes it, types of glaucoma and symptoms, detection and treatment. Links to related sites are provided.

Glaucoma Research Foundation

http://www.glaucoma.org/

Information on glaucoma, the Foundation and its activities. Features selected articles from eye care journals that are summarized in layperson's language.

Surgery

Radial Keratotomy Homepage
http://www-or.stanford.edu/~mob/RK/

Retinal Implant Project
http://www.ai.mit.edu/projects/implant/

This site describes the goal and theory behind a research project which seeks to develop a silicon-chip eye implant that can restore vision for patients suffering from retinitis pigmentosa and macular degeneration."

FAMILY MEDICINE

Covered in this section: Background Check; General Topics; Links; Patient Education/Fact Sheets.

Background Check

Medi-Net
http://www.askmedi.com/

Receive background information on every physician licensed to practice medicine in the United States. Service tells medical school, year of graduation, residency, medical specialty certifications, licensure data, and records of sanctions or disciplinary actions taken against a physician. The cost is $15 for information about the first doctor and $5 for subsequent doctors.

General Topics

Cyberspace Telemedical Office
http://www.telemedical.com/Telemedical

Duke University Community and Family Medicine Home Page
http://dmi-www.mc.duke.edu/cfm/cfmhome.html

Family Health on the Net
http://www.tcom.ohiou.edu/family-health.html

Daily series of 2-1/2 minute long audio programs for a general audience. Answers most of the frequently asked health and medical-related questions, including information on ADD, bee stings and whiplash.

Family-L Archives
gopher://spiner.gac.edu:80/1/pub/E-mail-archives/family-l

Family health-related issues.

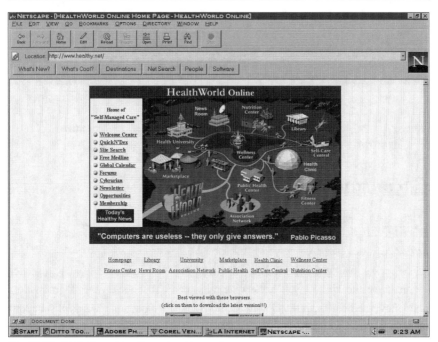

Health World Online. http://www.healthy.net/

Family Medicine Resources on the World Wide Web
http://www.uwo.ca/fammed/resource.html

Family Practice/Primary Care Working Group Newsletter
http://www.med.ufl.edu/medinfo/pcnews/

GlobalMedic
http://www.globalmedic.com/

Online software that results in recommendations for self-care and managed care when information is provided.

Health Answers
http://www.healthanswers.com/index.htm

Health Links
http://www.hslib.washington.edu/

Information and references about family health, basic science, clinical specialties, public health and informatics. Includes links to journals and legislation updates.

HealthWorld Online

http://www.healthy.net/

This site seeks to be a comprehensive global health network providing integrative health, wellness, and medical information, products and services. It provides links to medical libraries, and offers a marketplace, a healing center, nutrition, fitness, professional, educational and self-care resources.

Mayo Clinics Health O@sis

http://www.mayo.ivi.com/

Information for health care consumers, including access to an online library, cancer center, and heart center. Includes information on diet and nutrition, pregnancy and children's health care.

MedAccess On-Line

http://www.medaccess.com/

Health and wellness information, including newsletters, personalized health goals, and databases of hospitals, physicians and HMOs.

MedWeb's Family/Consumer Health

http://www.gen.emory.edu/MEDWEB/Keyword/consumer-health.html

Pareras Online

http://www.pareras.com/online/home.htm

Medical information for patients.

Pharmaceutical Care Associates

http://www.wnwcorp.com/pharmca/

Type in personal information such as allergies, diagnoses, current medications, and a description of your medical history and condition to receive medical advice via the internet.

POL Health Information Network

http://www.polhealth.net/html/polhealth/

Provides information to educated health consumers. Includes access to MEDLINE, searchable drug databases, medical news, discussion groups and other web resources. Monthly fee.

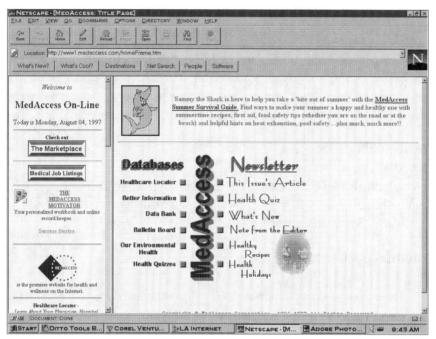

Med Access On-Line. *http://www1.medaccess.com/homeFrame.htm*

Self-Help Sourcebook Online

http://www.cmhc.com/selfhelp/

Thrive @ Pathfinder

http://thriveonline.com/

   Healthy lifestyle information and advice.

University of Iowa Family Practice Handbook

http://indy.radiology.uiowa.edu/Providers/ClinRef/FPHandbook/
FPContents.html

   Electronic clinical reference source that places an emphasis on the diagnosis
and treatment of common medical illnesses. Chapters study different medical
specialties, with a special section on AIDS.

University of Texas' Health Explorer

http://dpalm2.med.uth.tmc.edu/ptnt/tocptnt.htm

   Health and healthy lifestyle information, suggestions and links.

Links

Health Mall
http://www.hlthmall.com/
> Links to sites of companies that sell natural products.

MEDguide
http://www.medguide.net/
> Guide to medicine and health care links on the internet.

VOLC-R Family Medicine Related Internet Sources
http://griffin.vcu.edu/views/fap/volc-r.html
> Links to primary care resources.

Patient Education/Fact Sheets

Annotated List of Patient Educational Materials
http://www.vh.org/Patients/PatientsAnnotatedList.html
> From anesthesia to surgery, a great deal of information for patients.

CareSheets
http://www.infolane.com/pamp/
> New patient education sheets every month. Order form available at web site.

Family Practice Information Fact Sheets
http://www.uiowa.edu/~famprac/med.html
> Fact sheets on everything from asthma to urinary tract infections.

Patient Education Materials
http://lib-sh.lsumc.edu:80/fammed/pted/pted.html
> Health problems, health maintenance, and information on drugs.

Rural Health Village: Patient Education Information
http://www.vtmednet.org/diner/home.htm
> Covers topics such as alcohol abuse, allergies, asthma, cancer, cardiovascular health, diabetes and much more.

FITNESS

Aerobics

Aerobics Page
http://www.turnstep.com/

Bonnie's Jazzercise Page
http://users.ccnet.com/~bonnie/

Answers to frequently asked questions about jazzercise, tips for beginners and web links.

Boxerobics
http://ourworld.compuserve.com/homepages/ianmeck/boxhome.htm

Basic questions about boxerobics, which developed from boxing fitness training combined with aerobics. Includes a home workout page.

Jazzercise
http://www.jazzercise.com/

Includes jazzercise news and articles, as well as specifics about the jazzercise industry.

Bicycling

Bicycle Discussion Lists on Internet
http://eksl-www.cs.umass.edu/~westy/cycling/cycling-on-internet.html

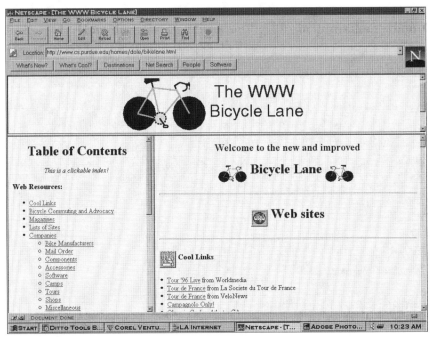

The WWW Bicycle Lane. *http://www.cs.purdue.edu/homes/dole/bikelane.html*

Bicycle Terms

gopher://draco.acs.uci.edu.:1071/00/glossary/

Long list of biking terminology. Excludes the obvious and the commercial.

Bicycles FAQ

http://www.cis.ohio-state.edu/hypertext/faq/usenet/bicycles-faq/top.html

Bike Culture Quarterly and Encycleopedia Website

http://bikeculture.com/home/

Cyberider Cycling WWW Site

http://blueridge.infomkt.ibm.com/bikes/

This site provides cyclists with information about all aspects of bicycles and bicycling, including advocacy, training routes, equipment, food, news, places, events and links to hundreds of other cycling-related sites.

GearHead Mountain Bike Cyberzine

http://gearhead.com/toc.html

Global Cycling Network

http://cycling.org/

E-mail lists, links and bike groups.

Rec.Bicycles FTP Archives

gopher://draco.acs.uci.edu:1071/

Roger Marquis' Cycling Page

http://www.roble.com/jarquis/

Trento Bike Pages

http://www-math.science.unitn.it/Bike/

These pages contain information on mountain biking in Europe and the Mediterranean.

WOMBATS on the Web

http://www.wombats.org/

The WOmen's Mountain Bike And Tea Society.

WWW Bicycle Lane

http://www.cs.purdue.edu/homes/dole/bikelane.html

Links, bike commuting and advocacy, magazines, companies, catalogs, bike clubs, bike races, bike safety, mountain bikes, and more.

Exercise

Abdominal Training FAQ-Index Page

http://www.dstc.edu.au/TU/staff/timbomb/ab/

American Council on Exercise Online

http://www.acefitness.org/

Fact sheets on nutrition and exercise, hotline and online publication.

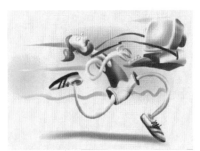

Perpetual Motion.
http://www.teleport.com/~pmotion/

Cybercise

http://www.cybercise.com/

Includes the cybercise forum on fitness-related issues; cybercise sound room (with music to exercise by); fitness supplies and fitness events around the world. Nutrition information provided as well.

Guidelines for Personal Exercise Programs

http://www.hoptechno.com/book11.htm

Perpetual Motion World Wide Web Sites

http://www.teleport.com/~pmotion/

Links to other fitness-related sites; archive and subscription information on "Don't Stop Moving," their newsletter.

Stretching and Flexibility

http://www.cs.huji.ac.il/papers/rma/stretching_toc.html

General Topics

Balance

http://hyperlink.com/balance

Online fitness magazine with search engine.

Calculate Your Body Fat Percentage, Circumference Method

http://www.he.net/~zone/prothd2.html

Continuing Education Web

http://www.cewl.com/

Links for athletic health care professionals.

Department of Kinesiology and Health Science W3

http://www.tahperd.sfasu.edu/sfakin.html

At the Stephen F. Austin State University.

Department of Kinesiology, Kansas State University

http://www.ksu.edu/kines/

Programs, courses, faculty and research information, and application for admission.

Elaine's Physical Fitness and Health Links

http://www.elainecase.com/ecfit.html

Fit Talk

http://www.mypage.net/fittalk/

Physical fitness discussion group.

Fitness

http://segment.ucsf.edu/brent/fitness/fitness.htm

Links to fitness, weight lifting and body building sites.

Fitness Files

http://rcc.webpoint.com/fitness/index.htm

Fitness Matters

http://lifematters.com/fitnesn.html

Fitness, nutrition and weight management. Includes book reviews, news and feature articles.

Fitness Partner Connection Jumpsite

http://primusweb.com/fitnesspartner/

FitnessLink

http://www.fitnesslink.com/

Offers articles and tips on fitness; lists books, magazines, newsgroups, mailing lists and related internet links.

Health and Fitness World Guide Forum

http://www.worldguide.com/Fitness/hf.html

Subjects include anatomy, strength training, cardiovascular exercise, eating well, and sports medicine.

Internet Fitness Resource

http://rampages.onramp.net/~chaz/

Information on exercise and fitness. Lots of links.

Introduction to Kinesiology

http://kines/99.kines.uiuc.edu/

University of Illinois at Urbana-Champaign class description and lecture notes.

New Balance Cyberpark

http://newbalance.com/

Site focuses on running, health and fitness.

On-Line to Fitness

http://www.thegallery.com/fitness.html

Shape Up America

http://shapeup.org/sua/

Provides information on safe weight management and physical fitness. Determine your body-mass index (BMI), and develop a meal plan suitable for your health. Take a health and fitness quiz; download information. Has a special page for health and fitness professionals.

Stepping Stones: Practical Tools for Achieving Your Goals

http://www.flpinstitute.com/steppingstones/

Monthly newsletter providing advice and support on how to change your lifestyle and reach fitness, health and emotional goals.

Texas Association of Health, Physical Education, Recreation and Dance

http://www.tahperd.sfasu.edu/

Waist/Hip Ratio Calculator

http://www.amhrt.org/news/fact/whcalc.html

World Fitness

http://www.worldfitness.org/

Hiking and Walking

Dirty Sole Society
http://www.barefooters.org/

A site for people who love going barefoot all the time, or who are barefoot hikers, dancers, etc.

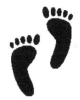

Gorp Regional Trail Guides
http://www.gorp.com/gorp/activity/hiking/hik_guid.htm

Great Outdoor Recreation Pages
http://www.gorp.com/

Dirty Sole Society. http://www.

Hiking and Walking Homepage
http://www.teleport.com/~walking/hiking.html

Offers information on hiking and walking clubs, places to go hiking, appropriate gear, philosophy and trail guides.

Koby's Hiking Information Center
http://www.cs.usask.ca/undergrads/jdk132/

Information and tips on backpacking; questions and answers, links.

National Recreation Trails
http://www.gorp.com/gorp/activity/hiking/natrectr.htm

These trails range from one to 40 miles long.

National Scenic Trails
http://www.gorp.com/resource/us_trail/nattrail.htm

Descriptions of great long-distance footpaths such as the Appalachian Trail, the Pacific Crest, and the Continental Divide.

National Historic Trails
http://www.gorp.com/gorp/resource/us_trail/historic.htm

Power Walking Home Page
http://members.aol.com/PowerWalkr/index.html

Volksmarch and Walking Index

http://www.teleport.com/~walking/

Volksmarch is a non-competitive, 6-mile walk, around which numerous volkssport clubs are based. Site provides information on how to join, upcoming events and walks, articles, and e-mail groups.

Walking Extra

http://www.wellnesscenter.com/Walking/NWalkingMain.htm

Walking Wellness On-Line

http://www.wellnesscenter.com/WWBook/Ndefault.htm

Includes a description of race-walking races, events and clubs.

Walklist and Walklist-digest

http://www.teleport.com/~walking/walklist.htm

To join these two discussion groups, send e-mail to: Majordomo@lists.teleport.com and in the message, write either "subscribe walklist" or "subscribe walklist-digest."

Running

Cool Running

http://www.coolrunning.com/

News and races, race results, editorials, forums and mail.

Dead Runners Society

http://storm.cadcam.iupui.edu/drs/drs.html

Information on the listserv and numerous links to other related sites. Contrary to its name, this is a discussion group for runners who are very much alive. To subscribe, send e-mail to: listserv@listserv.dartmouth.edu with the message: "SUB DRS yourname."

Marathon Listing Page

http://sunsite.unc.edu/drears/running/marathon/marathon.html

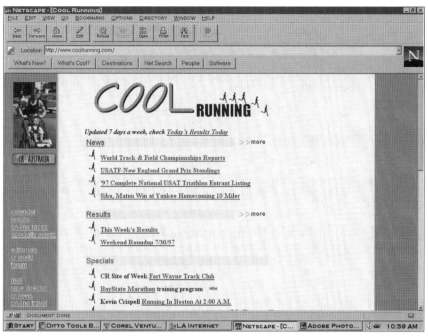

Cool Running. http://www.coolrunning.com/

Peak Performance

http://www.siteworks.co.uk/pperf/conts.htm

This is a scientific newsletter devoted to improving stamina, strength and fitness. Sample articles and subscription information are provided.

Road Runners Club of America

http://rrca.org/

Runners World Online

http://www.runnersworld.com/

Daily news and articles. Departments include running for beginners, running injuries, women and running, nutrition, travel and training shoes.

Running Clubs

http://sunsite.unc.edu/drears/running/clubs/clubs.html

Running Network

http://www.runningnetwork.com/index.html

Information clearinghouse on running. Huge amount of information.

Running Page

http://sunsite.unc.edu/drears/running/running.html

Running Research News

http://www.gisd.com/rrn/

Written by exercise physiologists. Information about subscribing.

Ultramarathon World

http://Fox.stn.ca:80/~dblaikie/

For athletes who run distances longer than the standard marathon of 52.195 kilometers, or 26 miles.

U.S.A. Track and Field Road Running Information Center

http://www.usaldr.org/

Sports

CyberQueer Lounge Sports Page

http://www.cyberzine.org/html/GLAIDS/Sports/sportspage.html

From body building to wrestling.

Gay Games

http://www.dds.nl/~gaygames/index2.html

The 1998 Gay Games are to be held in Amsterdam, August 1-8. Site provides information on registration, festivities, sports, culture and volunteering.

Go, Girl! Magazine

http://www.gogirlmag.com/

Free, biweekly magazine dedicated to getting women of all ages and fitness levels involved in sports.

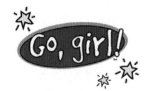

Go, Girl! Magazine.
http://www.gogirlmag.com/

LBG-Sports Home Page

http://www.kwic.net/lgb-sports/index.html

Information of interest to gay and bisexual sports fans and athletes. Includes organizations, sports events, book lists and web links.

International Gay and Lesbian Aquatics

http://www.kwic.net/igla.html

Internet Athlete

http://www.athlete.com/

Snowboarding FAQ

http://www.nyx.net/~mwallace/sb_faq.html

WWW Women's Sports Page

http://fiat.gslis.utexas.edu/~lewisa/womsprt.html
    General and sports-specific pages for women.

Sports Medicine

American Academy of Podiatric Sports Medicine

http://www.clark.net/pub/aapsm.html

Dr. Pribut's Running Injuries Page

http://www.clark.net/pub/pribut/spsport.html

Links to Physical Therapy

http://www.hia.net/pdesmidt/physicaltherapy.htm

MedFacts' Sports Doc

http://www.medfacts.com/sprtsdoc.htm
    Twenty-four virtual patient examinations.

Medicine in Sports Pages on the Web

http://www.mspweb.com/
    Broken down into organizations, schools and universities; magazines and online journals; clinics and practices; and other points of interest.

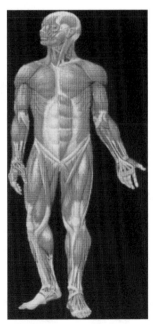

The Medisport Interactive Getting Better Guide.
http://www.medisport.co.uk/siteof.htm

Medisport Interactive Getting Better Guide

http://www.medisport.co.uk/

Includes the "Site of Pain Index" self-treatment guidelines.

Sports Medicine and Orthopedic Surgery

http://www.sports-medicine.com/

Submit a question relating to sports medicine to Dr. Stuart Zeman.

Steadman Hawkins Website

http://www.ortho-con.com/steadman-hawkins/

Hospital grand rounds for sports medicine.

Weight Training/Body Building

Biofitness Health Club

http://www.biofitness.com/

Sample plans for weight training and aerobic training.

Body Mechanics

http://www.imgsys.com/bodymech/index.html

Information on fitness, nutrition and body building.

Bodybuilders Around the World

http://www.solace.mh.se/~alpha/bbpics.htm

Faith Sloan's Bodybuilding Site

http://www.frsa.com/bbpage.shtml

Includes female and male body building galleries, articles, discussion forum, business directory, competitions and results, links and statistics on Faith Sloan, a professional competitor and the creator of this site.

Lewis Wolk's A-Z Fitness and Bodybuilding Links

http://www.axess.com/users/lewis/index.htm

Performance Zone

http://triemme.com/performance/

Weight training, nutrition and fitness for both serious and weekend athletes.

Welcome to the Platform

http://www.waf.com/bin/windex.pl/

Olympic weight lifting rules, as well as advice on mental training and nutrition, weight lifting calendars and a weight lifter's calculator.

Yoga

American Yoga Association

http://members.aol.com/amyogassn/index.htm

Information about the AYA and yoga in general.

Benefits of Yoga to Modern Life

http://www.genius.net/indolink/Health/yoga.html

The Dhyanyoga Centers

http://www.dyc.org/

Learn about Kundalini Maha Yoga and the mental and physical benefits of meditation.

Kundalini Resource Center

http://www.hmt.com/kundalini/

Kundalini articles, events, frequently asked questions (FAQs) and mailing list.

Shoshoni: A Yoga Retreat Center

http://shell.rmi.net/~shoni/index.html

A yoga and meditation retreat center in the Colorado Rockies.

Sivananda Yoga "Om" Page

http://www.sivananda.org/

Yoga Central

http://www.yogaclass.com/welcome.html

YogaNet

http://www.yogajournal.com/

Online magazine about Yoga.

GRANTS & FUNDING FOR RESEARCH

AHCPR Funding Opportunities
http://www.ahcpr.gov/news/funding.htm

The Agency for Health Care Policy and Research supports research projects that examine the availability, quality, and costs of health care services; ways to improve the effectiveness and appropriateness of clinical practice, including the prevention of disease; and other areas of health services research, such as services for persons with HIV infection. AHCPR also supports small grants, conference grants, and training through dissertation grants and National Research Service Awards to institutions and individuals. This site provides an overview of the funding process, policy notices and an application.

Biomedical Sciences Funding Information
http://www.arisnet.com/biomed.html

This site describes some governmental and non-governmental funding sources available for the field of biomedicine, and it includes contacts and deadlines for application. It lists federal and private sources of grants, fellowships, scholarships, contracts and awards to colleges and universities, research centers, and individuals that can be found in the *Biomedical Sciences Report*, which is available every six weeks from ARIS publications (link provided).

Database: NIH Guide to Grants and Contracts
http://www.med.nyu.edu/nih-guide.html

The *NIH-Guide* is distributed weekly via e-mail and contains detailed information on the programs supported by the National Institutes of Health. This site contains the current and back issues of the guide. A gopher menu is available at: *gopher://gopher.nih.gov:70/11/res/nih-guide/*.

DIH: Division of Research Grants

http://www.drg.nih.gov/

The Division of Research Grants is part of the National Institutes of Health and assists in the formulation of grant application review policies and procedures. It aids in assigning NIH grant applications to supporting institutes, and provides for scientific review of most NIH research grants.

FEDIX

http://web.fie.com/fedix/

Federal Information Exchange Funding Opportunities. This is a database providing information on the funding opportunities available to the educational and research communities from a dozen federal agencies. Participating agencies include the National Institutes of Health, the Agency for International Development, the Department of Agriculture, the Department of Veterans Affairs and the Environmental Protection Agency.

Grants and Funding Guide

http://info.yale.edu/library/reference/publications/grants.html

Grants Web

http://web.fie.com/cws/sra/resource.htm

Lists many U.S., Canadian and international government and private grants funding resources, and offers policy information, circulars and legislation information. Includes some grant forms online and offers links to related sites.

Medical Research Council of Canada

http://www.hinetbc.org/information/2fmed.htm

Operating (research) grants, major equipment grants, research scholarships, fellowships, studentships, and workshop support are offered to qualified Canadian recipients working in the field of health sciences.

MOLIS Scholarship Search

http://www.fie.com/molis/scholar.htm

Search this database for information on scholarships available to minorities. Qualified applicants include high school seniors, college and graduate school students from the United States.

National Science Foundation Grants & Awards

http://www.nsf.gov/home/grants.html

The National Science Foundation is an independent U.S. government agency responsible for promoting science and engineering through programs that invest over $3.3 billion per year in almost 20,000 research and education projects in science and engineering. This site describes funding opportunities, proposal criteria and preparation, and other information required to apply for financial support.

NLM Extramural Programs

http://www.nlm.nih.gov/ep/extramural.html

Describes the grants and other assistance mechanisms available from the National Library of Medicine. Research and resource grants, individual fellowships, institutional training grants, publication and conference grants are awarded to selected domestic public and private, nonprofit institutions involved in health science research, education or practice.

Robert Wood Johnson Home Page

http://www.rwjf.org/main.html

The Robert Wood Johnson Foundation claims to be the largest philanthropic organization in the United States exclusively devoted to health and health care. Grants are awarded in support of three goal areas: assuring that all Americans have access to basic health care at reasonable cost; improving the way services are organized and provided to people with chronic health conditions; and reducing the personal, social and

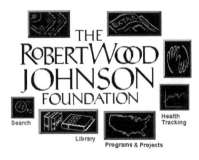

The Robert Wood Johnson Foundation Home Page. *http://www.rwjf.org/main.html*

economic harm caused by substance abuse (tobacco, alcohol, and illicit drugs). This site describes the Foundation's principles and projects, and provides instructions for applying for a grant. The gopher site may be found at *gopher://gopher.rwjf.org:4500.*

University of Wisconsin Medical School Research Resources

http://www.biostat.wisc.edu/research/research.html

This site provides links to many medical research resources, as well as access to databases of interest to biomedical researchers.

HEALTH ADMINISTRATION

American College of Healthcare Executives

http://www.ache.org/

    General information about this professional society for health care executives. Site provides access to ACHE publications, membership information, and a description of upcoming ACHE educational programs. The career resource center describes workshops, and offers a career guide and links to related sites.

Health Administration and Management Resources

http://www.execpc.com/~stjos/admin.html

    Clinical outcomes, clinical practice guidelines, health economics and finance, health services administration, quality improvement, electronic journals and government resources.

Health Administration Discussion Lists

http://mel.lib.mi.us/health/health-hospital-lists.html

Health Administration Resources

http://www.mercer.edu/health/

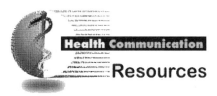

Health Communication Resources.
http://www.emerson.edu/acadepts/cs/healthcom/Resources/HOME.html

Health Care Administration on the World Wide Web

http://www.geocities.com/ResearchTriangle/1221/health.htm

Health Communication Resources

http://www.emerson.edu/acadepts/cs/healthcom/Resources/HOME.HTM

    How to effectively communicate health-related information to the public. Monthly updates to this site include articles and editorials. Maintained by Emerson College and Tufts University School of Medicine.

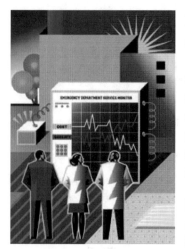

Healthcare Financial Management Association. *http://www.hfma.org/*

Health Hippo

http://www.winternet.com/~hippo/

A collection of policy and regulatory materials related to health care. From Antitrust to Vaccines, links are listed by topic and type of reference. Additional topics include: insurance, policy and administration, antitrust laws, fraud and abuse issues, medical devices, reproductive rights and tax exempt status.

Healthcare Financial Management Association

http://www.hfma.org/

The HFMA is comprised of over 34,000 financial management professionals employed by hospitals, managed care organizations, medical group practices, and other health care organizations. It offers members educational programs, professional guidance, career development, and inter-field communication. This site describes the organization's activities and publications, posts job announcements and classified ads, and provides information on HFMA chapters and how to join.

Knowledge Inc.

http://www.knowledgeinc.com/

Conferences, upcoming events and information about Knowledge Inc., which offers executives information on how to enhance knowledge, technology and performance. The company publishes a newsletter, available for a fee.

HEALTH CARE CAREERS & EDUCATION

Dental Education

American Association of Dental Schools
http://www.aads.jhu.edu/

Dental Student Educational Resources
http://www.hsdm.med.harvard.edu/pages/dentstud.htm
>Biomedical sites of interest to dental students.

International Dental Schools Directory
http://www.dentalsite.com/dentists/intsch.html

Pre-Dental Page
http://www.cet.com/~kgray/Predental.HTM
>All about dentistry and applying to dental schools. Includes a list of U.S. dental schools with links and additional resources.

Professional Connection
http://www.oralb.com/connect/index.html
>Articles, journal abstracts and clinical abstracts for dental health professionals.

So, You Want to Be a Dentist?
http://www.vvm.com/~bond/home.html
>Kirk Bond, D.D.S. created this site to answer some basic questions individuals who are considering entering the field of dentistry may have. It describes the different kinds of dentists, provides dental images and interesting web sites.

U.S. Dental Schools Directory

http://www.dentalsite.com/dentists/densch.html

Web Sites for Dental Students

http://www.dentalsite.com/dentists/denstu.html

Links to dental student pages and resources, dental school sites, histology sites and publications.

General Topics

Health Careers On Line

http://www.ers-online.com/

Health care employment database.

Healthcare Careers Online

http://www.ers.com/

Visitors may view employment opportunities, apply to positions online, or use the career resources offered at this site.

Office of Medical Education, University of Vermont

http://salus.med.uvm.edu/ome/conf.html

Information on medical education conferences, fellowships and society meetings.

SearchCME

http://www.searchcme.com/

Continuing medical education (CME) information on more than 3,000 medical conferences indexed by medical specialty, geographic lcation and date.

Support Site for Educators in the Health Professions

http://www.uchsc.edu/CIS/

This site provides resources to enhance the health professional's educational, research, leadership and management skills, and offers resources for career and personal development. Information on educational journals, conferences and workshops as well as fellowship and funding opportunities are also offered.

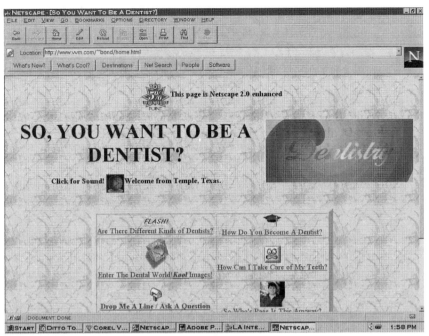

So, You Want to Be a Dentist? *http://www.vvm.com/~bond/home.html*

WebDoctor Continuing Medical Education Resources
http://www.gretmar.com/webdoctor/cme.html

Index of CME resources, multi-media text books and patient simulations available on the internet.

Nursing Education

Continuing Education for RNs and Other Health Professionals
http://www.rnceus.com/

Cybernurse.com
http://www.cybernurse.com/

Good information for those interested in becoming nurses.

EDNET Online
http://www.ed-net.com/

Online continuing education for nurses.

Healthcare Education and Resources for Nurses

http://www.swandesign.com/LRC.html

Nursing Student WWW Page

http://WWW2.CSN.NET/~tbracket/htm.htm

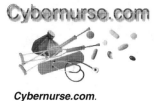

Cybernurse.com.
http://www.cybernurse.com/

NurseOne

http://www.nurseone.com/

This company offers online continuing education courses aimed to improve or refresh the knowledge base of interested nurses. While these courses are available forfree through the internet to anyone equipped to read URL document, with payment of $10 per unit and satisfactory completion of tests, an official CEU certificate will be mailed.

Student Nursing Lists

http://free.websight.com/Miller5/

Osteopathic Schools

Colleges of Osteopathic Medicine

http://www.aacom.org/com.htm

Maintained by the American Association of Colleges of Osteopathic Medicine.

List of Schools of Osteopathic Medicine

http://www.collegenet.com/geograph/osteo.html

Peterson's Osteopathic Medical Schools List

http://www.petersons.com/graduate/select/633020se.html

Pharmacology Schools

Schools of Pharmacy in the U.S.
http://www.li.net/~edhayes/rxschool.html
> List of schools of pharmacy that includes addresses and phone numbers.

World List of Schools of Pharmacy
http://www.cpb.uokhsc.edu/SoP/SoPListHomePage.html

Public Health Schools

Association of Schools of Public Health
http://www.asph.org/

Schools of Public Health in the United States
http://weber.u.washington.edu/~larsson/sphcm94/phealth/schools.html

HEALTH CARE POLICY & ECONOMICS

Covered in this section: General Topics; Government; Statistics.

Related sections: Health Administration; Public Health.

General Topics

Agency for Health Care Policy and Research
http://www.ahcpr.gov/cgi-bin/allsrch.pl
    Search engine.

Alpha Center
http://www.ac.org/
    Non-profit, non-partisan health care policy center offering information and analysis.

C. Everett Koop Institute
http://www.dartmouth.edu/acad-inst/koop/
    The Institute designs and implements strategies to enhance the health of individuals, families and communities. Currently the Institute is undertaking a number of projects, one of which will be the Koop Village, a WWW-based conference and discussion center addressing issues of health care issues. In cooperation with Dartmouth college.

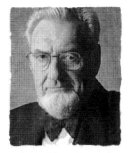

C. Everett Koop Institute.
http://www.dartmouth.edu/
acad-inst/koop/

Center for Health Care Strategies, Inc.
http://www.chcs.org/CHCS/welcome.htm

Center on Budget and Policy Priorities

http://epn.org/cbpp.html

Non-partisan research organization and policy institute that focuses on analysis of government policies and programs, especially those affecting low and middle-income populations.

Electronic Policy Network

http://epn.org/

Articles and reports on health care policy and related issues.

EPN's Recommended Health Policy Links

http://epn.org/idea/hciclink.html

Glossary for Healthcare Standards

http://dmi-www.mc.duke.edu/dukemi/acronyms.htm

Health Care Information Resources on the Web

http://www.xnet.com/~hret/statind.htm

Health Care Liability Alliance

http://www.wp.com/hcla/

National advocacy coalition representing physicians, hospitals, blood banks, liability insurers, health device manufacturers, health care insurers, businesses, producers of medicines, and the technology industry.

Health Economics

http://papers.uni-bayreuth.de/departments/vwliv/hec.html

A great number of links to managed care, health economics, health policy, public health and related internet sites.

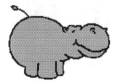

Health Hippo

http://www.winternet.com/~hippo/

Collection of policy and regulatory materials related to health care.

Health Hippo. *http://www.winternet.com/~hippo/*

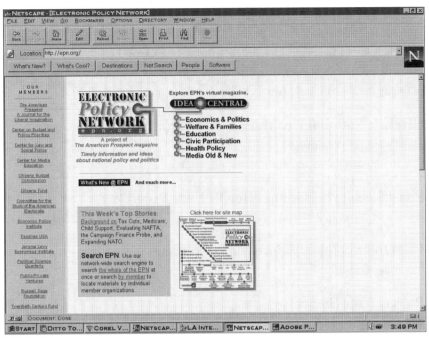

Electronic Policy Network. *http://epn.org/*

Health Services Research

http://www.xnet.com/~hret/

Bimonthly journal of the Association for Health Services Research. Contains a ten-year index by subject and author, as well as articles and abstracts from more recent issues.

Idea Central: Health Policy Page

http://epn.org/idea/health.html

Online journal.

Intergovernmental Health Policy Project

http://www.ncsl/ihpp/

Devoted to conducting research and reporting on health care policy in the United States.

Journal of Health Politics, Policy and Law

http://www.pitt.edu/~jhppl/jhppl.html

National Coalition on Health Care

http://www.americashealth.org/

    This site claims that the Coalition is the largest non-partisan group working to improve America's health care. It is comprised of businesses, labor unions, religious groups, primary care providers, and educators.

NHeLP: National Health Law Program, Inc.

http://www.healthlaw.org/

    Health care advocacy for low-income people.

Physicians for a National Health Care Program

http://www.pnhp.org/

PIE Online: Policy Information Exchange

http://www.pie.org/

Project Vote Smart

http://www.vote-smart.org/

    Tracks the voting records, issue positions, and other information on over 13,000 political leaders.

Government

Agency for Health Care Policy and Research

http://www.ahcpr.gov/

FedWorld Information Network

http://www.fedworld.gov/

    Searching through the bureaucracy of the federal government.

HCFA Fact Sheets

http://www.hcfa.gov/facts/facts.htm

    These fact sheets cover issues such as Medicare, Medicaid, home health care, and the Health Insurance Portability and Accountability Act of 1996.

Information for State Health Policy

http://www2.umdnj.edu/shpp/homepage.htm

THOMAS. *http://thomas.loc.gov/*

National Health Security Plan

http://kumchttp.mc.ukans.edu/service/dykes/RRPAGES/hlthpol.html

Executive Summary that includes President Clinton's 1993 health care reform plan and supporting documents.

THOMAS

http://thomas.loc.gov/

"In the spirit of Thomas Jefferson," this is a service of the U.S. Congress that provides legislative information available via the internet.

U.S. Department of Labor, Occupational Safety and Health Administration

http://www.osha.gov/

White House Virtual Library

http://www1.whitehouse.gov/WH/html/library.html

Contains press releases, radio addresses, photographs, executive orders, and web pages for the White House and staff, as well as links to all governmental sites and some historic national documents. Searchable.

Statistics

Dartmouth Atlas of Health Care in the United States

http://www.dartmouth.edu/~atlas/

Describes the geographic distribution of health care resources in the United States.

Social Statistics Briefing Room

http://www.whitehouse.gov/fsbr/health.html

Data and information in chart format about vital statistics, health services, health status and health care expenditures.

HEART & VEINS / CARDIOVASCULAR

Cholesterol

Doctor's Guide to Elevated Cholesterol

http://www.pslgroup.com/ELEVCHOL.HTM

Information and resources on high cholesterol and what to do about it.

How to Lower Your Cholesterol

http://www.coolware.com/health/medical-reporter/cholesterol.html

Article.

Lowdown on High Cholesterol

http://www.cholestfacts.com/

Medicine Net: Cholesterol and the Heart

http://www.medicinenet.com/mainmenu/encyclop/ARTICLE/ART_C/choleste.htm

Very Low Fat Diet FAQ

http://www.fatfree.com/FAQ/fatfree-faq/

Congenital Heart Anomalies

CHASER: Congenital Heart Anomalies Support, Education and Resources

http://www.csun/edu/~hfmth006/chaser/

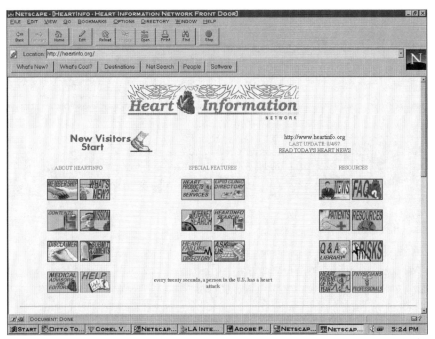

Heart Information Network. *http://heartinfo.org/*

Congenital Heart Disease Mailing List

http://www.csun.edu/~hcmth011/heart/

Good listing of mail groups, for adults and children with congenital heart disease.

Discussions

HEART-LIST Mailing Group

All aspects of heart disease are discussed, for patients and professionals. Send E-mail to: heart-list@BIOMED.MED.YALE.EDU with the message: "Subscribe Heart-List firstname lastname."

Heart Surgery Forum

http://www.hsforum.com/heartsurgery/home.hsf

For cardiothoracic professionals, includes forums, articles and links.

General Topics

American College of Cardiology

http://www.acc.org/

Information for clinicians regarding patient education, ACC programs and membership information.

American College of Cardiology Publications, Programs and Products

http://www.acc.org/pubs/index/

Large number of audiotapes, books, CD-ROMs, journals, slides, videotapes, journals, position and policy statements, practice guidelines, and patient education materials.

Cardiac HealthWeb

http://www.bev.net/health/cardiac/

Features "Ask the Cardiologist" database and direct question submission.

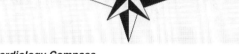

Cardiology Compass.
http://osler.wustl.edu/~murphy/cardiology/compass.html

Cardiac Rehabilitation

http://www.wpi.edu/~gerg/

CARDIAX

http://www.med.umich.edu/lrc/cardiax/cardiax.html

CARDIAX is a computer-aided instructional program of 20 planned cases in basic cardiology. It uses text, digital images, audio and videos to teach cardiac diagnosis.

Cardio-Consult

http://pharminfo.com/conference/cconslt.html

E-mail group for cardiovascular professionals to discuss case studies, research and clinical experiences. To subscribe, send e-mail to: LISTSERV@ SHRSYS.HSLC.ORG with the message: "SUBSCRIBE CARDIO-CONSULT Firstname Lastname."

Cardiology Compass
http://osler.wustl.edu/~murphy/cardiology/compass.html

Extensive compilation of cardiovascular information resources. Well organized. Includes a large section on education resources.

Cardiology INDEX
http://www.ability.org.uk/cardiolo.html

Long list of sites, alphabetized. Also includes chat rooms.

Cardiovascular Disease in the Black Population
http://www.uvm.edu/~vdouglast/project.htm

Healthy Heart Handbook
http://www.medaccess.com/workbook/health_heart/HHH_TOC.htm

Heart at Work
http://www.amhrt.org/hhf/corporate/heartatwork/calccvd.htm

Estimate the number of employees at your company with modifiable risks for heart disease or stroke.

Heart History
http://sln.fi.edu/biosci/history/history.html

Informative and entertaining site geared to children.

Heart Homepage
http://www.hearthome.com/

Includes 20 of the most frequently asked questions about the heart.

Heart Information Network
http://www.heartinfo.org/

Loads of information including: articles on cardiovascular diseases, a drug database, CPR instructions, frequently asked questions (FAQs) about heart disease, heart products and services, lipid clinic, news, risk assessment, and an "Ask Us" area for e-mail question and response from qualified physicians.

Heart Preview Gallery
http://sln2.fi.edu/biosci/preview/heartpreview.html

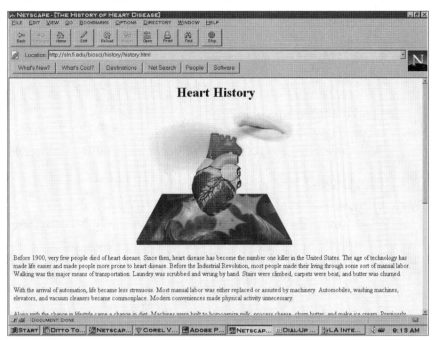

Heart History. *http://sln.fi.edu/biosci/history/history.html*

HeartWeb

http://webaxis.com/heartweb/

Online peer-reviewed cardiology journal.

MedWeb's Cardiology Sites

http://www.gen.emory.edu.medweb/medweb.cardiology.html

Many links to heart-related sites.

Meta-List Site

http://www.arcade.uiowa.edu/hardin-www/ind-cardio.html

Contains cardiology-related links.

National Heart, Lung and Blood Institute

http://www.nhlbi.nih.gov/nhlbi/nhlbi.htm

This site describes the NHLBI's research and educational activities, including cardiovascular, lung, blood and sleep disorders information.

NHLBI Gopher

gopher://fido.nih.gov/

The gopher for the National Heart, Lung and Blood Institute contains government reports, abstracts, news and activities.

Synapse's Heart Sounds

http://www.medlib.com/beats/00b10000.htm

Listen to normal heart sounds, "innocent murmurs" and defective heart sounds.

UCI Heart Disease Prevention Program

http://www.reg.uci.edu/UCI/CARDIOLOGY/PREVENTIVE/

At this site, find information on coronary artery, heart disease and stroke; heart disease research and risk factors, prevention and related resources.

WebDoctor: Cardiology Links

http://www.gretmar.com/webdoctor/Cardiology.html

General resources, associations and societies; clinical practice guidelines, teaching files; journals and computers in cardiology.

Heart Disease

Aneurysm Information Project

http://www.columbia.edu/~mdt1/

Frequently asked questions (FAQs), lectures and papers; research and support.

Aneurysm Support Page

http://www.westga.edu/~wmaples/aneurysm.html

Includes a number of narratives from patients, and direct 3-mail connection to "Talk to a Surgeon."

Aortic Aneurysm: 3-D Visualization and Measurements

http://everest.radiology.uiowa.edu/DPI/nlm/apps/aorta/aorta.html

Includes an overview of aortic aneurysms, images and patient scan protocol.

Atherosclerosis and Thrombosis Index

http://www-medlib.med.utah.edu/WebPath/ATHHTML/ATHIDX.html

Images of arteries and veins, healthy and damaged.

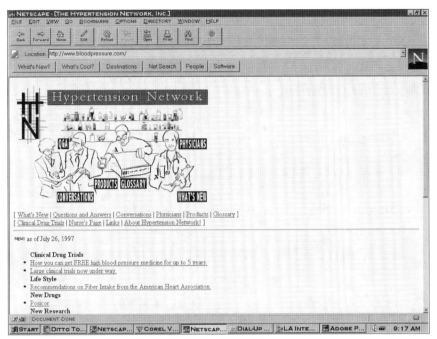

Hypertension Network. *http://www.bloodpressure.com/*

Heart and Stroke A-Z Guide

http://www.amhrt.org/heartg.ha.html

Consumer information from the American Heart Association.

Heart Attack (Myocardial Infarction)

http://www.medicinenet.com/mainmenu/encyclop/ARTICLE/Art_H/heartak.htm

Medicine Net highlights key points and answers basic questions with several hypertext links.

Heart Attack Survival Calculator

http://www.mediqual.com/library/amicalc/heart.htm

Enter patient information to receive the probability of his or her survival.

Heart Attacks, Bypass Surgery and Depression

http://www.hsc.ufl.edu/hs/bypass.htm

Prevention of Stroke, Heart Attack and the Symptoms of Alzheimer's Disease

http://www.webcom.com/ldvonch/

You've Had a Heart Attack - What Now?
http://weber.u.washington.edu/~bmperra/heart_help.html

Heart Murmurs

Heart Murmurs
http://www.aomc.org/HOD2/general/heart-HEART-4.html
> Information on heart murmurs and when they might be a concern.

When Your Child's Doctor Hears a Heart Murmur
http://www.cnmc.org/heart.htm
> An article with helpful information for parents.

Hypertension

American Society of Hypertension
http://www.pharminfo.com/ash/ashmnu.html
> Contains information relating to the Society's mission, member benefits, and highlights from their annual scientific meetings.

Hypertension
http://www.mayo.edu/hypertension/hyper1.htm
> Information on the Mayo Clinic's Division of Hypertension.

Hypertension Articles
http://www.cardio.com/categories/hypertensionarticles.htm

Hypertension Educational Material
http://www.mediconsult.com/noframes/hypertension/shareware/contents.html
> Basic information and articles for patients.

Hypertension Network
http://www.bloodpressure.com/
> Information about the latest research on hypertension, basic questions and answers, discussion forums, physician registry, glossary and product description.

Primary Care Teaching Module: Treatment of Hypertension

http://www.med.stanford.edu/school/DGIM/Teaching/Modules/HTN.html

Outline of an online course.

Primary Pulmonary Hypertension

http://fido.nhlbi.nih.gov:70/1/nhlbi/health/cardio/hbp/prof/pph/

Downloadable text of a report (too large for online viewing) about Primary Pulmonary Hypertension, a rare lung disorder.

Virtual Hospital: Hypertension

http://indy.radiology.uiowa.edu/Providers/ClinRef/FPHandbook/Chapter02/06-2.html

Part of the Virtual Hospital, this site offers an overview on hypertension, its causes, evaluation and treatment.

Organizations

American Heart Association

http://www.amhrt.org/

Includes AHA information, news, and the *Heart and Stroke Guide from A-Z.*

Cardiovascular Institute of the South

http://www.cardio.com/

This is a library of reports on cardiovascular topics for physicians. Article categories include arrhythmia, cardiac treatment, heart frequently asked questions (FAQs), hypertension, preventing heart disease, peripheral vascular disease, research, women and heart disease, stroke, and "words of caution."

National Heart, Lung and Blood Institute

http://www.nhlbi.nih.gov/nhlb/nhlbi.htm

Contains medical alerts, research and training, and heart-related information for health professionals and the public.

National Stroke Association

http://www.stroke.org/

Stroke prevention, treatment, rehabilitation, research and support for stroke survivors and their families. Also includes a quiz and links to additional resources.

Raynaud's Disease

Facts about Raynaud's Phenomenon
gopher://fido.nhlbi.nih.gov:70/00/educprog/other/gppubs/raynaud.txt

Power Points about Raynaud's Phenomenon
http://www.medicinenet.com/mainmenu/encyclop/article/art_r/raynaud.htm

Raynaud's Disease Home Page
http://www.atlantic.edu/Raynaud/rayhompg.htm

General information, resource links, questions and personal stories about patients who suffered from Raynaud's disease.

Raynaud's Phenomenon
http://ovchin.uc.edu/htdocs/arthritis/ray.html

Information from the Arthritis Foundation about this condition in which poor blood flow results in pain and skin color changes in affected parts, most commonly the fingers, toes, ears, or tip of the nose

Stroke

Stroke: Cerebrovascular Accident
http://www.clearlight.com/~morph/present/strk0.htm

Information about strokes for patients and their families.

Stroke Support and Information
http://members.aol.com/scmmlm/main.htm

This site offers an opportunity to share experiences and information about stroke treatment, rehabilitation and job resources. Information about stroke support chat group as well as e-mail support for caregivers are provided.

Stroke Support Web Site
http://www.tpoint.net/creative/

Software to help sufferers of stroke recover language skills.

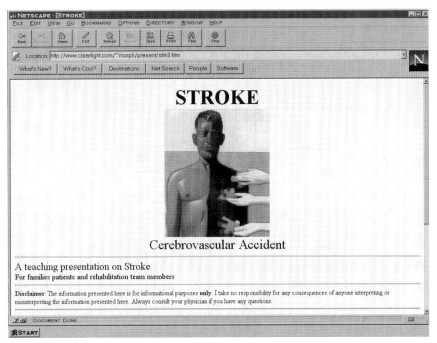

Stroke. *http://www.clearlight.com/~morph/present/strk0.htm*

Thrombosis and Homeostasis Resources for the Public

http://www.temple.edu/departments/SSTRC/public.htm

  Stroke information.

Treatment

Cardiac Rehabilitation and Prevention - Patient Information

http://www.jhbmc.jhu.edu/cardiology/rehb/patientinfo.html

  Lifestyle information on exercise, nutrition, smoking, stress, emotions and behavior modification. Medical information and heart-health information sheets, online newsletter and links. This site emphasizes ways individuals can take charge of their own health.

Drugs for Treating Cardiovascular Disease

http://www.heartinfo.org/card_db.html#drugs

  Check out what your doctor has prescribed.

Varicose Veins

MediData Varicose Vein Information
http://www.medi-data.co.uk/

What varicose veins are, why they occur, how to test for them and different methods of treating them.

Vein Disorder Education Center
http://www.veinsonline.com/

Information about venous disorders for the general public. This site offers physician referral, as well as answers frequently asked questions about varicose veins, spider veins and treatment options available.

Venous Treatment Center for Varicose Veins
http://girch301.med.uth.tmc.edu/thoracic/venous.html

HISTORY OF MEDICINE

Ancient Medicine

Ancient Medicine/Medicina Antiqua
http://web1.ea.pvt.k12.pa/us/medant/

A resource for the study of Greco-Roman medicine and medical thought from Mycenaean times until the fall of the Roman Empire.

Childbirth

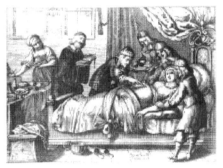

Brief History of Nurse-Midwifery in the U.S.
http://www.acnm.org/focus/
history.htm

Century of Obstetrics
http://www.obgyn.upenn.edu/History/
Index.html

Cesarean Section - A Brief History.
http://www.nlm.nih.gov/exhibition/cesarean/
cesarean_1.html

Cesarean Section - a Brief History
http://www.nlm.nih.gov/exhibition/cesarean/cesarean_1.html

Chinese Medicine

Chi Med: The History of Chinese Medicine Web Page
http://www.soas.ac.uk/Needham/Chimed/

History of Traditional Chinese Medicine
http://www.mic.ki.se/China.html

Egyptian Medicine

Ancient Egyptian Medicine
http://www.Iri.ucsf.edu/public_html/egypt.html

Life in Ancient Egypt
http://www.sentex.net/~aquarius/mags/harts/iss96/egypt.html

General Topics

Aesclepion
http://www.indiana.edu/~ancmed/intro.HTM
   Web page devoted to the study of ancient medicine.

American Association for the History of Medicine
http://www.utb.edu/mml/aahm/contents.htm
   Newsletter.

Ancient Medicine Hypertexts
http://web1.ea.pvt.k12.pa.us/medant/hyprtxts.htm
   Hypertext translations of significant ancient medical texts, including those written by Hippocrates and Galen.

Faces of Science: African Americans in the Sciences
http://www.lib.lsu.edu/lib/chem/display/faces.html

Florence Nightingale

http://www.dnai.com/~borneo/nightingale/

Country Joe McDonald's tribute to Florence Nightingale.

From Quackery to Bacteriology

http://www.cl.utoledo/canaday/quackery/
quackery1.html

An exhibit from the University of Toledo Libraries on the emergence of modern medicine in 19th century America.

Galaxy's History of Medicine

http://galaxy.einet.net/galaxy/Medicine/
History-of-Medicine.html

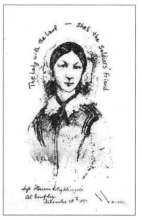

Florence Nightingale.
http://www.dnai.com/~borneo
/nightingale/

History of Science, Technology and Medicine

http://www.asap.unimelb.edu.au/hstm/hstm_ema.htm

E-mail lists and newsgroups.

HISTLINE

http://www.nlm.nih.gov/pubs/factsheets/histline.html

The National Library of Medicine's online bibliographical database covering the history of medicine.

History of Biomedicine

http://www.mic.ki.se/History.html

Good starting point to jump to other sites about medicine and health care from ancient to present-day.

History of Cadaver Dissection

http://meded.com.uci.edu/~anatomy/willed_body/dissect.html

History of Science Society

http://weber.u.washington.edu/~hssexec/index.html

History of Science, Technology andMedicine Electronic Journals

http://www.asap.unimelb.edu.au/hstm/hstm_jou.htm

History of the Condom and Technical Developments

http://www.durex.com/study/history.html

This site is interesting, but also commercial.

History of the Light Microscope

http://www.duke.edu/~tj/hist/hist_mic.html

"If You Knew the Conditions"

http://www.nlm.nih.gov/exhibition/if_you_knew/if_you_knew_01.html

Exhibition showing the history of health care for Native Americans.

Images from the History of Medicine

http://wwwihm.nlm.nih.gov/

Nearly 60,000 photographs, artwork and printed texts drawn from the large collection at the NLM History of Medicine Division. Search for images or browse.

Index of Medieval Medical Images in North America

http://www.mednet.ucla.edu/dept/neurobio/immi/immi/immihtm.htm

Johns Hopkins University Institute of the History of Medicine

http://www.welch.jhu.edu/ihm/

Medicine and Biology: Ancient Theories, Modern Bodies

http://141.142.3.130/SDG/Experimental/vatican.exhibit/f-medicine_bio/medicine_bio.html

MedWeb's History of Medicine

http://www.gen.emory.edu/medweb/medweb.history.html

19th Century Scientific American Online

http://www.history.rochester.edu/Scientific_American/

Online Medical Heritage Center

http://bones.med.ohio-state.edu/heritage/

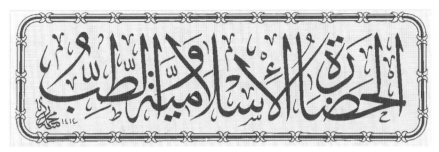

Islamic Culture and the Medical Arts.
http://www.nlm.nih.gov/exhibition/islamic_medical/catalog_00.html

Overview of HealthCare's History
http://www.infinityheart.com/overview.html

Physics Around the World
http://www.tp.umu.se/TIPTOP/paw/

Scientific and Medical Antiques
http://www.duke.edu/~tj/sci.ant.html

Scientific and Medical Antiques Links
http://www.utmem.edu/personal/thjones/sci_ant.htm

Surfing the Internet for the History of Medicine
gopher://una.hh.lib.umich.edu:70/00/inetdirsstacks/medhist%3ahirtle/

Vast Sea of Misery
http://www.cee.indiana.edu/gopher/Turner_Adventure_Learning/
Gettysburg_Archive/Primary_Resources/Vast_Sea_of_Misery
Eyewitness reports from Gettysburg, 1863.

X-Ray Century
http://www.cc.emory.edu/X-RAYS/century.htm

Islamic Medicine

Historical View of Islamic Medicine
http://www.coastal.bc.ca/cmc.holistic.college/persian.html

Islamic Culture and the Medical Arts

http://www.nlm.nih.gov/exhibition/islamic_medical/islamic_00.html

Islamic Medicine

http://www.safaar.com/im1.html

Libraries and Museums

Bakken Library and Museum

http://bakkenmuseum.org/

The Bakken Library and Museum is devoted to teaching and understanding the history, cultural context, and applications of electricity and magnetism to the fields of science and medicine.

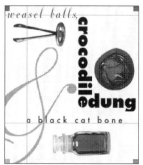

**The Museum of
Contraception.**
*http://www.salon1999.com/
07/features/contra.html*

Czech Pharmaceutical Museum

*http://www.faf.cuni/cz/welcome/
wheretostart_museum.htm*

Freud Museum

http://www.nltl.columbia.edu/students/DBA/freud/

Institute and Museum of History and Science

http://galileo.imss.firenze.it/index.html

Leonardo da Vinci Museum

http://cellini.leonardo.net/museum/main.html

Museum of Contraception

http://www.salon1999.com/07/features/contra.html

Museum of the History of Science

http://info.ox.ac.uk/departments/hooke/

Yale Historical Medical Library
http://info.med.yale.edu/library/historical/

Specialties

Dental History
http://www.catalog.com/dentist/denhis.html

History of Neurosurgery
http://neurosurgery.mgh.harvard.edu/history.htm

History of Psychology
http://www.yorku.ca/dept/psych/orgs/apa26/newslet.htm
   Newsletter.

Marvin Samson Center for the History of Pharmacy
http://pharminfo.com/gallery/pcps.html

Women in Medicine

4000 Years of Women in Science
http://www.astr.ua.edu/4000WS/4000ws.html

Brief History of Women in U.S. Medical Schools
http://www-med.stanford.edu/lane/specColl/medwomen.html

Diotima: Materials for the Study of Women and Gender in the Ancient World
http://www.uky.edu/ArtsSciencies/Classics/biblio/medicine.html

Distinguished Women of Past and Present: Health and Medicine
http://www.netsrq.com/~dbois/health.html

The History of Women and Science, Health and Technology
gopher://gopher.adp.wisc.edu/11/.browse/.METAGLSHW/

Selection of Letters Written by Florence Nightingale

http://222.kumc.edu/service/clendening/florence/about.html

HIV/AIDS

Antibody Testing

HIV Exposure: The Waiting Game
http://ng.netgate.net/~adamsclan/hiv.htm
> Test anxiety.

HIV Home Test
http://www.hivhometest.com/

HIV Home Test Information
http://www.koool.com/hivtest.html

Home Access
http://www.homeaccess.com/
> HIV testing and HIV/AIDS information.

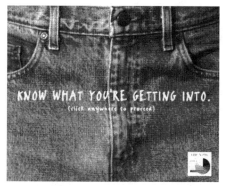

ImmunoScience, Inc.
http://www.immunoscience.com/
> Site from the makers of SALIVAX HIV test.

Home Access. *http://www.homeaccess.com/*

Testing for HIV
http://www.HIVpositive.com/f-TestingHIV/TestingMenu.html
> Information on HIV testing and viral load testing; counseling checklist for physicians; FDA approved HIV tests.

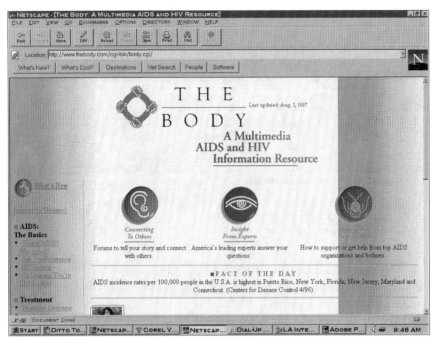

The Body. *http://www.thebody.com/cgi-bin/body.cgi/*

General Topics

AEGIS
http://www.aegis.com/

"The largest HIV knowledgebase in the world." Fully indexed and searchable. Includes a daily summary of AIDS news, articles, statistics, life cycle, and library.

AIDS Channel of the Cyber Queer Lounge
http://www.cyberzine.org/html/GLAIDS/AIDS/aidspage.html

AIDS Fact Sheets
http://www.aidsnyc.org/network/sf.html

Simple fact sheets on HIV and AIDS tests, treatment and conditions.

AIDS FAQ/Gopher
gopher://gpagopher.who.ch/11/aidsfaq/

AIDS Glossary of Medical, Statistical and Clinical Research Terminology

http://www.teleport.com/~celinec/glossary.htm

AIDS Information

gopher://odie.niaid.nih.gov/11/aids

AIDS Reader

http://www.medscape.com/SCP/TAR/public/journal.TAR.html

A peer-reviewed, clinical journal devoted exclusively to HIV disease and its complications.

AIDS Virtual Library

http://planetq.com/aidsvl/index.html

Alert! News about AIDS

http://www.mcs.net/~garyh/alert.html

AIDS news from a Christian group.

CAPS: Center for AIDS Prevention Studies

http://www.epibiostat.ucsf.edu/capsweb/

CAPS program information includes prevention fact sheets, bibliographies, sections on how to develop new prevention programs, a survey for use in needs assessment, abstracts of selected relevant articles, and an overview of current behavior research on risk-taking. Links to other sites.

CDC National AIDS Clearinghouse

http://www.cdcnac.org/

There is more information here than first appears. Numerous publications, and information on CDC AIDS services such as the AIDS Hotline, references and referrals, databases and more. Includes CDC fact sheets, government reports and health statistics.

Critical Path AIDS Project, Hypertext Edition

http://www.critpath.org/

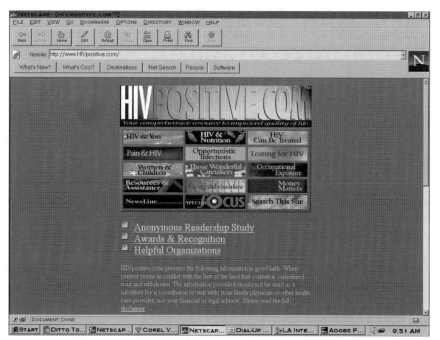

HIVPOSITIVE.COM. *http://www.HIVpositive.com/*

Deadly Medicine

http://www.nmia.com/~mdibble

Articles that discuss the transmission of HIV/AIDS through blood transfusion and products.

Global AIDS Resource Directory

http://web-1.interliant.com/immunet/inetgard.nsf?OpenDatabase/

Glossary of HIV/AIDS-Related Terms

http://www.hivatis.org/glossary/

HIV/AIDS Internet Information Index

http://www.arens.com/hiv/

HIV/AIDS Resources

http://www.mcphu.edu/~AIDSinfo/

HIV Insite

http://hivinsite.ucsf.edu/

From the University of California at San Francisco's AIDS Research Institute. Daily information on medical, and social aspects of AIDS, as well as prevention and resources. Also has state-by-state information on AIDS and HIV subjects and key topics. Includes articles, news, opinions, documents, abstracts, bibliographies and contacts. Some topics include adolescent, medical marijuana, women with AIDS, AIDS in prison, and needle exchange programs.

HIV.NET

http://hiv.net/hiv/intern/us.htm

The English language version of the European Information Center for HIV and AIDS. Analysis of the European AIDS epidemic and selected internet HIV/AIDS links. The Information Exchange Desk allows visitors to leave messages, ask questions and point others to important articles and publications.

HIVPOSITIVE.COM

http://www.HIVpositive.com/

Great resource for information on HIV and nutrition, drug advisories, money issues, news, resources, women and children, and HIV testing.

Internet Grateful Med/AIDSLINE

http://igm.nlm.nih.gov/

Grateful Med through the internet. Online computer file containing references to published literature on HIV and AIDS. Indexes journals from biomedical, epidemiological, health care administration, oncologic, social and the behavioral sciences. Citations and abstracts to articles, monographs, meeting papers, government reports, newspaper articles and theses, from 1980 to the present. Online access is free, but there is a charge for each search.

Links, Links, Links: AIDS Prevention Project

http://www.metrokc.gov/health/apu/links.htm

Selected sites from the huge number of AIDS/HIV resources available online.

Links to HIV/AIDS

http://www.hivnet.org/english/e-links.html

Marty Howard's HIV/AIDS Home Page

http://www.smartlink.net/~martinjh/

Important and thorough information. Hard to read but definitely a great resource.

Medscape: AIDS

http://www.medscape.com/Home/Topics/AIDS/AIDS.html

Peer-reviewed clinical articles and literature reviews.

MedWeb's AIDS and HIV

http://www.gen.emory.edu/medweb/medweb.aids.html

Many links.

National Commission on AIDS Gopher

gopher://odie.niaid.nih.gov:80/11/aids/hca/

Several reports from the NCA.

NOAH: AIDS & HIV Resources

http://www.noah.cuny.edu/illness/aids/aidsrsrc.html

Advocacy, medical institutions, government organizations, education, AIDS in daily life, and internet links.

On-Line Interactive HIV/AIDS Continuing Medical Education

http://www.healthcg.com/cme.html

Paradiselost's HIV/AIDS Resources

http://www.paradiselost.com/hivaids/

Links to a numer of AIDS/HIV sites. Includes news and research, general information, education, memorials, hospices, fundraisers, and a section for women with AIDS.

sci.med.aids

http://persephone.hampshire.edu/aids/sci.med.aids.faq1.html

General information on this newsgroup. Links to frequently asked questions.

The Body: A Multimedia AIDS and HIV Information Resource

http://www.thebody.com/cgi-bin/body.cgi/

This site includes the basics on AIDS and AIDS prevention, treatment updates, and research efforts. Also covers conferences, quality-of-life issues, AIDS forums,

Q&A, and how to get support from AIDS organizations and hotlines. Search engine helps to sort through the enormous amount of information here. Addresses the impact of AIDS on emotions and mental health, as well as the legal, workplace and sports ramifications.

UNAIDS
http://www.us.unaids.org/

The Joint United Nations Programme on HIV/AIDS offers fact sheets, statistics, and conference information.

University of California at Berkeley Gopher of AIDS
gopher://uclink.berkeley.edu:1901/11/other/aids/

Yahoo's AIDS/HIV Links
http://www.yahoo.com/Health/Diseases_and_Conditions/AIDS_HIV/

History

Deja Vu: AIDS in Historical Perspective
http://www.radio.cbc.ca.radio/programs/current/ideas/syphilis.html

So Little Time: An AIDS History
http://www.aegis.com/topics/timeline/index.html

Interesting site traces that the history of AIDS from 1978 to the present. In 1997, 6.4 million deaths (total) had thus far been attributed to AIDS, and the approximate number of HIV-positive people worldwide is 22 million.

Needle Safety

North American Syringe Exchange Network
http://www.nasen.org/

List of syringe exchange programs, HIV/AIDS information, safe sex information, drug policy and drug treatment and a mailing list.

Safe Injection/Vein Care Page

http://www.safeworks.org/injection/

Images and text carefully demonstrate the safest way to shoot up, if you are going to do it anyway.

Safe Works AIDS Project

http://safeworks.org/

Needle exchange, condoms and safe sex distribution program in Minneapolis/St. Paul area. Links to sites on the web with needle-exchange programs, by region. A lot of information on how to set up a program.

Safer Injection Manual

http://cures-not-wars.org/junkie/inject.html

Organizations

International Association of Physicians in AIDS Care

http://www.iapac.org/

Dialogue and discussion of AIDS issues.

Pathology

AIDS Pathology Images

http://www-medlib.med.utah.edu/WebPath/AIDSPATH.pdf

Public Policy

White House National AIDS Strategy 1997 - Text

http://www.cdcnac.org/strategy.pdf

You will need Acrobat Reader to download the main text of this White House statement.

Publications

AIDSWEEKLY PLUS
http://www.newsfile.com/x1a.htm
> Order a sample copy or check out current issue. Subscription information.

HIV: Electronic Media Information Review
http://florey.biosci.uq.edu.au/hiv/HIV_EMIR.html

Journal of AIDS/HIV
http://www.CCSPublishing.com/J_AIDS.htm
> This monthly journal includes information in outline-format on general care and opportunistic infections. Also includes a medical library and links to other online journals. While some articles require registration, others do not.

Magazines, Periodicals and Libraries of HIV/AIDS
http://gopher.hivnet.org:80/1/magazines/

Morbidity and Mortality Weekly Reports on AIDS
http://www.cdc.gov/nchstp/hiv_aids/pubs/mmwr.htm
> Monthly publication from the Centers for Disease Control. Abstracts available, and full text with Adobe Acrobat Reader.

Positive Nation - Web Edition
http://www.positivenation.co.uk/
> Monthly print and electronic magazine offers features, regular articles and news updates. Strives to represent all people affected by HIV and AIDS in the UK.

Research

AmFAR: American Foundation for AIDS Research
http://www.amfar.org/

AVERT: AIDS Education and Research Trust
http://www.oneworld.org/avert/
> Education, information, UK statistics, news and publications.

CDC Statistics on New AIDS Cases in the U.S. Per Year
http://www.sunlabs.com/~shirriff/java/statsgraph.html

HIV Sequence Database
http://hiv-web.lanl.gov/
HIV genetic sequence data collection, annotation, analysis and publication.

JAMA HIV/AIDS Information Site
http://www.ama-assn.org/special/hiv/hivhome.htm
Resources for physicians, other health professionals and the public. Offers clinical updates, news, articles and information on social and policy issues. Links to the National Library of Medicine's AIDS databases, and CME for physicians.

Office of AIDS Research Home Page
http://www.nih.gov/od/oar/oar_home.htm
OAR is responsible for the scientific, budgetary, legislative and policy elements of the NIH AIDS research program.

Support/Advocacy

ACT-UP New York
http://www.actupny.org/
Direct action to end the AIDS crisis. Information, links, and what to do to help. Includes daily updates and weekly cyber-broadcast features and archives.

AIDS Memorial Quilt Website
http://www.aidsquilt.org/
The AIDS Memorial Quilt is a patchwork quilt of many 3-by-6-feet panels (the size of a human grave), each devoted to the memory of a person who died from AIDS. This site discusses how to make and submit a panel. View sample panels and find AIDS information and support.

AIDS Project Los Angeles
http://www.apla.org/apla/

ArtAIDS
http://www.illumin.co.uk/artaids/

Day One

http://www.aegis.com/day-one.html

Site for people who have just discovered they are HIV positive.

Estate Project for Artists with AIDS

http://artistswithaids.org/

Gay Men's Health Crisis on the Web

http://www.gmhc.org/

Internet home to the New York-based group at the forefront of AIDS advocacy and support, this site offers AIDS news, support, resources, prevention and advocacy.

Student Organization for AIDS Research

http://www.princeton.edu/~chris2/SOFAR.html

United in Anger

http://www.panix.com/~boyfren/

Photo documentary of AIDS activists by photographer Bill Bytsura.

Treatment

AIDS Alternative Treatment

http://www.critpath.org/alt.htm

AIDS Patent Project

http://aps.cnidr.org/

Full text and images of all international patents relating to AIDS.

AIDS Treatment Data Network

http://www.aidsnyc.org/network/index.html

Treatment education and counseling for individuals with AIDS and HIV. Extensive, up-to-date information databases on AIDS treatments, research studies, services, and how to access care. Includes a directory of clinicians, a drug glossary, a glossary of opportunistic infections and conditions and alternative treatments. Information also available in Spanish.

AIDS Treatment News/Internet Directory

http://www.aidsnews.org/

AIDSTRIALS and AIDSDRUGS

http://www.nlm.nih.gov/pubs/factsheets/aidstdfs.html
Fact sheet about these two NLM databases.

HIV/AIDS Treatment Information Service

http://www.hivatis.org/
Information on federally approved treatment guidelines for HIV and AIDS.

Immunet

http://www.immunet.org/
Treatment information on AIDS/HIV; updates, resources and a forum.

Marijuana As a Medicine

http://www.calyx.com/~olsen/MEDICAL/
Includes information on AIDS and marijuana.

Viral Load Measurement

http://www.iapac.org/consumer/vload/
The ability to measure the viral load represents a new advance in HIV treatment and management.

Yoga Group: Yoga for HIV/AIDS

http://www.yogagroup.org/

Women and AIDS

Cindy's Women and AIDS

http://www.vuse.vanderbilt.edu/~suerkeck/aids.html

Guidelines for Women with HIV/AIDS

http://www.projinf.org/fs/woman.html

Minnella's Alphabetical List of Women & HIV/AIDS URLs

http://www.fas.harvard.edu/~minnella/ws375urls.html

HOSPICE CARE

Related sections: _Aging/Gerontology; Pain & Pain Management._

All About Hospice: A Consumer's Guide

http://www.nahc.org/Haa/guide.html

American Academy of Hospice and Palliative Medicine

http://www.aahpm.org/

All about the Academy, membership and events. Links to other hospice and palliative care sites.

Choosing a Good Death

_http://www.boston.com/globe/specialreports/
1996/june/hospice/home.htm_

One woman's story about her decision to receive hospice care.

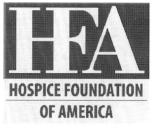

Hospice Foundation of America. _http://www. hospicefoundation.org/_

Dr. Stall's Hospice Home Care

http://www.acsu.buffalo.edu/~drstall/hospice.html

Homecare Online

http://www.nahc.org/home.html

Service of the National Association for Home Care. Includes home care and hospice locator and other information.

Hospice: A Photographic Inquiry

_http://pathfinder.com/@@dBX3ywcAQKkR0*eZ/twep/artslink/exhibitions/
hospice/_

Hospice and Palliative Care Resources

http://wings.buffalo.edu/faculty/research/bioethics/hospice.html

Hospice Foundation of America

http://www.hospicefoundation.org/

General information on hospices and specific information about the Foundation. Learn how to find a hospice, and read publications, books, and stories about hospice situations.

Hospice Hands

http://hospice-cares.com/

Links and information.

HospiceNet

http://members.aol.com/HospiceNet/homepage.htm

Medicare Hospice Benefits

http://www.zianet.com/connealy/hospice/medicare.html

Basic questions with answers; contact information.

National Hospice Organization

http://www.nho.org/

Zen Hospice Project

http://www.zenhospice.org/

Projects, reading lists and a newsletter.

INFECTIOUS DISEASES

E. Coli

E. Coli Genetic Stock Center

http://cgsc.biology.yale.edu/

Database of *E. coli* information, including *E. coli* genotypes, gene names, properties, linkage maps, and gene product information. Direct queries of database are possible.

E. Coli Genome Project

http://www.genetics.wisc.edu/Welcome.html

Site created by the E. Coli Genome Center at the University of Wisconsin at Madison, whose project goal is to completely sequence the *E. coli* genome and several *E. coli* phages. FTP files showing the sequence decoded thus far may be downloaded.

EcoCyc: Encyclopedia of E. Coli Genes and Metabolism

http://www.ai.sri.com/ecocyc/ecocyc.html

Databank describing the genes and intermediary metabolic activity of *E. coli*. Written for the scientific community.

Ebola

Dr. Frederick A. Murphy Talks About the Ebola Virus

http://outcast.gene.com/ae/WN/NM/interview_murphy.html

Dr. Murphy was the first to view Ebola through an electron microscope.

Centers for Disease Control and Prevention. *http://www.cdc.gov/*

Ebola Information

http://www.ebay.com/ebola.html

News related to the Ebola virus and Ebola outbreaks worldwide. Sources include CNN, National Public Radio (audio capability required) and journal articles.

Ebola Outbreaks - Updates

http://www.bocklabs.wisc.edu/outbreak.html

Citations for articles and other documents relating to recent Ebola outbreaks, as collected from World Health Organization (WHO), Centers for Disease Control and Prevention (CDC), CNN, AP Newswire, Reuters news service, and other sources. Links to documents appearing on the web.

Ebola Recommended Reading List

http://www.bocklabs.wisc.edu/ebola.html

Lists documents about the Ebola virus. Collected from scientific journals, news publications, various television media, Centers for Disease Control (CDC) reports and books.

Ebola Virus Hemorrhagic Fever: General Information

http://www.cdc.gov.ncidod/publications/brochures/ebola/html

General and straightforward information about the Ebola virus offered in question and answer format.

Ebola Virus Links on the Web

http://www.iohk.com/UserPages/amy/ebola.html

Kerry Townsend's Homepage

http://www.ru.ac.za/departments/journ/awol/ebola.html

Short article on the Ebola virus and virus outbreaks, written by Kerry Townsend of Rhodes University in South Africa.

News on the Ebola Viruses

http://www.uct.ac.za/microbiology/ebopage.html

Lists and links to ProMED articles, popular print media, and World Health Organization (WHO) releases providing news updates and general information on the Ebola virus.

Emerging Diseases

Emerging Infectious Diseases Resource Link

http://www.cdc.gov/ncidod/id_links.htm

General and specific information on emerging diseases. Includes links to related web sites, journals, online newsletters and other publications.

Outbreaks

http://www.who.ch/outbreak/outbreak_home.html

Access to news on outbreaks as reported to the World Health Organization (WHO) disease fact sheets, and other links.

Program for Monitoring Emerging Diseases Electronic Conference

http://www.healthnet.org/programs/promed.html

Global system of early detection and timely response to disease outbreaks that was proposed by the Federation of American Scientists. You can subscribe to seven different mail groups here.

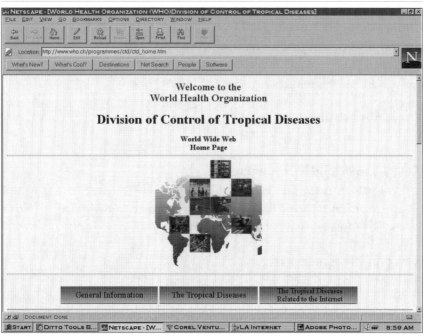

WHO Division of Control of Tropical Diseases.
http://www.who.ch/programmes/ctd/ctd_home.htm

ProMED: Program for Monitoring Emerging Diseases

http://www.fas.org/promed/

ProMED was formed by the Federation of American Scientists to establish global monitoring of emerging diseases. It also operates as an information source and subscription mailing list for scientists, public health officials, journalists and laypeople.

World Health Organization's Emerging and Other Communicable Diseases Surveillance and Control (EMC)

http://www.who.ch/programmes/emc/emc_home.htm

Describes EMC activities for monitoring and controlling diseases in different countries and professional fields, with links to the Weekly Epidemiological Record and news summaries of outbreaks and disease incidence world-wide.

General Topics

Bad Bug Book

http://vm.cfsan.fda.gov/~mow/toc.html

This FDA site is oriented to laypeople and offers information on foodborne pathogenic microorganisms and natural toxins.

CDC Homepage

http://www.cdc.gov/

This home page for the Centers for Disease Control and Prevention offers health information, publications, traveler's information, training and employment, as well as data collection and statistics.

CDC Wonder

http://wonder.cdc.gov/

Start here to access CDC reports, text- and numeric-based public health data.

CELLS Alive!

http://www.comet.chv.va.us/quill/

This beautiful and user-friendly site contains commentary and images of microbiology in action. Includes scanning electron microscope photographs and computer animation of how cells fight infection, and how viruses and bacteria behave.

Centre for the Epidemiology of Infectious Diseases

http://www.ceid.ac.uk/

This site from the Department of Zoology, University of Oxford, offers technical information on infectious diseases, including publications, research, news, seminars, and a dictionary of epidemiology.

Communicable Diseases Fact Sheets

http://www.charm.net/~epi1/diseases.html

The Maryland Department of Health has prepared fact sheets on a large number of diseases.

Communicable Disease Fact Sheets for Consumers

http://www.health.state.ny.us/nysdoh/consumer/commun.htm

Over 50 different infectious organisms and communicable diseases are discussed, in **.pdf* (Adobe Acrobat) file format.

Epidemiology

http://www.epibiostat.ucsf.edu/epidem/epidem.html

Provides epidemiological information and numerous links world-wide.

Global Health Network

http://www.pitt.edu/HOME/GHNet/

An international alliance of health experts assembled from government, global organizations, businesses and academia, the Global Health Network is working towards developing programs for the world-wide prevention of disease. Available in Japanese, Spanish, and Portuguese.

Infectious Diseases

http://www.slackinc.com/matrix/SPECIALT/INFECT.HTML

A Medical Matrix site offering many links to news, articles, abstracts, reports, meetings, organizations, etc., relating to infectious diseases. Summaries provided.

Medical Microbiology Home Page

http://biomed.nus.sg/microbio/home.html

This site for medical doctors, medical students and scientists was created by microbiologist Raymond Lin and is full of microbiology links to other sites, journals, and organizations on the web.

Microbial Underground (U.K.)

http://www.qmw.ac.uk/~rhbm001/index.html

Everything relating to microbiology on the internet, including news, web sites, courses, newsgroups, bulletin board services, culture and stain data, and online publications.

Microbial Underground (U.S.)

http://www.lsumc.edu/campus/micr/mirror/public_html/index.html

This companion site to The Microbial Underground (U.K.) offers a collection of web pages with medical, micro- and molecular biological links, as part of a project to build an online course in medical microbiology.

National Electronic Telecommunications System for Surveillance

http://www.cdc.gov/epo/other/netss.html#general

Information for the general public on the NETSS, a computerized health surveillance system that provides weekly morbidity data on the 52 nationally notifiable diseases.

OUTBREAK

http://www.outbreak.org/cgi-unreg/dynaserve.exe/index.html

An online information source addressing the emerging diseases. Offers an overview of emerging diseases, articles and other information on specific diseases and recent outbreaks, as well as a glossary of related terms.

Virtual Library of Diseases

http://www.medscape.com/NFID/lib/lib.html

This site created by the National Foundation for Infectious Diseases offers fact sheets and clinical updates as well as links to infectious diseases resources on the internet, including information on AIDS, hepatitis and ebola.

What You Should Know About Infectious Diseases

http://www.ucsf.edu/research/science_made/infectious.html

This is an adaptation from UCSF Magazine article in October, 1995 answering basic questions about the flu, susceptibility, antibiotics and drug resistance.

WHO's Weekly Epidemiological Record

http://www.who.who.ch/wer_home.htm

Distributed every week, this free electronic publication containing epidemiological information on cases and outbreaks of all diseases listed under the International Health Regulations, as well as other infectious diseases and health problems. Requires Acrobat Reader to receive electronically.

World Wide Web Communicable Diseases Resources

http://www.open.gov.uk/cdsc/links.htm

Links to mailing lists, public health and disease sites across the globe.

Lyme Disease. http://www.uri.edu/artsci/zool/ticklab/Lyme.html

Immunizations/Vaccinations

See also: Children's Health/Pediatrics - Immunizations; Public Health - Travel Recommendations.

CDC Immunization Information Page

http://www.cdc.gov/diseases/immun.html

Basic information on immunization theory, diseases, transmission, and vaccination, as well technical recommendations from the Immunization Practices' Advisory Committee.

CDC Travel Information

http://www.cdc.gov/travel/travel.html

Users select their region of travel and receive a summary of health risks, precautions and vaccinations recommended for travelers.

CDC's Immunization Schedule

http://www.bvrhc.org/cdcimmuni.htm

The Centers for Disease Control and Prevention schedule for immunization.

Clinician's Handbook of Preventive Services

*http://vh.radiology.uiowa.edu/Providers/ClinGuide/PreventionPractice/
TableOfContents.html*

Start from the table of contents to find immunization information for specific diseases, including references, patient resources and recommendations. Several chapters discuss the immunization of children, other chapters discuss the immunization of adults.

Diseases and Immunizations

http://www.medaccess.com/cdcimun/General/Gen_toc.htm#toc

Table of contents on immunization provided by the online informational service, MedAccess Corp. Includes theory of immunization, standards for vaccination, immunization goals, and morbidity and mortality information for selected diseases.

Facts About Childhood Immunization

http://www.metronet.com/~thearc/laqs/vaccineq.html

Concise information on vaccinating children for prevention of the nine major illnesses, as well as national health and educational resources available online.

Global Programme for Vaccines and Immunization

http://www.who.ch/programmes/gpv/GPV_Homepage.html

World Health Organization (WHO) site developed to expand immunization programs and to advance vaccine development, supply and quality. Offers the latest news, as well as graphs, updates on eradication of diseases, weekly epidemiological data, meetings, links, and a catalog of materials.

Global Programme for Vaccines - Poliomyelitis Eradication

http://www.who.ch/programmes/gpv/gEnglish/avail/polio.htm

Update on the efforts of this WHO program to eradicate polio by the year 2000, including country-by-country statistics. Good general information source; includes graphs and maps.

Immunization Action Coalition/Hepatitis B Coalition

http://www.immunize.org/

Information on the Coalition and its publications, *NEEDLE TIPS* and *The Hepatitis B Coalition News*. Ready-to-print documents about vaccines, adult immunization, Hepatitis A and B, legal issues and lawsuits.

Immunization Information
http://vh.radiology.uiowa.edu/Patients/IowaHealthBook/Immunization/
Immunization.html
    Site directs users to information sheets on specific diseases and vaccines.

NIP: National Immunization Program for Children and Adults
http://www.dynares.com/nip/index.htm
    Site offers news, links, frequently asked questions (FAQs), publications and immunization schedule.

Traveler's Medical and Immunization Service
http://www.tmis.com/

Vaccine Information and Awareness Web Site
http://www.ihot.com/~via/

Vaccine Weekly
http://www.newsfile.com/1v.htm
    News briefs and article summaries are offered on vaccine-related research topics world-wide. Full access to the text of articles available with subscription.

Vaccines and Diseases News
http://www.biol.tsukuba.ac.jp/~macer/NBBV.html
    References to books, research articles and other published and governmental texts discussing vaccines and related topics. Compiled by the Eubios Ethics Institute.

WHO's Global Programme for Vaccine and Immunization
http://www.who.ch/programmes/WHOProgrammes.html

Influenza

Influenza Bibliography
http://www.nimr.mrc.ac.uk/Library/flu/
    Lists recently published journal articles on influenza. Includes general and clinical articles, articles on prevention and control, epidemiology, epizootiology, immunology, pathology, influenza genetics and viruses. Updated 6 times each year.

Influenza Surveillance
http://www.who.ch/programmes/emc/flu.htm

Information and graphics on influenza activity in the current season by country, as reported to the World Health Organization (WHO). Also connect to institutes for studying influenza and vaccine manufacturers.

Lyme Disease

American Lyme Disease Foundation, Inc.
http://www.w2.com/docs2/d5/lyme.html

Informative site designed for both professionals and the general public to advance awareness of Lyme disease throughout the U.S. Areas covered include ecology and environmental management, precautions, recommendations, and information on vaccines.

Lyme Disease
http://www.uri.edu/artsci/zool/ticklab/Lyme.html

Attractive site offering general information on Lyme disease and the biomonics (i.e., life cycle and spread) of black-legged deer ticks. Provides links to other relevant sites and research studies. Site is maintained by The Rhode Island Tick Pickers at the Tick Research Laboratory, University of Rhode Island.

Lyme Disease
http://next.cambridge.ma.us/vineyard/health/lyme/

Symptoms, treatment, prevalence, and protection from Lyme disease are described, as well as the life cycle of the ticks that carry it.

Lyme Disease Information Resource
http://www.sky.net/~dporter/lyme1.html

Clearinghouse for information about Lyme disease. Offers many links and information on conferences, meetings, organizations, clinical studies and research.

Lyme Disease Network/Lyme Net Online
http://www.lymenet.org/

Keep up on the events and activities of the Lyme community, including the latest research study results and treatment recommendations, illustrations of ticks, contact information for Lyme disease support groups, and links to related web sites.

LymeNet Newsletter

http://www.lehigh.edu.lists/lymenet-l/

Information on the internet newsletter of the same name. To subscribe, send e-mail to: listserve@lehigh.edu and type the message: "subscribe LymeNet-L Yourfirstname Yourlastname."

Poison Center Answer Book/Lyme Disease

http://edison.ucdmc.ucdavis.edu/poison_control/lyme_dis.html

Describes the symptoms, prevention and treatment of Lyme disease, as well as general information on ticks.

Malaria

Disease Sheet: Malaria

http://www.who.ch/programmes/ctd/diseases/mala/malamain.htm

This site, maintained by WHO/Division of Control of Tropical Diseases, offers information on malaria, including a description, epidemiological data, and malaria control efforts, as well as links to additional sites.

Doctors' Answers to "Frequently Asked Questions": Malaria

http://www.druginfonet.com/faq/faqmalar.htm

Site addresses drug-related questions on malaria.

Malaria Database

http://www.wehi.edu.au/biology/malaria/who.html

Information resource for scientists working in malaria research. Includes malaria genome sequencing, nucleotide and protein information and jobs available in the field.

Malaria Discussion Mail Server

http://www.wehi.edu.au/biology/malaria/listserv.html

To subscribe to the malaria discussion group, send e-mail to: listserv@wehi.edu.au with the following message: "subscribe malaria Yourname."

Malaria Information

http://www.who.ch/whosis/malinfo/malinfo.html

Provides epidemiological data on the incidence of malaria around the world, as assembled by the WHO Statistical Information System.

Malaria Weekly

http://www.newsfile.com/1m.htm

Online news source covering malaria, mosquito control, drug resistance, vaccines, blood screening and related topics. Brief summaries of news and journal articles offered; full text available with subscription.

Organizations

National Center for Infectious Diseases

http://www.cdc.gov/ncidod/ncid.htm

Information about the prevention and control of traditional, new, and reemerging infectious diseases in the United States and around the world.

National Foundation for Infectious Diseases Homepage

http://www.medscape.com/NFID/

This NFID site provides infectious diseases fact sheets, information on adult immunization, additional web sources, brochures, and an online publication *The Double Helix.*

National Institute of Allergy and Infectious Diseases

gopher://gopher.niaid.nih.gov/1/

This is the National Institute of Health's NIAID gopher that allows queries and offers information for researchers and administrators on infectious diseases.

Parasitology

Bacterial and Fungal Diseases

http://www.mic.ki.se/Diseases/c1.html

Information on specific diseases, bacterial organisms, eye infections, skin diseases, fungi, and zoonoses, as well as links to numerous related web resources.

Karolinska Institute's Linkages to Parasitic Sites
http://www.mic.ki.se/Diseases/c3.html

Connections to images and research studies on particular parasites and the diseases they cause, as well as to other parasitology sites on the internet.

Parasite Links
http://www-museum.unl.edu/asp_image/links.html

Provides numerous links to places of parasitological interest on the web. Includes information on food poisoning and infections in domesticated animals.

Parasitology Page
http://www.pasteur.fr/Bio/parasito/Parasites.html

A narrated list of sites specifically related to parasitology and molecular biology. Includes journals, institutes, global organizations and government sites.

Peter Pappas' Graphic Images of Parasites
http://www.biosci.ohio-state.edu/~zoology/parasite/graphic2.html

Illustrations of common parasites, with brief descriptions of the organisms.

Plague

CDC Plague Information Page
http://www.cdc.gov/diseases/plague.html

Information about the disease for the public and for health care workers. Includes description, diagnosis, treatment, spread, vaccines and prevention.

Plague
http://www.ento.vt.edu/IHS/plague.html

Well-organized presentation on the plague, including information on causal agents, vectors, forms, and life cycle in humans. Also offers histories of past plague epidemics. Part of a virtual presentation on "Insects and Human Society" delivered by Dr. Tim Mack of the Entomology Department at Virginia Tech.

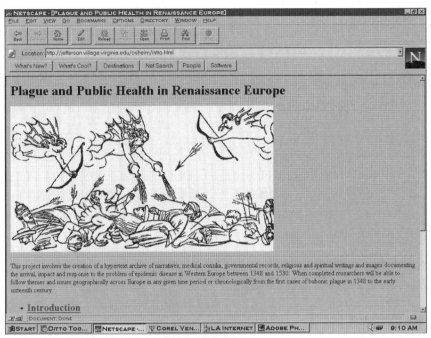

Plague and Public Health in Renaissance Europe.
http://jefferson.village.virginia.edu/osheim/intro.html

Plague and Public Health in Renaissance Europe

http://jefferson.village.virginia.edu/osheim/intro.html

Hypertext archive offers narratives, medical counsel, government records, religious and spiritual writings and images documenting the arrival, impact and response to the bubonic plague in Western Europe, 1348-1530. Created by the Institute for Advanced Technology in the Humanities.

Plague Links

http://ccme-mac4.bsd.uchicago.edu/CCMEDocs/Plague/

Impressive compilation of information on the plague and other infectious and emerging diseases, including HIV, tuberculosis, Ebola, cholera and leprosy. Journal articles, studies, and research on antibiotic resistance and vaccines.

Plaguescape

http://www.plaguescape.com/home.html

Artistic web version of an article by John S. Marr, M.D., M.P.H., and Curtis D. Malloy, M.P.H., presenting an epidemiological analysis of the biblical ten plagues of Egypt.

Publications

Bug Bytes

http://www.ccm.lsumc.edu/bugbytes/

Bi-weekly publication on infectious diseases.

Disease Weekly Plus

http://www.newsfile.com/1i.htm

This weekly electronic publication is devoted to human diseases ranging from AIDS to tuberculosis. Articles focus on disease prevention, diagnosis, drug treatment and vaccines. Summaries of the articles are accessible to browsers; full text is available with subscription.

Emerging Infectious Diseases (Journal)

http://www.cdc.gov/ncidod/EID/eid.htm

Peer-reviewed, online journal published by the National Center for Infectious Diseases. Index and abstracts of articles in present and past issues. Articles may be downloaded. Spanish language version also available.

Infectious Disease News

http://www.slackinc.com/general/idn/idnhome.htm

This electronic publication devoted to infectious diseases offers articles and bulletins, as well as online forums, seminars, and a chat room.

Infectious Disease Newsletter

http://www.zilker.net/~medair/newslet.html

An electronic newsletter summarizing recent research on epidemiology and infectious disease treatment as published in journals in the field. Article titles and summaries are provided, as well as links to related sites.

Morbidity and Mortality Weekly Report

http://www.cdc.gov/epo/mmwr/mmwr.html

The online version of MMWR, a weekly publication based on Centers for Disease Control and Prevention data as reported by state health departments. Contains provisional weekly disease morbidity and mortality data, reports, news, and survey results.

Tuberculosis

Ask NOAH About: Tuberculosis
http://noah.cuny.edu/tb/tb.html

Site offers basic information on tuberculosis and AIDS-related tuberculosis, including care and treatment. Part of the New York Online Access Health (NOAH) site.

Division of Tuberculosis Elimination
http://www.cdc.gov/nchstp/tb/dtbe.html

For the general public, patients and health care providers, this site provides information on tuberculosis prevention and eradication, including frequently asked questions (FAQs) and access to an online newsletter and the Tuberculosis Information Management System (TIMS). TIMS is a software program allowing entry into and queries to a national database on the administration of TB prevention, surveillance and control programs.

Facts About... Tuberculosis
http://www.pbs.org/ppoo/tbfacts.html

The American Lung Association addresses simple questions about tuberculosis: such as, what it is, symptoms, spread, treatment, and drug-resistance.

Multidrug-Resistant Tuberculosis (MDR-TB) Annotated Bibliography
http://uhs.bsd.uchicago.edu/uhs/topics/resist.tb.bib.html

Bibliographical and Medline information accompany a summary of each article. List of articles is grouped by the following topics: reviews, epidemiology and high risk groups, diagnosis, treatment strategies and outcomes, public health, the law, and editorials.

National Tuberculosis Center
http://www.umdnj.edu/~ntbcweb/ntbchome.htm

This site offers patients and the general public questions and answers on tuberculosis, as well as a brief history of the disease. Maintained by the New Jersey Medical School National Tuberculosis Center, of the University of Medicine and Dentistry of New Jersey.

People's Plague Online

http://www.pbs.org/ppol/

This site was created to accompany the Public Broadcasting System's program on tuberculosis in America. It offers health and educational resources and includes an interactive area, with audio and video excerpts from the program and a self-administered quiz. Spanish language version available.

TB/HIV Research Laboratory

http://www.brown.edu/Research/TB-HIV_Lab/

Offers an overview of Brown University's TB/HIV Research Laboratory and current projects, and provides information on all aspects of tuberculosis, from famous people who died from TB, to clinical data on the disease.

TB Weekly

http://www.newsfile.com/1t.htm

"The latest" information on TB control, programs, drug resistance, vaccines and related topics. Abstracts of articles in current and past issues available; full text accessible only with subscription.

Tuberculosis: Prevention and Treatment

http://www-med.stanford.edu/school/DGIM/Teaching/Modules/TBcases.html

This site is addressed to health care professionals and teaches about the prevention and treatment of tuberculosis. Case studies are provided.

Tuberculosis Resources

http://wash.cpmc.columbia.edu/tbcpp/

Tuberculosis detection, prevention and treatment information for both patients and health care professionals, in the form of easy-to-use electronic pamphlets. Spanish language and kiosk (screen button) versions also available.

Virology

All the Virology on the WWW

http://www.tulane.edu/~dmsander/garryfavweb.html

Very thorough list of links includes institutes, servers, societies and organizations, publications, government resources, patents and technology, online courses and virus images. Helpful and complete table of contents.

Electron Micrographs of Viruses

http://www.gene.com/ae/AB/GG/examples_of_viruses.html

Illustration of three viruses: the tobacco mosaic virus, the T4 bacteriophage, and the Human Immunodeficiency Virus (HIV.)

Microbiology and Virology

http://golgi.harvard.edu/biopages/micro.html

More web sources and microbiology, bacteriology and virology links, as gathered by Harvard Biological Laboratories.

Pathology and Virology Center

http://www-sci.lib.uci.edu/~martindale/MedicalPath.html

Martindale's Health Science Guide offers world daily reports on travel warnings and immunization updates, as well as multimedia web courses on virology and pathology, databases, case and teaching files.

Ray's Virology Home Page

http://fiona.umsmed.edu/~yar/home.html

Ray provides his lecture notes covering arboviruses to viral zoonoses, as well as links to CDC fact sheets and selected virus sites.

Virology Newsgroup Archive

http://www.bio.net:80/hypermail/VIROLOGY/

Post your own query or article, or read the latest in virology sorted by subject or by date.

Virus Diseases

http://www.mic.ki.se/Diseases/c2.html

The Karolinska Institute in Sweden has provided browsers with a long list of virology web links. Everything from lecture notes, tutorials, and student papers, to U.S. FDA and Department of Health information sheets. List of sites that focus on specific viruses and virus-caused diseases is extensive.

KIDNEYS / NEPHROLOGY & UROLOGY

> *Covered in this section: Dialysis; General Topics; Hemolytic/Uremic Syndrome; Kidney Stones; Nephrotic Syndromes; Organizations; Pathology; Polycystic Kidney Disease; Publications.*
>
> *Related sections: Cancer/Oncology; Transplantation.*

Dialysis

Dialysis On-line Support Discussion Group

http://cybermart.com/aakpaz/support.html

To subscribe, send e-mail to: listproc@mail.wustl.edu and in message body type: "subscribe dialysis Yourname." AOL users must type "subscribe" in the subject header of the e-mail; in other cases it may be left blank.

Hypertension Dialysis Clinical Nephrology

http://www.medtext.com/hdcn.htm

Renal diseases electronic journal. Provides information on renal disorders and their treatment, as well as information on hypertension, dialysis, and clinical nephrology. Includes frequently asked questions and answers, summaries of news and articles, and information on relevant medical products, services and drugs.

Kidney Dialysis Center

http://connect.colorado.edu/health/chn/dialysis/dia/main/html

Information on and links to kidney dialysis programs and issues. Includes Medicare eligibility rules, support services, statistics, a research library, and links.

Nephrology Research and Training Center

http://nephaux.dom.uab.edu/

The Center studies kidney disease and physiology, focusing on research and clinical aspects. Site describes the Center's research.

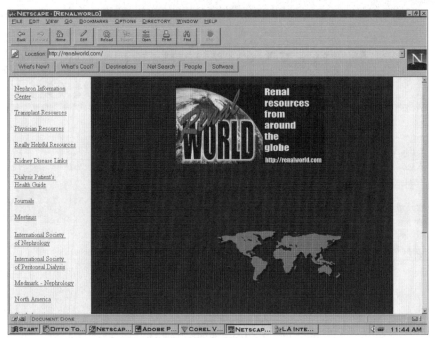

Renal World. *http://renalworld.com/*

General Topics

Alport Syndrome Home Page
http://www.cc.utah.edu/~cla6202/ASHP.htm

Site covers Alport Syndrome, a hereditary disease that affects renal functioning and hearing.

Basics of the Kidney
http://www.clark.net/pub/nhp/med/kidney/basics.html

This site answers the questions: What are the human kidneys? What do they do? And how do they work?

Emory NephrOn Line
http://web.cc.emory.edu/RENAL/home.html

A clinical site which offers lectures, slides and audio clips on renal-related medical conditions. Includes clinical case studies of nephrotic syndrome, lupus nephritis and acute renal failure. Also provides access to recent publications and research activities.

HDCN Urea Kinetics Calculators

http://www.medtext.com/dzer.htm

This site helps browser to determine a patient's Kt/V, PCRn, and V values by completing a form about the patient and treatment data.

IgA Nephropathy Home Page

http://www.hooked.net/users/rgeorge/iga.html

Information on the diagnosis and treatment of IgAN (also known as IgA nephropathy or IgA glomerulonephritis) for patients, their family, the general public and health care professionals. The site is part of an internet project which seeks to facilitate the development and sharing of research on the disease. A listserver is also available.

Internet Kidney Failure Meta-FAQ

http://www.dynamite.co.uk/renal/

Starting point to reach a variety of kidney and kidney failure resources available on the web. Includes web sites, newsgroups, and mailing lists.

Kidney

http://chorus.rad.mcw.edu/index/53html

Start on this page if you want to get concise information about a specific kidney disorder. Everything from acute kidney transplant rejection to xanthogranulomatous pyelonephritis. Part of CHORUS, Collaborative Hypertext of Radiology, an online service for physicians and medical students.

Kidney and Urologic Health

http://www.healthtouch.com/level1/leaflets/106107/106107.htm

Site provides a large number of leaflets on subjects such as urinary tract infection, incontinence, kidney stones, cysts, transplants, dialysis, benign prostatic hyperplasia and penile disorders.

Kidney Disease

http://www.diabetes.org/ada/c70f.html

General information addressing kidney disease and diabetes, written for patients and their families. Discusses symptoms and treatment of kidney disease, diabetes, and various forms of dialysis.

Kidney Patients' Resources

http://www.cc.utah.edu/~cla6202/KPR.htm

Lists with comments on books, brochures, conferences, documents, hyperlinks, magazines, newsgroups, organizations, support groups and videos. All sorts of kidney-related topics are addressed, including pediatric kidney disease, personal stories of kidney disease patients, organ donation, transplantation and travel for kidney patients.

National Kidney and Urologic Diseases Information Clearinghouse

http://www.aerie.com/nihdb/nkudic/kudbase.html

Search database that provides titles, abstracts, and availability information for documents on kidney and urologic diseases.

NEPHROL

http://synapse.uah.ualberta.ca/isn/000i001r.htm

Information about an online discussion group about nephrology for nephrology professionals. Subscribe by sending e-mail to: majordomo@majordomo.srv.ualberta.ca and type in text: "subscribe NEPHROL."

Nephron Information Center

http://nephron.com/

A good starting place for information about the variety of kidney disease links and web resources available for both health care professionals and patients. Offers quick references for diabetic nephrology, hypertensive nephropathy, glomerulonephritis, polycystic kidney disease, interstitial nephritis, end-stage renal disease and many other kidney disorders. Also offers links to organizations, physician resources, quality improvement, and transplant information.

NephroNet

http://www.nephronet.com/stannet/nephro/welcome.html

Images, general information and a search engine, as well as links to organizations, institutions and publications about nephrology, pediatric nephrology, the renal diseases and transplantation. Nephrology classified ads and "yellow pages" offered as well.

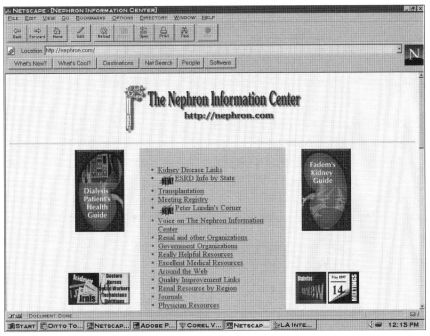

Nephron Information Center. http://nephron.com/

NIDDK WWW Server

http://www.niddk.nih.gov/

The National Institute of Diabetes and Digestive and Kidney Diseases of the National Institutes of Health Homepage. Information for the public, patients and health care providers about digestive, endocrine, hematologic, kidney and urologic diseases, including diabetes and obesity. Searchable databases offered.

Patient Information Documents on Kidney Diseases

http://www.niddk.nih.gov/kidneyDocs.html

Description, treatment options, and other patient information about end-stage renal disease (ESRD), diabetes, kidney stones, and polycystic kidney disease.

Patient Information Documents on Urologic Disease

http://www.niddk.nih.gov/UrologicDocs.html

RENALNET Information Service

http://ns.gamewood.net/renalnet.html

Clearinghouse for information on the cause, treatment and management of kidney disease and end-stage renal disease (ESRD). Site serves educational, research and treatment purposes. Extensive and easy-to-use. Nephrology resources, ESRD resources, information and other links offered.

Renalworld
http://renalworld.com/

United States Renal Data System
http://www.med.umich.edu/usrds/

The USRDS is a national data system which collects, analyzes and distributes information about end-stage renal disease in the United States. A research guide offers information for using USRDS standard analysis files. Statistics provided show incidence, prevalence, treatment, transplants, outcome and demographic data on ESRD.

Urologic and Male Genital Diseases
http://www.mic.ki.se/Diseases/c12.html

Urology Page: Kidney
http://home.pi.net/~noordzij/kidneyO.html

Anatomy, function, diseases, examination and treatment of the kidney. Written for patients who want to find out more about kidney disease.

Hemolytic Uremic Syndrome

Canadian Pediatric Kidney Research Centre
http://www.cpkdrc.org/

The CPKRC coordinates communication and research efforts devoted to fighting pediatric kidney disorders across Canada. There is special emphasis on hemolytic uremic syndrome (also known as Hamburger disease), an infection often transmitted to children through the consumption of contaminated meat. Links to related web sites, scientific associations, universities and hospitals.

Lois Joy Galler Foundation for Hemolytic Uremic Syndrome
http://www.comed.com/galler/

This site was created to raise public awareness of HUS and to promote research on developing preventive and treatment strategies. It provides a description of HUS, its symptoms, mode of transmission, treatment, statistics and new research.

Kidney Stones

Enlightenment Given Me By My Kidney Stone

http://pulsar.cs.wku.edu/~travibr/kidney.html

Kidney stones, fact and humor. Lighthearted presentation of a collection of information on kidney stones, as well as advice from fellow sufferers. Links provided as well.

Kidney Stones Network Newsletter

*http://www.readersndex.com/
imprint/000000d/newslett.html*

Approximately one million Americans are affected by kidney stones each year. This is a quarterly newsletter with information and support groups.

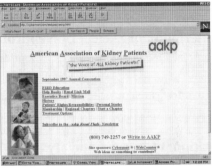

American Association of Kidney Patients.
http://cybermart.com/aakpaz/aakp.html

Nephrotic Syndrome

Nephrotic Syndrome Information

http://www.familyinternet.com/peds/scr/000490sc.htm

Good information describing the causes, symptoms, prevention and treatment of Nephrotic syndrome, a group of signs and symptoms including protein in the urine, low blood protein, and swelling (edema).

Nephrotic Syndrome/Parentsplace

http://titan.glo.be/bombernf/ns/nsindex.htm

Parents' network and users' pages with a description of the pathology of this genetic disease syndrome.

Organizations

American Association of Kidney Patients
http://cybermart.com/aakpaz/aakp.html

The AAKP is a national patient advocacy and support organization. Site offers online support, end-stage renal disease education, description and philosophy of the organization, patient stories and treatment options.

International Society of Nephrology Homepage
http://synapse.uah.ualberta.ca/isn/000i0000.htm

Offers access to the academic world of kidney and kidney-related disorders, with information on national and international societies, congresses, commissions, meetings, workshops, and research studies.

National Enuresis Society
http://www.peds.umn.edu/Centers/NES/

Addresses bedwetting in children, which is not an emotional problem, but may develop into one if the child is punished.

National Kidney Foundation 1997 Calendar of Events
http://www.kidney.org/cal97.html

Dates, conference title, and meeting places for various conferences held by the National Kidney Foundation.

National Kidney Foundation Homepage
http://www.kidney.org/index.html

Overview of kidney disease, the Kidney Transplant Games, newsletter, conferences, professional councils, and other Foundation news and events.

Renal Physicians Association
http://kdp-sparc.kdp-baptist.louisville.edu/rpa/

This sites offers information about the RPA, an organization composed of nephrologists and related staff. The RPA mission is to promote the care of patients suffering from renal and related diseases, and to serve as a information source and a representative for physicians engaged in the care of these patients. Quality improvement issues, research, health care financing and liaison activities are addressed.

Pathology

Renal Pathology Index
http://www-medlib.med.utah.edu/MedPath/RENAHTML/REALIDX.html

Polycystic Kidney Disease

Polycystic Kidney Disease
http://www.coolware.com/health/medical_reporter/kidney2.html

Article by Joel R. Cooper of *The Medical Reporter* describes this genetic disease, its symptoms and associated problems. Some links provided.

Polycystic Kidney Disease (PKD)
http://www.clark.net/pub/nhp/med/pkd.html

Describes polycystic kidney disease in terms of anatomy, symptoms, progression, prevalence, diagnosis, treatment and related questions. Glossary available, and link to the Polycystic Kidney Research Foundation.

Publications

Digital Urology Journal
http://www.duj.com/

Journal covers adult and pediatric urology.

Electronic Kidney
http://www.kidney.org/eleckid.html

Online newsletter of the National Kidney Foundation.

LIVER / HEPATOLOGY

> *Covered in this section: Alpha 1-Antitrypsin Deficiency; Cirrhosis; General Topics; Hepatitis; Organizations; Pathology.*
>
> *Related section: Transplantation.*

Alpha 1-Antitrypsin Deficiency

Alpha 1-Antitrypsin Deficiency
http://www.alphalink.org/

Frequently asked questions, and links to related web sites about alpha-1 antitrypsin deficiency. Access to a free, international mailing list for sufferers of the disease world wide. To join, send a message stating so to: alpha-1-request@home.ease.lsoft.com.

Alpha 1-Antitrypsin National Association
http://www.alpha1.org/

Informative site devoted to promoting an understanding of alpha 1-antitrypsin deficiency, a rare liver disease afflicting the lung and liver of less than 100,000 Americans. Provides information for patients and personal stories, as well as medical and product information, internet and other resource links.

Cirrhosis

CIRRHOSIS
http://www.medicinenet.com/mainmenu/encyclop/article/art_c/cirrho.htm

Cirrhosis: Many Causes
http://sadieo.lucsf.edu/alf/alffinal/infocirrh.html

Cirrhosis of the Liver
http://www.niddk.nih.gov/Cirrhos/Cirrhos.htm

PBC Foundation

http://www.nhtech.demon.co/uk/pbc/index.html

This organization offers support to individuals who suffer from PBC (Primary Biliary Cirrhosis) and to their families.

Primary Biliary Cirrhosis Patient Support Network

http://www.superaje.com/~pbc/index.htm

What is Primary Biliary Cirrhosis (PBC)?

http://cpmcnet.columbia.edu/dept/gi/PPC.html

Read this article to find out.

General Topics

100 FAQs on Liver Disease

http://sadieo.ucsf.edu/alf/alffinal/toplivdisfaqs.html

American Association for the Study of Liver Disease

http://hepar-sfgh.ucsf.edu/

Publications, conferences, research studies, and other information. for physicians and scientists who study and treat liver diseases.

American Liver Foundation Delaware Valley Chapter

http://www.netaxs.com/~emagroup/alfdelva.htm

Lots of links.

Diseases of the Liver

http://cpmcnet.columbia.edu/dept/gi/disliv.html

Alphabetical list of dozens of liver diseases and conditions with hypertext links to relevant files. Links to current research papers in liver disease as well. Maintained by Columbia-Presbyterian Medical Center.

American Association for the Study of Liver Diseases. http://hepar-sfgh.ucsf.edu/

Hepatitis

Brian's Chronic Hepatitis Home Page

http://ourworld.compuserv.com/homepages/BGARENS

Fact sheets about chronic hepatitis. Information on clinical drug trials, blood tests, support groups, transplant information, meetings and events.

Get Hip to Hep: Hepatitis Information

http://www.hep-help.com/

Hepatitis information for patients. Includes the basics of liver function, hepatitis A, B, and C, links and more.

Hepatitis A to E

http://www.cdc.gov/nicdod/diseases/hepatitis/slideset/httoc.htm

An overview of the epidemiology and prevention of viral hepatitis forms A through E. Presented in slide-show format with accompanying text. Bibliography also provided.

Hepatitis B Foundation

http://www.libertynet.org80/~hep-b/

Non-profit organization dedicated to the elimination of hepatitis B through public education and research progress. The site has fact sheets on hepatitis B, offering description of the virus, risk groups, symptoms and vaccine information. Provides advice to carriers and to parents of child carriers. Among other data, this site provides a directory of liver specialists by state.

Hepatitis Branch

http://www.cdc.gov/nicdod/diseases/hepatitis/hepatitis.htm

The National Center for Infectious Diseases' Hepatitis Branch web site offers fact sheets and general information on the transmission of hepatitis viruses A through E, as well as health guidelines for patients and health care workers.

Hepatitis C Information and Support

http://planetmaggie.pcchs.saic.com/hepc.html

Begins with a list of support groups and organizations, as well as personal stories of Hepatitis C patients. Lists links to recent articles concerning treatment and research and fact sheets and related web resources around the world. Also offers references to alternative treatments.

Hepatitis Foundation International

http://www.hepfi.org/home.htm

Numerous online pamphlets and newsletter articles covering all aspects of hepatitis, from hepatitis in children to support groups to health insurance. Treatment and prevention information and links to other web sites related to hepatitis as well.

Hepatitis Haven

http://www.tiac.net/users/birdlady/hep.html

Designed for those who have chronic hepatitis, this site contains personal stories and pictures of individuals suffering from the disease, as well as a directory of doctors, tips for receiving social security, suggestions of support groups and liver transplant information.

Hepatitis Weekly

http://www.homepage.holowww.com/1h.htm

The Hepatitis Information Network. *http://www.hepnet.com/*

Weekly electronic publication on hepatitis viruses A,B, C, D, E and G; and on non-A/non-B (NANB) hepatitis. News and research summaries offered, including discussions of vaccines, government regulations, transmission, incidence, prevention and treatment. Full-text is available only with subscription.

Hepatitis, Viral, Human

http://www.ohsu.edu:80/cliniweb/c2/c2.440.html

This page from the Oregon Health Sciences University provides information about all of the hepatitis viruses (A-E) and provides links to government and academic resources.

HepNet

http://www.hepnet.com/

The Hepatitis Information Network. Updates on patient care issues, serology, new clinical papers and news releases, as well as links to other hepatitis-related web sites. Slides, surveys and survey results, frequently asked questions (FAQs), information on continuing education and on high risk-populations also provided.

HEPV-L

http://www.tiac.net/users/birdlady/listinfo.html

A hepatitis discussion mailing list for those who have or are treating chronic hepatitis. To subscribe, send e-mail to: listserv@sjuvm.stjohns.edu with the following message: "SUB HEPV-L yourfirstname yourlastname."

Human Viral Hepatitis

http://doradus.einet.net:8000/galaxy/Medicine/Diseases-and-Disorders/Virus-D iseases/Human-Viral-Hepatitis.html

A good starting place for articles relating to viral hepatitis.

Organizations

American Liver Foundation Home Page

http://sadieo.ucsf.edu/alf/alffinal/homepagealf.html

Consumer-oriented information on the Foundation as well as on the liver and liver diseases. Includes description, disease symptoms, treatment, frequently asked questions, publications, and additional educational resources.

Pathology

Atlas of Liver Pathology

http://vh.radiology.uiowa.edu/Providers/Textbooks/LiverPathology/Text/ TitlePage.html

A multimedia textbook of liver pathology by Frank A. Mitros, M.D., of the University of Iowa College of Medicine.

Hepatic Pathology Index

http://www-medlib.med.utah.edu/WebPath/LIVEHTML/LIVERIDX.html

Over 60 images of normal and diseased livers and liver cells.

LUNGS / RESPIRATORY & PULMONARY

Asthma

ALA's Breath Easy/Asthma Digest
http://www.lungusa.org/noframes/global/contact/newsletter.html

Sign up to receive the American Lung Association's free monthly electronic newsletter on asthma.

Allergy and Asthma FAQ Home Page
http://www.cs.unc.edu/~kupstas/FAQ.html

This site describes itself as an informal gathering of all of the net wisdom on allergies and asthma. There is a special (but not exclusive) emphasis on children's health. Site offers general information, resources, book reviews, recipes and many related web links.

Allergy and Asthma Network/Mothers of Asthmatics, Inc.
http://www.podi.com/health/aanma/

The AAN/MA calls itself as grassroots patient education association. This site offers organization information and activities, an online survey, general asthma and allergy information, research news, and a bulletin board of events.

Allergy and Asthma/Rochester Resource Center
http://205.247.58.12:80/aarrc/

This site describes the Center, its staff and activities. It provides information and advice on allergy triggers and asthma medication, as well as on research studies and results. Links for both physicians and patients are provided.

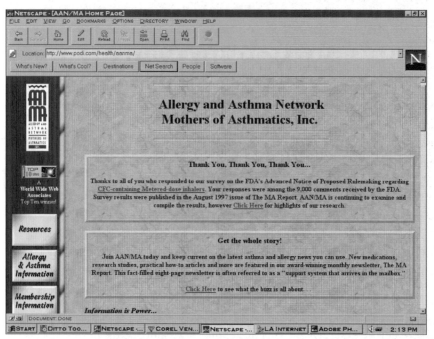

Allergy and Asthma Network/ Mothers of Asthmatics, Inc.
http://www.podi.com/health/aanma/

Asthma

http://galen.med.virginia.edu/~smb4v/tutorials/asthma/asthma1.html

Multimedia asthma tutorial for kids and their parents. Audio and images discuss what is asthma, why it occurs, what are the symptoms of asthma, and how it is treated.

Asthma and Allergy Triggers

http://www.hchp.org/html/clinpubs/fs-829.htm

This text file describes the most common triggers of an allergy attack and how to avoid them.

Asthma and Lung Specialists

http://www.cpgs.com/als/

This medical group provides information for patients and the general public about some of the major lung problems, particularly asthma. Frequently asked questions are helpful and to-the-point, and while the so-called "in-depth topic of the month" may not change that frequently, it is well-written and informative.

Asthma Electronic Discussion Groups

http://nytsyn.com/asthma/0005.html

Sign-up information for asthma electronic discussion groups.

Asthma Information Center

http://www.ama-assn.org/special/asthma/asthma.htm

Stories, guidelines, resources and recommended web sites.

Asthma Zero Mortality Coalition Breathing Free Room

http://www.asthma.com/pag2.html

Find out, "What is asthma?" An asthma survey at this site reveals how much control the patient has over asthma. Also find a description of different asthma organizations and how to join. Statistics about the prevalence, mortality and public perception of asthma are also provided.

Doctor's Guide to Asthma Information and Resources

http://www.pslgroup.com/ASTHMA.HTM

Includes medical news and alerts, asthma and drug information, discussion groups and newsgroups and related web sites. Emphasis on drug and product news.

Healthy Kids

http://KidsHealth.org/parent/healthy/

This section of Kids Health web site offers information on asthma and allergies, including frequently asked questions and advice on asthma management.

National Institute of Allergy and Infectious Diseases Home Page

http://www.niaid.nih.gov/

As part of the National Institute of Health, this institution has created a web site that provides news, research and fact sheets on allergies and asthma, as well as on many other infectious diseases and disorders of the immune system.

Teach Your Patients About Asthma

http://www.meddean.luc.edu/lumen/Medicine/Allergy/Asthma/asthmatoc.html

A clinician's guide containing ten teaching units on asthma management. It includes learning records and patient worksheets that may be printed and used by the physician and his or her patient. The guide is part of the National Asthma Education Program at the National Institute of Health.

Wee Willie Wheezie Asthma Education Web Site

http://www.newcomm.net/ies/

This web site describes an educational interactive computer game created for asthma sufferers ages 5 through 12. Information on ordering the game is provided, as are related asthma information links.

Chronic Bronchitis

Chronic Bronchitis - ALA

http://www.lungusa.org/learn/lung/lunchronic.html

This American Lung Association text file addresses the most basic questions about chronic bronchitis, including what it is, who gets it, treatment options and more.

COPD

http://osler.med.und.nodak.edu/CDIM/curric/copd.html

Lecture notes describing the etiology of chronic obstructive pulmonary diseases and how to treat patients who suffer from it.

Cystic Fibrosis

Canadian Cystic Fibrosis Foundation

http://www.ccff.ca/~cfwww/intro/pub.htm

Reports, newsletter articles, brochures and other publications offer patients and their families valuable information on cystic fibrosis.

CF-Web

http://www.ai.mit.edu/people/mernst/cf/

Online information about cystic fibrosis. This site offers a collection of cystic fibrosis links to support and research organizations world-wide, as well as general information, frequently asked questions, articles, resources for patients, physicians and researchers.

Cystic Fibrosis Foundation Home Page

http://www.cff.org/

Site addresses what's new in cystic fibrosis. Offers a description of cystic fibrosis and of the Foundation's mission and activities, information on public policy and clinical trials. Also offers links to publications and related web sites.

Cystic-L Community Page

http://www.ai.mit.edu/people/mernst/cf/cystic-l/index.html

Join the Cystic-L mailing list, read frequently asked questions, browse through archives and images, and hear personal stories about the disease.

UMHS Cystic Fibrosis Center Home Page

http://wwwhosp.umhc.umn.edu/cfcenter/

The University of Minnesota has created a guidebook for cystic fibrosis care, offering 21 chapters on diagnosis, treatment, complications, and follow-up for physicians who are treating patients with cystic fibrosis. In addition, this site offers a long list of related web links to pages created by individuals sharing personal stories, international organizations and others.

Emphysema

Emphysema

http://www.columbia.net/phys/emph/html

The surgical treatment of emphysema is discussed.

Emphysema

http://www.alignment.org/emph.htm

Emphysema - ALA

http://www.lungusa.org/learn/lung/lunemphysem.html

The American Lung Association's text file on emphysema offers answers to some of the most basic questions on emphysema: what it is, how serious it is, what causes it, and how it may be treated.

Emphysema - Getting your Second Wind

http://www.thoracic.org/

General Topics

Common Respiratory Viruses
http://wwwminer.lib.rochester.edu/wwwml/stevedfolder/med/lec4.html

This text file describes infections of the respiratory tract, including common colds, viral pneumonias, measles, rubella and numerous other viral respiratory infections and hemorrhagic rashes. It describes the diseases and how each infection progresses, as well as common complications.

RC-Web
http://www.hsc.missouri.edu/shrp/rtwww/rcweb/docs/rcweb.html

Created by the University of Missouri's Respiratory Therapy Program, this page serves students, educators, physicians and others interested in respiratory care. The AARC Clinical Practice Guidelines are linked. Special feature includes a Lung Sounds page.

Respiratory Care Home Page
http://www.theshop.net/kkuhlman/resp.htm

Find frequently asked questions (FAQs) relating to respiratory conditions such as asthma, bronchiolitis, bronchitis, allergies and hauntavirus. Also, patient-related links, schools and educational resources, organizations, hospitals, newsgroups, resources, employment opportunities, software and product information, and other related respiratory pages on the web.

Respiratory Care Related Links
http://www.hsc.missouri.edu/shrp/rtwww/rcweb/docs/rtlinks.html

Alphabetical listing of over 100 sites on the web related to respiratory care and lung health, both for health care consumers and for medical professionals.

Respiratory Hot Links
http://www.xmission.com/~gastown/herpmed/respi.htm

A long list of links to respiratory care and sleep disorder sites, loosely defined. Includes societies, publications, chat lines, hospitals, employment opportunities and educational sites, as well as industry and drug sites.

Organizations

American Association of Respiratory Care

http://www.aarc.org/

American Lung Association

http://www.lungusa.org/noframes/index.html

General information and news about asthma and other lung-related problems, as well as ALA activity at the national and local levels, and legislative and medical updates.

American Thoracic Society

http://www.thoracic.org/

The American Thoracic Society is the medical section of the American Lung Association. This site provides information for medical personnel on professional education programs and conferences, relevant legislative news and press releases, as well as ATS journals and other publications.

MANAGED CARE & INSURANCE

> Covered in this section: General Topics; Glossaries; Medicaid; Medicare; Quality Assurance.
>
> Related section: Health Care Policy & Economics.

General Topics

Aetna U.S. Healthcare

http://www.aetnaushc.com/

Consumer information about this large health care insurer.

AHCPR Research about Managed Care Organizations

http://www.ahcpr.gov/research/mgdnot1.htm

Information from the Agency for Health Care Policy and Research.

American College of Physicians' Managed Care Resources

http://www.acponline.org/mgdcare/mgdcare.htm

Association of Managed Care Providers

http://www.comed.com/amcp/

Business of Medicine/Managed Care

http://www.acponline.org/journals/news/busman.htm

Genetic Discrimination and Health Insurance: An Urgent Need for Reform

http://www.edoc.com/aaas/policy/genetics.html

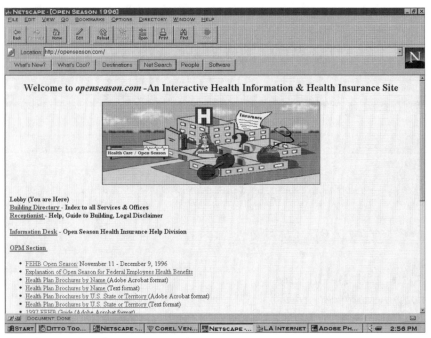

Open Season. *http://openseason.com/*

Health Fair On-Line

http://www.medaccess.com/gtehome/hfol.htm

Information for employees about health care benefits, with samples of personal cost scenarios and advice on how to choose and how to enroll in a health plan.

Healtheon

http://www.healtheon/

Online products and services for health care information and management. For insurers, employers who offer insurance benefits, employees and their dependents.

Healthscope

http://www.healthscope.org/

Consumer advice on how to choose and evaluate a health care plan, when to receive preventive care, and what health care services your managed care plan should provide.

HMO Group

http://www.hmogroup.com/index.html

Alliance of over 30 practice-based HMOs who exchange data and ideas.

HMO Page

http://www.hmopage.org/

Managed Care Update

http://www.managedcaremag.com/

Managed Care World Wide Web Resource Directory

http://www.themcic.com/mcweb.htm

MedConnect Managed Care Forum

http://www.medconnect.com/finalhtm/managedcare/managedhome.htm

OpenSeason

http://openseason.com/

An interactive health information and health insurance site.

VSB Corp

http://www.vrsc.com/

Financial resources for the seriously ill.

Your Money and Your Life: America's Managed Care Revolution

http://www.wnet.org/mhc/index.html

Web companion piece to the PBS report of the same name offers information and discussion forum on managed care issues.

Glossaries

Managed Care Glossary

http://www.bcm.tmc.edu/ama-mss/glossary.html

What is Managed Care? A Glossary

http://www.wnet.org/mhc/Info/Guide/Resglossary.html

Medicaid

The Families USA Medicaid Tool Kit
http://www.handsnet.org/handsnet2/medicaid/introtl.htm

HCFA's Welfare Reform and Medicaid
http://www.hcfa.gov/medicaid/wrethmpg.htm

Medicaid Clearinghouse
http://www.handsnet.org/handsnet2/medicaid/

Medicaid Managed Care Fact Sheets
http://www.healthlaw.org/mafact.html

NHeLP: Medicaid and Health Plan Consumer Education Brochures
http://www.healthlaw.org/casey.html

Free educational brochures to help agencies educate their clients about how to choose a health plan and how managed care may change the way Medicaid beneficiaries receive health care. Two brochures at this site are available in English, Spanish and Chinese, and may be downloaded.

Overview of the Medicaid Program
http://www.hcfa.gov/medicaid/mover.htm

Medicare

Facts On... Medicare
http://epn.org/library/agmedi.html#r-f01

HCFA Information on Medicare
http://www.hcfa.gov/medicare/medicare.htm

Information for consumers as well as professionals.

How Do I Use Medicare?
http://www.lbcommunity.com/plan/hpmususe.html

Medicare and You. *http://www.medicareinfo.com/*

How Medicare Works

http://www.house.gov/wise/medicare.htm

Basic information, courtesy of the U.S. House of Representatives.

Know Your Medicare Basics: Ten Tips

http://www.hcfa.gov/facts/f9609tps.htm

Managed Medicare and Medicaid News

http://www.ucg.com/health/mmm.htm

Sample subscriptions of this biweekly newsletter includes topics such as "How to dodge HMO tricks and strong-arm tactics," and "A 5-step guide for evaluating Medicaid HMO contracts."

Medicare and Managed Care Sites

http://www2.umdnj.edu/gpph/ira8.html

Medicare and You: Helpful Information for Medicare Beneficiaries

http://www.medicareinfo.com/

Contains news and events, Medicare pamphlets, question and answers, and detailed information for consumers.

Medicare Consumer Publications from HCFA

http://www.hcfa.gov/medicare/mcarpubs.htm

Covers issues such as hospice benefits, consumer fraud and dvance directives, as well as general Medicare information.

Medicare Information

http://ssa.gov/mediinfo.htm

Frequently asked questions (FAQs), information on premiums and HCFA, and a provider listing.

Medicare Rights Center

http://www.wwonline-ny.com/~faylin/homepage.htm#Homepage

Information about the non-profit organization MRC, which offers counseling services to Medicare beneficiaries. Programs include direct service, public education and public policy.

Section 7: Social Security

http://amf.org/text/index-7.htm

The General Index of Section 7 Social Security includes articles related to Medicare procedures, including assignment, billing, claims, and a suppliers directory. This site is part of the Retired Activity Office Files of the Airmen Memorial Foundation, and appears in large print format.

Your Medicare Handbook

http://www.hcfa.gov/pubforms/mhbktoc.htm

Published by HCFA.

Quality Assurance

Joint Commission on Accreditation of Healthcare Organizations
http://www.jcaho.org/

National Committee for Quality Assurance
http://www.ncqa.org/

An independent, nonprofit organization dedicated to assessing and reporting on the quality of managed care plans, including health maintenance organizations. Accreditation and performance measurements are addressed.

QualiNET
http://www.qualinet.com/

Information and discussion forums for quality assurance professionals.

Quality Resources Online
http://www.quality.org/

MEDICAL EQUIPMENT

DIRECTory: Medical, Dental and Hospital Equipment and Supplies Wholesale
http://okdirect.com/(sic)/sic-5/5047.html

Global Medical Instrumentation, Inc.
http://www.medres.com/
   Refurbished medical and laboratory equipment.

InVisionnet: Access to Medical Equipment Resources
http://www.invisionet.com/
   This site is for medical professionals who actively buy, sell or service medical equipment. It provides directories of manufacturers, links, and reference material for all medical equipment.

MedNet Locator
http://mednetlocator.com//equip.html
   Direct source for buying and selling used medical equipment, especially in the fields of otolaryngology and ophthalmology.

MedStore
http://www.medstore.com/index.html
   Listing of companies that offer new, used and refurbished medical equipment for sale, repair or recalibration.

Online Medical Exchange Doctors and Related Services
http://www.medicalexchange.com/
   Marketing for doctors, hospitals and other health care-related businesses or services.

Online Medical Sales Network
http://www.medsales.com/
   New and used medical equipment, surgical instruments, and hospital products.

MedStore. *http://www.medstore.com/index.html*

Pharmaceutical Products and Supplies

http://www.world-trading.com/prodcomp/pharmacy.html

Listing of company profiles. Can view list of compnies by name or category. Also provides links to other sites that may be useful for information on trade, exports, finance, business, government bodies andinternational organizations.

Physician 2 Physician Online Reviews

http://ncemi.org/reviews/p2p_home.html

A medical product reviews repository for medical software, medical books/textbooks, emergency medical equipment, and computer hardware.

MEDICAL HUMOR

Covered in this section: Addiction; Emergency Medicine; General Topics; Nursing; Sleep; Weight Loss.

Addiction

Humor and Addiction
http://www.users.cts.com/crash/e/elmo/funindex.htm

Emergency Medicine/Critical Care

Critical Care Medicine Humorpage
http://www.ccm-l.med.edu/jokes/

Emergency Medical Humor
http://home.cwnet.com/catspaw/emshumor.htm
> For the emergency room crowd.

General Topics

American Association for Therapeutic Humor
http://www.callamer.com/itc/aath/

Articles from Therapeutic Humor Literature
http://www.callamer.com/itc/aath/lit.html

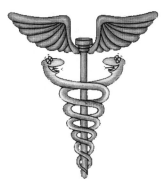

Medical Humor Page. *http://dacc. uchicago.edu/medhumor.html*

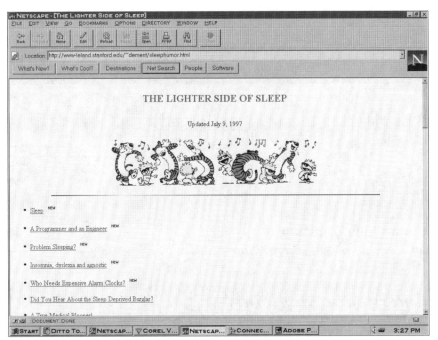

The Lighter Side of Sleep. *http://www-leland.stanford.edu/~dement/sleephumor.html*

Humor Page: Medical
http://www.swcbc.com/medical.html

Humor Potential, Inc.
http://www.stressed.com/

HUMOR Project, Inc.
http://www.wizvax.net/humor/

HUMORx
http://www.callamer.com/itc/humorx/

Insert humor into a health care professional's personal and professional life.

Jest for the Health of It!
http://www.mother.com/JestHome/

Journal of Irreproducible Results

http://www.reutershealth.com/jir/

Self-described as presenting "timeless satirical and critique articles emanating from and about the scientific and medical community that have enraged, confounded, amused and fascinated thousands of subscribers."

Medical Humor Page

http://dacc.uchicago.edu/medhumor.html

RxLaughs

http://www.rxlist/comix/

Nursing

Home Health Humor

http://www.whidbey.com/ihn/humor.html

Journal of Nursing Jocularity

http://www.jocularity.com/

Weird Nursing Tales

http://users.twave.net/texican/

Sleep

Lighter Side of Sleep

http://www-leland.stanford.edu/~dement/sleephumor.html

Weight Loss

Dieter's Guide to Weight Loss During Sex

http://www.maui.net/~jms/weight.html

Have some fun!

MEDICAL IMAGING / TELEMEDICINE

Gamma Knife

Center for Image-Guided Neurosurgery
http://www.neuronet.pitt.edu/groups/ctr-image/welcome.html
> Information about gamma knife surgery from the University of Pittsburgh.

General Topics

American Institute of Ultrasound in Medicine
http://www.well.com/user/aium/

Andrew Barclay's Medical Imaging Pages
http://www.emory.edu/CRL/abb/
> Radiology and nuclear medicine images.

Center for Human Simulation
http://www.uchsc.edu/sm/chs/about.html
> Describes the projects going on at the University of Colorado's Center for Human Simulation.

Chiropractic Radiology WebPage
http://web.idirect.com/~xray/chiro.html

CHORUS

http://chorus.rad.mcw.edu/

CHORUS = Collaborative Hypertext of Radiology. This site for medical students and physicians is a quick reference to more than 1,100 documents describing: diseases, radiological findings, differential-diagnosis lists ("gamuts"), pertinent anatomy, pathology, and physiology. CHORUS documents are indexed by organ system and are interconnected by hypertext link

Images and Imaging Science

http://www.sunshine.net/folkstone/anatomist/anatomy/images.html

Twenty-eight web sites related to medical imaging and medical illustration are listed and described. Access to collections and databases of radiological images, as well as to libraries, journals, and tutorials.

Medical Imaging Database

http://www.largnet.uwo.ca/med/i-way.html

Click on anatomic area to access database of cases containing radiologic images, case history and diagnosis.

Medical Imaging Resources on the Internet

http://agora.leeds.ac.uk/comir/resources/links.html

National Library of Medicine Quantitative Visualization/Teleradiology Project

http://everest.radiology.uiowa.edu/nlm/nlmhome.html

Obstetric Ultrasound

http://home.hkstar.com/~joewoo/joewoo2.html

Addresses basic questions about this technology and how it works, with hypertext links and an image gallery.

Radiologic Anatomy Interactive Quiz

http://www.gsm.com/resources/raquiz/

Radiological Society of North America Launch Pad

http://www.rsna.org/edu/internet/launchpad.html

Search the RSNA database, or browse through key categories related to the radiological sciences. Many web sites covering a huge variety of topics are

National Telemedicine Initiative. *http://www.nlm.nih.gov/research/telemedinit.html*

provided, including anatomy on the web, medical ethics, nuclear medicine and telemedicine.

Radiology Library
http://www.embbs.com/xray/xr.html

"Virtual" Medical Center: Medical Imaging Center
http://www-sci.lib.uci.edu/HSG/MedicalImage.html
Extensive links to MPEG movies and thousands of medical images.

Volume Slicer Applet Demos
http://www.cc.emory.edu/CRL/java/slicer/
Demo site for Java software technology.

Nuclear Medicine

Cases Related to Nuclear Medicine
http://mfs.med.u-tokai.ac.jp/radiology/index.html

Nuclear Medicine Browser
http://www.xs4all.nl/~dschonf/

What Is Nuclear Medicine?
http://www.mallinckrodt.nl/nucmed/nuclear.htm

Basic information from the Mallinckrodt Group, a company that sells nuclear medicine products.

Telemedicine

First International Telemedicine Trial to China: Zhu Ling's Case
http://www.radsci.ucla.edu/telemed/zhuling/

NLM National Telemedicine Initiative
http://www.nlm.nih.gov/research/telemedinit.html

The National Library of Medicine supports 19 telemedicine projects. This site offers information on each, its purpose, and other telemedicine programs.

Telemedicine Information Exchange
http://tie.telemed.org/

These pages provide basic information on telemedicine and its applications, a brief history of telemedicine, business and product news summaries, examples of historical and current uses, and articles and abstracts from journals. Particularly thorough list of links to telemedicine-related sites from medical images to videoconferencing. A TIE forum presents experts' answers to FAQs.

Telemedicine Resources
http://icsl.ee.washington.edu/~cabralje/tmresources.html

Offers a list of web resources and services related to telemedicine. Broken down into topics of general telemedicine, compression and teleconferencing standards, networking, and medical imaging.

MEDICAL LAW

Covered in this section: *Americans with Disabilities Act; General Topics; Health Insurance.*

Americans with Disabilities Act

ADA and Disability Information

http://www.public.iastate.edu/~sbilling/ada.html

Long list of ADA resources on the web, including accessibility guidelines, reference books, compliance handbooks, and a newsgroup devoted to ADA issues. Other links to general and specific disability material are offered.

Americans with Disabilities Act Home Page

http://www.usdoj.gov/crt/ada/adahom1.com

The U.S. Department of Justice maintains this site on the 1990 ADA. Information about the toll-free ADA phone line, ADA enforcement programs, ADA status reports, new or proposed regulations, and ADA Technical Assistance grants are provided.

Americans with Disabilities Act of 1990

gopher://wiretap.spies.com/00/Gov/disable.act/

Full text of the 1990 ADA passed by Congress to prohibit discrimination on the basis of disability.

General Topics

American College of Legal Medicine

http://execpc.com/~aclm/

Covers medico-legal affairs.

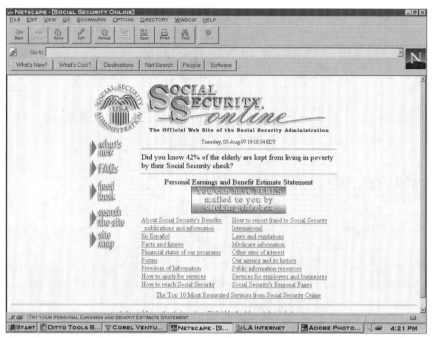

Social Security Online. *http://www.ssa.gov/SSA_Home.html*

Centre for Health Law Ethics & Policy
http://www.newcastle.edu.au/centre/home.html

Epilepsy Legal Rights/Legal Issues
http://www.efa.org/what/advocacy/legal.html

FindLaw Internet Legal Resources
http://www.findlaw.com/
> Links include sites devoted to health law.

Medical and Public Health Law Site
http://plague.law.umkc.edu/
> Online textbook for physicians.

Medical Protection Society
http://www.mps.org.uk/medical/
> International non-profit association offering medico-legal services.

Medical Record Privacy

http://epic.org/privacy/medical/

Site presents laws, articles and discussion about medical privacy law and policy, and consumer advice on safeguarding medical records.

Psychiatry and the Law

http://ua1vm.ua.edu/~jhooper/index.html

Selected Internet Resources in Health Law and Policy

http://lawlib.slu.edu/centers/hlthlawhlthlnk.htm

Health Insurance

COBRA Online

http://www.medlaw.com/

Online health law resource center for health care professionals, hospitals, risk managers and legal counsel. Information on COBRA/EMTACA, medical malpractice, health issues, health care economics and related subjects.

Social Security Online

http://www.ssa.gov/SSA_Home.html

Information and publications on Social Security entitlement programs.

MEDICAL REFERENCES / RESOURCES

Computers/Internet

Healthcare Information and Management Systems Society
http://www.himss.org/

Medicine by Modem
http://www.news.com/SpecialFeatures/0%2C5%2C7943%2C00.html?nd

This is a NEWS.COM special report that discusses benefits and cautions involved in the use of the internet by physicians and consumers seeking medical information. Site has a great deal of relevance for these individuals.

Support and Discussion Groups on the Internet
http://www.stud.unit.no/studorg/ikstrh/ed/ed_inet.htm

The Net: User Guidelines and Netiquette
http://www.fau.edu/rinjaldi/netiquette.html

It's good to be aware of the web protocol when you are surfing the net and entering into discussions online.

W3 Servers
http://www.w3.org/DataSources/WWW/Servers.html

Summary of a list of all registered WWW servers alphabetically by continent, country and state.

World Congress on the Internet in Medicine
http://www.mednet.org/uk/mednet/mednet.htm

World Wide Web FAQ
http://www.boutell.com/faq/

Select the site closest to you to have access to the World Wide Web's Frequently Asked Question database.

Databases

Cyberspace Clinic
http://www.unm.edu/~vuksan/mario/clinic.html

DynaMed Home Page: Medical Information System Database
http://home.earthlink.net/~alper/index.html

Clinical reference tool for patient encounters.

Edmund's Home Page
http://www.li.net/~edhayes/ed.html

Personal home page that provides many links to different medical specialties.

Firstmark Healthcare Providers and Facilities
http://www.firstmark.com/finkcat/03toc.htm/#hcproviders/

A collection of databases that includes AIDS treatment centers, dentists and nursing homes.

Health Web
http://healthweb.org/

A cooperative effort of a number of health sciences libraries to develop an interface which provides organized access to evaluated non-commercial, health-related, internet-accessible resources. Links and information on a number of health and medical topics.

MEdIC (Medical Education Information Center). http://dpalm2.med.uth.tmc.edu/

MedGate

http://www.healthgate.com/HealthGate/medgate/index.html

For a monthly fee, members can obtain access to nine different biomedical databases, as well as *Detwiler's Directory of Health and Medical Resources, Newswire,* and the *Morbidity and Mortality Weekly Report.*

MEdIC: Medical Education Information Center

http://dpalm2.med.uth.tmc.edu/

Medical information for professionals and consumers.

NLM Online Databases and Databanks

http://www.nlm.nih.gov/pubs/factsheets/online_databases.html

Describes 40 NLM online databases, including: AIDSDRUGS, AIDSLINE, AIDSTRIALS, CANCERLIT, HealthSTAR, MEDLINE, PDQ, TOXLINE and TOXNET.

Drug References

See also: Drugs/Pharmacology.

Merck Manual of Diagnosis and Therapy Online

http://www.merck.com:80/!!rABLW3Y3TrABLY0OmS/pubs/mmanual/

   Search the online version of this famous handbook of disorders and therapy.

PDRNET.COM

http://www.pdrnet.com/

   Online _Physicians' Desk Reference_ free to physicians. Also find access to Medline and to PDR prescription information.

Gateways

Achoo!

http://www.achoo.com/

   Online internet health care services.

CliniWeb

http://www.ohsu.edu/cliniweb/

   CliniWeb is maintained by Oregon Health Services University and offers an index to clinical information on the World Wide Web. Includes approximately 10,000 web site links.

Diseases, Disorders and Related Topics

http://www.mic.ki.se/Diseases/index.html

   Alphabetical list to links covering hundreds of diseases. From Sweden's Karolinska Institute.

Galaxy's Medicine

http://galaxy.einet.net/galaxy/Medicine.html

   Links to medical information, arranged by specialty and disease. Includes academic organizations, commercial organizations, directives, government agencies and private organizations.

Health/Medical Internet Entry Points

http://www.age.ne.jp/x/akagi/healthep.htm

Healthfinder

http://www.healthfinder.gov/

The United States government's consumer health site. Links to chosen online publications, databases, support groups, organizations, government sites and other health information resources on the net.

HealthWEB

http://hsinfo.ghsl.nwu.edu/healthweb/

Alphabetical list of health and medical-related subjects.

Healthwise

http://www.columbia.edu/cu/healthwise/

Includes *Go Ask Alice!* an interactive question-and-answer response service.

Martindale's Health Science Guide

http://www-sci.lib.uci.edu/~martindale/HSGuide.html

Medical Gophers

gopher://peg.cwis.uci.edu:7000/11/gopher.welcome/peg/MEDICINE/

MedMark

http://medmark.bit.co.kr/

Offers resources by specialty and free access to MEDLINE search index.

MedWeb: Emory University Health Sciences Center Library

http://www.cc.emory.edu/WHSCL/medweb.html

An excellent place to start a search. Provides many links on health, medicine and related topics. Easy to use.

MedWorld Best Sites

http://medworld.stanford.edu/medlinks

Selective listing of medical web sites.

Six Senses Review

http://www.sixsenses.com/

Resource providing reviews. Search or browse by topic.

WWW Virtual Library: Biosciences: Medicine
http://www.ohsu.edu/clinicweb/wwwvl/

General Topics

AMA Health Insight
http://www.ama-assn.org/insight/insight.htm
    Consumer health information. Includes specific conditions, general health information and medical care advice.

Avicenna
http://www.avicenna.com/
    Provides medical information for health care professionals. Includes free MEDLINE access and reference materials such as FDA Drug information, *Outlines in Clinical Medicine*, and information about clinical trials and medical professional associations. Also includes a lifestyle area, financial news and leisure information. Free registration.

Galen II
http://www.library.ucsf.edu/
    The digital library of the University of California at San Francisco.

Go Ask Alice!
http://www.columbia.edu/cu/healthwise/alice.html
    Submit questions about sexuality, sexual health, relationships, general health, emotional well-being, alcohol/drugs, and fitness and nutrition.

Hardin Meta Directory: Internet Health Sources
http://www.arcade.uiowa.edu/hardin-www/md.html
    Their slogan is, "We list the sites that list the sites." Then they arrange these lists according to length (long, medium or short.)

Health Information Resources
http://www.nih.gov/health/
    Describes what is available from the National Institutes of Health.

National Library of Medicine. *http://www.nlm.nih.gov/*

Health Resources

http://www.nova.edu/Inter-Links/medicine.html

Links to basic information resources in health and medicine.

HealthGate

http://www.healthgate.com/

Includes access to healthy living, drug and patient information. Search MEDLINE, CANCERLIT, AIDSLINE, AIDSDRUGS, AIDSTRIAL, HealthSTAR, and BIOETHICSLINE databases for free.

HealthSeek

http://www.healthseek.com/

Commercial, online service for health care professionals, consumers and companies providing news, information and links.

Healthtouch

http://www.healthtouch.com/

Provides links to drug information, pharmacy search, health resource directory, health and product information.

Internet Health Resources

http://www.ihr.com/

Access to health resources for consumers and health care providers.

Internet Medical Terminology Resources

http://www.gsf.de:80/MEDWIS/activity/

Mayo Health O@sis

http://www.mayo.ivi.com/ivi/mayo/common/htm/newsstand.htm

Includes health news and consumer resources. Sub-topics include a health library, cancer center, diet and nutrition, heart center, pregnancy and children, Medicare center, and women's health.

MedAccess On-Line

http://www1.medaccess.com/homeFrame.htm

Includes newsletter and databases, bulletin board, health quizzes, articles, family health information, and the "MedAccess Motivator," an interactive workbook to set and achieve health and wellness goals.

MedForum

http://www.migraine.com/

Medical forum for patients, physicians, journalists and the general public. Includes peer-reviewed journal, a section on the "Business of Medicine," information for patients, access to newsgroups, JobLine, MedWeb and other links. Membership fee required.

Medical Yellow Pages Online

http://www.publistar.com/myp/index.htm

Internet medical directory.

MedicineNet

http://www.medicinenet.com/

Provides health facts, "Ask the Experts" section, news, diseases and treatments, and pharmacy information.

Multimedia Medical Reference Library

http://www.med-library.com

Includes subjects such as software, audio and chat sites, as well as the usual breakdown of medical topics by specialty.

National Center for Research Resources

http://www.ncrr.nih.gov/

The Center creates and provides critical research technologies and shared resources.

New York Online Access to Health Main Menu

http://www.noah.cuny.edu/

Main menu is in English and in Spanish. Allows surfers to browse through health topics, or perform a word search.

Paper Chase

http://enterprise.bih.harvard.edu/paperchase/

Medical information resources composed of four major databases that can search biomedical journals back to 1966. Available for a monthly or yearly fee.

Patti Peeple's Guide to Health Economics, Medical and Pharmacy Resources on the Net

http://www.exit109.com/~zaweb/pjp/index.shtml

A great number of links to sites providing disease information and medical humor, and to associations, institutions and commercial medical companies, medical libraries and more.

Physicians' Choice

http://mdchoice.com/

Physician reviewers have evaluated these lists of internet sites on health and medicine-related topics.

Priory Journals

http://www.priory.com/journals/

Includes samples of *Dentistry On-Line*, *Psychiatry On-Line*, *Chest Medicine On-Line*, *General Practice On-Line*, *Anaesthesia On-line*, *Medicine On-Line*, and *Family Medical Practice On-Line*. Also includes a book shop and search engine.

Virtual Hospital

http://vh.radiology.uiowa.edu/

The Virtual Hospital provides patient care support and distance learning to practicing physicians and other health care professionals. The Iowa Health Book section provides information to the general public on a variety of health issues.

Virtual Medical Clinic

http:/www.mediconsult.com/

Choose from over 50 medical topics, ranging from AIDS to Strokes; and receive information, articles and links. Also includes medical information, support groups, products, and suggestions.

USC's List of Medical-Related Gophers

gopher://cwis.usc.edu:80/11/Other_Gophers_and_Information_Resources/
Gophers_by_Subject/Gopher_Jewels/medical/

Includes gophers on AIDS, disabilities and other medical-related subjects.

Wellness Web Patient's Network References

http://wellweb.com/refer/refer.htm

Links to references of medical and general use.

WWW Medical Indexes

http://www.intmed.mcw.edu/MedIndex.html

Long list of medical indexes gathered by the Medical College of Wisconsin.

Hospitals

Council of Teaching Hospitals

http://www.aamc.org/hlthcare/teach/

Lists hospitals alphabetically and geographically.

Hospital Locator

http://www.medaccess.com/hospitals/hosp01.htm

Hospital database. Offers advice on how to select a hospital.

HospitalWeb
http://neuro-www.mgh.harvard.edu/hospitalweb.nclk/

List of U.S. and international hospitals that have pages on the internet.

Libraries

Gopher Menu from the U.S. Library of Congress
gopher://marvel.loc.gov:70/11/global/med/general/

Internet Public Libraries
http://ipl.sils.umich.edu/svcs/greatlibs/

Collection of library web pages with a summary of resources on specific topics.

MedWeb's Medical Libraries
http://www.gen.emory.edu/medweb/medweb.medlibs.html

National Network of Libraries of Medicine
http://www.nnlm.nlm.nih.gov/

Access to world-wide biomedical information for U.S. health care professionals.

NIH Library
http://www.ncrr.nih.gov/home.html-ssi

Supports the biomedical and behavioral research needs of the NIH community with a comprehensive range of scientific, medical and administrative information and support.

NN/LM: National Network of Libraries of Medicine
http://clara.hslib.washington.edu/

U.S. National Library of Medicine
http://www.nlm.nih.gov/

This site provides information about the Library, as well as news, access to databases and special information programs, NLM publications (fact sheets, reports and ordering information), research programs, grant information, and many links.

Professional Resources

Achoo! Practice of Medicine
http://www.achoo.com/achoo/practice/medicine/fields/index.htm

Topics arranged by specialty, including areas such as audiology, midwifery, sports medicine, and toxicology.

ACP Online
http://www.acponline.org/

The American College of Physician's web site for internal medicine.

Alphabetical list of Specific Diseases/Disorders
http://www.mic.ki.se/Diseases/alphalist.html

Alphabetical list of specific diseases and disorders with related web links.

Doctor's Guide to the Internet
http://www.pslgroup.com/DOCGUIDE.HTM

Links to many sites offering information for physicians and for their patients.

Doctors' Independent Network
http://www.demon.co.uk/DIN/

A computer database and communication service uniting the health care professionals in the United Kingdom who are using internet technology.

HCN: Health Communication Network
http://www.ncn.net.au/

Australian-based site containing medical databases, indexes, publishing and bibliographic information, forums and other information for paying members.

Health Professionals' Online
http://www.hpol.net/hpol/welcome.html

Provides non-physician health professionals access to popular medical literature databases, drug databases, medical news, disease centers, discussion groups and directories of medical research for a monthly fee.

Journal Club on the Web
http://www.journalclub.org/

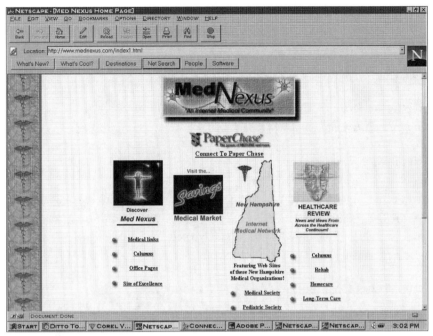

Med Nexus. *http://www.mednexus.com/index1.html*

Med Nexus

http://www.mednexus.com/

Medical news, information and commentary. Medical links, columns, art gallery, and conference information provided. Free registration.

MedConnect

http://www.medconnect.com/

Interactive education and jobs line, managed care forum, medical news and marketplace, meetings and conference information.

Medical Matrix

http://www.slackinc.com/matrix/

Clinical medicine resources online, including MEDLINE, journals, continuing medical education (CME) opportunities on the internet, news, prescription assistance, textbooks, forums, patient information and classified ads. Specialty and disease-categorized information lead users to internet links useful to health care professionals.

Medical Center Web

http://www.medcenter.com/

Contains links to the Physician and Surgeon Web Directory, ECG Web, Community Health Calendar, and Cardiac Cath Web.

Medicine Index - Biosciences on the Internet

http://www.ohsu.edu/cliniweb/wwwvl/

Medscape

http://www.medscape.com/

Features thousands of free, full-text, peer-reviewed articles, medical news, AIDSLINE, TOXLINE, MEDLINE, and interactive quizzes. For health professionals and interested consumers. Updated daily. Although registration is necessary, it is free and access is immediate.

MedWeb's Biomedical Internet Resources

http://www.cc.emory.edu/WHSCL/medweb.html#TOC/

Emory University's catalog of internet sites.

North American Primary Care Research Group

http://views.vcu.edu/views/fap/napcry.html

Online Clinical Calculator

http://www.intmed.mcw.edu/clincalc.html

This calculator finds the Bayesian Analysis of prevalence, sensitivity and specificity; and clinical calculations of estimated blood level, body surface/body mass ratio, weight and measurement conversions.

Physician's Guide to the Internet

http://www.webcom.com/pgi/

Physicians' HomePage

http://php2.silverplatter.com/php/mt-lib.htm#about

Membership allows you access to *MD Digests*, Internet Library, *MD Opinions* (primary care questions), *MD Drugs*, medical journals, and more. Flat rate fee is reduced for medical residents.

Physicians Network

http://www.njnet.com/~embbs.pn.html

For physicians and health care professionals. Includes radiology library, e-mail directory, job listings, EKG analysis/case studies, residents forum, and Best Picks of the Medical Web.

Physician's Online

http://www.po.com/Welcome.html

Members receive free access to MEDLINE and other medical and drug databases, an e-mail account, stock quotes, continuing medical education (CME) opportunities, physicians-only discussion groups, non-medical resources, and more. To join, you must install the Physicians' Online (POL) software (instructions provided at site).

Primary Care Baseline

http://www.med.ufl.edu/medinfo/baseline/

Contains clinical care algorithms and drug list.

Secret Source/Medical Secrets

http://www.secretsource.com/medical/

Strictly for medical professionals.

WebDoctor

http://www.gretmar.com/

Contains a peer-reviewed index of internet medical resources, by specialty and disease. Particularly large section on Rural Medicine.

What's New at the American Medical Association

http://www.ama-assn.org/what_new/what_new.htm

Association updates, registration and policy information, the current month's edition of *JAMA*, conference announcements, etc.

Search Tools

DocNet

http://www.docnet.org.uk/medis-frames.html

Health A to Z

http://www.HealthAtoZ.com/

Search engine to seek health sites on the internet.

Health Explorer

http://www.healthexplorer.com/

Over 3,000 health-related web sites. Search by topic or keyword.

Internet Sleuth Health Database Search Engine

http://www.isleuth.com/heal.html

Choose up to six health databases to search by keyword or topic.

Med Hunt

http://www.hon.ch/

Search the internet with this Health on the Net Foundation search engine. Includes library, media gallery, and free Medline access.

Medical World Search

http://pride-sun.poly.edu/

MedWeb

http://www.gen.emory.edu/MEDWEB/search.html

One of the best health and medicine search engines.

MedWorld: MEDBOT Searching Tool

http://medworld.stanford.edu/medbot/

This "Super Search" tool allows you to access information from four different indices at once.

Net Medicine

http://www.netmedicine.com/

Search the internet. Site includes a Cyberpatient Simulator, Medfinder search engine, EKG of the Month, Radiology Rounds, Pediatric Topics and much more.

OMNI

http://omni.ac.uk/

This is a UK gateway to biomedical resources on the internet.

U.S. National Library of Medicine

http://wwwindex.nlm.nih.gov/index/nlmindex.html

Search for information.

Statistics

Cancer Statistics Review

http://www-seer.ims.nci.nih.gov/Publications/CSR7394/index.html

Center for International Health Information

http://www.cihi.com/

This organization's purpose is to provide information on the Population, Health, and Nutrition (PHN) sector in developing countries that are assisted by USAID (United States Agency for International Development).

Combined Health Information Database

http://chid.nih.gov/

Country Health Profiles (The Americas)

http://www.paho.org/english/country.htm

Describes the general health trends, specific health problems and risks, and the health care resources and services available in approximately 40 countries in the Americas. From the Pan American Health Organization.

Health Insurance Statistics from the U.S. Census Bureau

http://www.census.gov/hhes/www/hlthins.html

Health Statistics

http://www.lib.umich.edu/libhome/PubHealth.lib/bib.statistics.html

Medicare and Medicaid Statistics and Data

http://www.hcfa.gov/stats/stats.htm

Mental Health and Substance Use/Abuse Statistical Data

http://www.samhsa.gov/oas/oasftp.htm

National Center for Health Statistics
http://www.cdc.gov/nchswww/nchshome.htm

Scientific Data, Surveillance, Health Statistics, and Laboratory Information
http://www.cdc.gov/scientific.htm

Statistical Tables: Information from the Centers for Disease Control
http://www.cdc.gov/nchswww/datawh/statab/pubd.htm

    Statistical information on behavioral risk factors (i.e. overweight, high cholesterol, smoking habits), chronic diseases, infant and child health, sex education and sexual activity.

Statistics on Drug Abuse from the National Institute on Drug Abuse
http://www.nida.nih.gov/NIDACapsules/NCIndex.html

WHOSIS
http://www.who.ch/whosis/whosis.htm

    WHO Statistical Information System.

MEDICAL SCHOOL WEB SITES & INFORMATION

U.S. Medical Schools

Alabama

University of Alabama School of Medicine (Birmingham)
http://www.uab.edu/uasom/

University of South Alabama, College of Medicine (Mobile)
http://southmed.usouthal.edu/com/index.html

Arizona

University of Arizona College of Medicine (Tucson)
http://www.ahsc.arizona.edu/com.shtml

Arkansas

University of Arkansas College of Medicine (Little Rock)
http://www.uams.edu/

California

Charles Drew University of Medicine & Science (Los Angeles)
http://www.cdrewu.edu/home.htm

Loma Linda University School of Medicine (Loma Linda)
http://www.llu.edu/llu/medicine/

Stanford University School of Medicine (Palo Alto)
http://www-med.stanford.edu/school/

University of California, Davis, School of Medicine (Davis)
http://www-med.ucdavis.edu/

University of California, Irvine, College of Medicine (Irvine)
http://meded.com.uci.edu/

University of California, Los Angeles, School of Medicine (Los Angeles)
http://www.mednet.ucla.edu/som/

University of California, San Diego, School of Medicine (San Diego)
http://medicine.ucsd.edu/

University of California, San Francisco, School of Medicine (San Francisco)
http://www.som.ucsf.edu/

University of Southern California School of Medicine (Los Angeles)
http://www.usc.edu/hsc/med-sch/

Colorado

University of Colorado School of Medicine (Denver)
http://www.uchsc.edu/sm/sm/

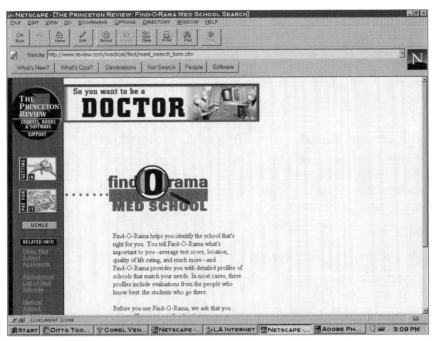

Find-O-Rama: Med School.
http://www.review.com/medical/find/med_schools_search.html

Connecticut

University of Connecticut Medical School (Farmington)
http://www9.uchc.edu/index.html

Yale University School of Medicine (New Haven)
http://info.med.yale.edu/medical/

District of Columbia

George Washington University Medical Center (Washington)
http://www.gwu.edu/~gwumc/

Georgetown University School of Medicine (Washington)
http://www.dml.georgetown.edu/schmed/

Howard University College of Medicine (Washington)

http://www.cldc.howard.edu/~bhlogan/hucm-cat.html

Florida

College of Medicine at the University of Florida (Gainesville)

http://www.med.ufl.edu/

Florida State University/University of Florida College of Medicine (Tallahassee)

http://www.fsu.edu/~pims/pims.html

University of Miami School of Medicine (Miami)

http://www.med.miami.edu/

University of South Florida College of Medicine (Tampa)

http://www.med.usf.edu/med.html

Georgia

Emory School of Medicine (Atlanta)

http://www.emory.edu/WHSC/MED/med.html

Medical College of Georgia School of Medicine (Augusta)

http://www.mcg.edu/SOM/Index.html

Mercer University School of Medicine (Macon)

http://www.mercer.edu/www/medicine.htm

Morehouse School of Medicine (Atlanta)

http://www.msm.edu/

Hawaii

University of Hawaii John A. Burns School of Medicine (Honolulu)

http://medworld.biomed.hawaii.edu/

Illinois

Finch University of Health Sciences/The Chicago Medical School (Chicago)

http://www.finchcms.edu/

Loyola University of Chicago, Stritch School of Medicine (Maywood)

http://www.meddean.luc.edu/

Northwestern University Medical School (Chicago)

http://www.nums.nwu.edu/introtext.htm

Rush-Presbyterian-St. Luke's Medical Center (Chicago)

http://www.rush.edu/

Southern Illinois University School of Medicine (Springfield)

http://www.siumed.edu/

University of Chicago Pritzker School of Medicine (Chicago)

http://www.uchicago.edu/u.acadunits/BSD.html

University of Illinois at Chicago Medical Center (Chicago)

http://www.uic.edu/depts/mcam/

*University of Illinois College of Medicine at Rockford (Rockford)

http://www.rockford.uic.edu/

*University of Illinois College of Medicine at Urbana-Champaign (Urbana-Champaign)
http://www.med.uiuc.edu/

Indiana

Indiana University School of Medicine (Indianapolis)
http://www.iupui.edu/it/medschl/home.html

Iowa

University of Iowa, College of Medicine (Iowa City)
http://www.medadmin.uiowa.edu/

*University of Osteopathic Medicine and Health Sciences/College of Osteopathic Medicine and Surgery (Des Moines)
http://www.aacom/org/uomhs.htm

Kansas

University of Kansas School of Medicine (Kansas City)
http://www.kumc.edu/som/som.html

Kentucky

University of Kentucky College of Medicine, Chandler Medical Center (Lexington)
http://www.comed.uky.edu/Medicine/welcome.html

University of Louisville School of Medicine (Louisville)
http://www.louisville.edu/medschool//

Louisiana

Louisiana State University Medical Center (New Orleans)
http://www.lsumc.edu/

Louisiana State University Medical Center (Shreveport)
http://lib-sh.lsumc.edu/

Tulane University Medical Center (New Orleans)
http://www1.omi.tulane.edu/

Maine

*University of New England College of Osteopathic Medicine (Biddeford)
http://www.aacom.org/unecom.htm

Maryland

Johns Hopkins University School of Medicine (Baltimore)
http://infonet.welch.jhu.edu/som/

Uniformed Services University of the Health Sciences (Bethesda)
http://www.usuhs.mil/

University of Maryland School of Medicine (Baltimore)
http://www.umm.edu/school/sm-home.html

Massachusetts

Boston University School of Medicine (Boston)
http://med-amsa.bu.edu/BUSM/

Harvard Medical School (Boston)
http://www.med.harvard.edu/

Tufts University School of Medicine (Boston)
http://www.nemc.org/tusm/

University of Massachusetts Medical Center (Worcester)
http://www.ummed.edu/

Michigan

Michigan State University College of Human Medicine (East Lansing)
http://www.chm.msu.edu/

University of Michigan Medical School (Ann Arbor)
http://www.med.umich.edu/medschool/

Wayne State University School of Medicine (Detroit)
http://www.phypc.med.wayne.edu/newpage.htm

Minnesota

Mayo Medical School (Rochester)
http://www.mayo.edu/education/mms/MMS_Home_Page.html

University of Minnesota at Duluth, School of Medicine (Duluth)
http://www.d.umn.edu/medweb/

University of Minnesota Medical School (Minneapolis)
http://www.med.umn.edu/

Mississippi

University of Mississippi Medical Center (Jackson)
http://umcnews.com/

Missouri

*Saint Louis University School of Medicine (Saint Louis)
http://www.slu.edu/colleges/med/

University of Missouri, Columbia, School of Medicine (Columbia)
http://www.hsc.missouri.edu/som/

University of Missouri, Kansas City, School of Medicine (Kansas City)
http://research.med.umkc.edu/

Washington University School of Medicine (St. Louis)
http://medinfo.wustl.edu/

Nebraska

Creighton University School of Medicine (Omaha)
http://medicine.creighton.edu/

University of Nebraska College of Medicine (Omaha)
http://www.unmc.edu/UNCOM/index.html

Nevada

University of Nevada, Reno, Medical School and Biosciences (Reno)
http://www.med.unr.edu/

New Hampshire

Dartmouth Medical School (Hanover)
http://www.dartmouth.edu/dms/

New Jersey

New Jersey Medical School (Newark)
http://www.umdnj.edu/academe/njms.html

Robert Wood Johnson Medical School (Piscataway)
http://www2.umdnj.edu/rwjms.html

New York

Albany Medical College (Albany)
http://www.amc.edu/html/medical_college.html

Albert Einstein College of Medicine of Yeshiva University (Bronx)
http://www.aecom.yu.edu/

Columbia University College of Physicians and Surgeons (New York)
http://cait.cpmc.columbia.edu/dept/ps/

Cornell University Medical School (New York)
http://www.med.cornell.edu/

Mount Sinai School of Medicine (New York)
http://www.mssm.edu/

New York Medical College (Valhalla)
http://nymc.edu/

New York University School of Medicine (New York)

http://www.med.nyu.edu/training.html

State University of New York at Stony Brook, School of Medicine (Stony Brook)

http://www.informatics.sunysb.edu/som/

State University of New York, Health Science Center at Brooklyn, College of Medicine (Brooklyn)

http://www.hscbklyn.edu/COM/

State University of New York, Health Science Center at Syracuse (Syracuse)

http://www.hscsyr.edu/

University of Buffalo School of Medicine and Biomedical Sciences (Buffalo)

http://www.smbs.buffalo.edu/

University of Rochester School of Medicine and Dentistry (Rochester)

http://www.urmc.rochester.edu/SMD/

North Carolina

Bowman Gray School of Medicine of Wake Forest University and the North Carolina Baptist Hospitals, Inc. (Winston-Salem)

http://isnet.is.wfu.edu/

Duke University Medical School and College of Allied Health (Durham)

http://www2.mcduke.edu/som/

East Carolina University School of Medicine (Greenville)

http://www.med.ecu.edu/DEPTMENU.HTM

University of North Carolina at Chapel Hill, School of Medicine (Chapel Hill)

http://www.med.unc.edu/welcome.htm

North Dakota

University of North Dakota School of Medicine & Health Sciences (Grand Forks)

http://www.med.und.nodak.edu/

Ohio

Case Western Reserve University School of Medicine (Cleveland)

http://mediswww.meds.cwru.edu/

Medical College of Ohio, School of Medicine (Toledo)

http://www.mco.edu/smed/smedmain.html

Northeastern Ohio Universities College of Medicine (Rootstown)

http://www.neoucom.edu/

Ohio State University College of Medicine (Columbus)

http://www.med.ohio-state.edu/

University of Cincinnati College of Medicine (Cincinnati)

http://www.med.uc.edu/htdocs/medicine/uccom.htm

Wright State University School of Medicine (Dayton)

http://www.med.wright.edu/

Oklahoma

University of Oklahoma Health Sciences Center (Tulsa)

http://w3.uokhsc.edu/home/default.html

Oregon

Oregon Health Sciences University, School of Medicine (Portland)

http://www.ohsu.edu/temp_som.htm

Pennsylvania

MCP•Hahnemann School of Medicine, Allegheny University of the Health Sciences (Philadelphia)

http://www.auhs.edu/medschool/medschl.html

Pennsylvania State University College of Medicine (Hershey)

http://www.hmc.psu.edu/hmc/colmed.htm

Temple University School of Medicine (Philadelphia)

http://www.temple.edu/medschool/

Thomas Jefferson University, Jefferson Medical College (Philadelphia)

http://jeffline.tju.edu/CWIS/JMC/jmc.html

University of Pennsylvania School of Medicine (Philadelphia)

http://www.med.upenn.edu/

University of Pittsburgh School of Medicine (Pittsburgh)

http://www.omed.pitt.edu/~omed/

Puerto Rico

University of Puerto Rico School of Medicine (San Juan)
http://wwwrcm.upr.clu.edu/school.htm

Rhode Island

Brown University Division of Biology and Medicine (Providence)
http://BioMedCS.biomed.brown.edu/

South Carolina

Medical University of South Carolina, College of Medicine (Charleston)
http://www2.musc.edu/medicine.html

University of South Carolina School of Medicine (Columbia)
http://www.med.sc.edu/

South Dakota

University of South Dakota School of Medicine (Vermillion)
http://www.usd.edu/med/

Tennessee

East Tennessee State University College of Medicine (Johnson City)
http://www.etsu-tn.edu/medcom/

Meharry Medical College (Nashville)
http://web.fie.com/htbin/Molis/MolisSummary?FICE=003506

University of Tennessee, Health Science Center (Memphis)
http://utmgopher.utmem.edu/utm.html

Vanderbilt University School of Medicine (Nashville)
http://www.mc.vanderbilt.edu/medschool/

Texas

Baylor College of Medicine (Houston)
http://www.bcm.tmc.edu/

College of Medicine at Texas A&M University (College Station)
http://hsc.tamu.edu/

Texas Tech University School of Medicine (Lubbock)
http://www.ttuhsc.edu/

University of Texas Health Science Center at San Antonio (San Antonio)
http://www.uthscsa.edu/som/som_main.htm

University of Texas Medical Branch at Galveston (Galveston)
http://www.utmb.edu/

University of Texas Medical School (Houston)
http://www.med.uth.tmc.edu/

University of Texas Southwestern Medical School (Dallas)
http://www.swmed.edu/home_pages/publish/sms_catalog/1smscat.html

Utah

University of Utah School of Medicine (Salt Lake City)
http://www.som.med.utah.edu/

Vermont

The University of Vermont College of Medicine (Burlington)
http://salus.med.uvm.edu/

Virginia

Eastern Virginia Medical School (Norfolk)
http://www.evms.edu/

School of Medicine, Medical College of Virginia/Virginia Commonwealth University (Richmond)
http://views.vcu.edu/html/schofmed.html

University of Virginia Health Sciences Center (Charlottesville)
http://www.med.virginia.edu/schools/medschl.html

Washington

University of Washington School of Medicine (Seattle)
http://www.washington.edu/medical/som/index.html

West Virginia

Marshall University School of Medicine (Huntington)
http://hopkins.med.jhu.edu/

West Virginia University School of Medicine (Morgantown)
http://www.hsc.wvu.edu/som/

Wisconsin

Medical College of Wisconsin (Milwaukee)
http://www.mcw.edu/

The University of Wisconsin Medical School (Madison)
http://www.biostat.wisc.edu/

Canadian Medical Schools

Alberta

University of Alberta Medicine and Oral Health Sciences (Edmonton)
http://www.med.ualberta.ca/

University of Calgary Faculty of Medicine (Calgary)
http://www.ucalgary.ca/UofC/faculties/Medicine/

British Columbia

University of British Columbia Faculty of Medicine (Vancouver)
http://www.med.ubc.ca/home.html

Manitoba

University of Manitoba Faculty of Medicine (Winnepeg)
http://www.umanitoba.ca/home/banner.html

Newfoundland

Memorial University of Newfoundland Faculty of Medicine (St. John's)

http://aorta.library.mun.ca/med/

Nova Scotia

Dalhousie University Medical School (Halifax)

http://www.mcms.dal.ca/index.html

Ontario

McMaster University Faculty of Health Sciences (Hamilton)

http://www-fhs.mcmaster.ca/

Queen's University at Kingston, Faculty of Medicine (Kingston)

http://meds-ss10.meds.queensu.ca/medicine/

University of Ottowa Faculty of Medicine (Ottawa)

http://www.uottawa.ca/academic/med/

University of Toronto Faculty of Medicine (Toronto)

http://utl1.library.utoronto.ca/www/medicine/index.htm

University of Western Ontario Faculty of Medicine (London)

http://www.med.uwo.ca/

Quebec

McGill University Faculty of Medicine (Montreal)

http://www.med.mcgill.ca/

Universite Laval Faculty of Medicine (Ste-Foy)
http://www.fmed.ulaval.ca/fmed/fmed.html

University of Montreal Faculty of Medicine (Montreal)
http://medes3.med.umontreal.ca/

University of Sherbrooke Faculty of Medicine (Sherbrooke)
http://www.usherb.ca/Programmes/fmed.htm

Saskatchewan

University of Saskatchewan College of Medicine (Saskatoon)
http://www.usask.ca/medicine/index.html

Medical Schools: Lists

Accredited Medical Schools of the U.S. and Canada
http://www.aamc.org/meded/medschls/start.html
> Compiled by the Association of American Medical Colleges.

Medical Schools
http://www.collegenet.com/geograph/medical.html
> Lists medical schools with addresses, enrollment, tuition and, when available, internet links.

Medical Schools and Medical Centers
http://cause-www.colorado.edu/member-dir/carnegie/med_institutions.html

Peterson's Guide to Medical Schools (Allopathic Medicine)
http://www.petersons.com/graduate/select/633005se.html

Tore B. Sjoboden's Medical School Links!
http://www.anat.dote.hu/~tore/medfak/
> Links to international and U.S. schools of medicine.

United States and Canada Medical Schools

http://www.mc.vanderbilt.edu/~aubrey/medstu/medical_schools.html

Vanderbilt University List of U.S. and Canadian Medical Schools

http://www.mc.vanderbilt.edu/~aubrey/medstu/medical_schools.html

Yahoo's List of Medical Schools

http://www.yahoo.com/health/medicine/medical_schools/

General Medical Education Information

ChronoNet

http://www.he.net/~chronow1/

"The Electronic Voice of the Medical Student and Applicant." Includes information on getting into medical school, an online medical bookstore, the Hippocratic Oath, and a forum for discussion.

Harvard Medical Web

http://www.med.harvard.edu/

List of links to medical institutions.

Interactive Medical Student Lounge

http://www.geocities.com/Heartland/1756/lounge.html

Lots of resources for medical and pre-medical students.

Johns Hopkins Medical Institutions Information

http://infonet.welch.jhu.edu/

Includes the School of Medicine, School of Hygiene, School of Nursing, and the Bayview Medical Center at Johns Hopkins.

Loyola University Medical Education Network

http://www.meddean.luc.edu/lumen/

Mature Medical Student

http://falcon.cc.ukans.edu:80/~cwpowell/

One individual's story of attending medical school at an older age.

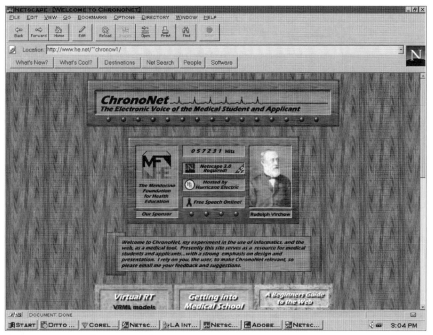

ChronoNet. *http://www.he.net/~chronow1/*

MEdIC: Medical Education Information Center

http://dpalm2.med.uth.tmc.edu/home.htm

Information for professionals and consumers.

Medical Education Page

http://www.scomm.net:80/~greg/med-ed/

Links to medical schools, news sources, frequently asked questions (FAQs), ftp sites and medical indexes.

Medical Education Software Homepage

http://www.webcom.com/~wooming/mededuc.html

Compilation of reviews of medical education software.

Medical Schools, Libraries and Catalogs

http://www.med.sc.edu/MEDLIB.HTM

Maintained by the University of South Carolina School of Medicine.

MedSearch: Healthcare Careers

http://www.medsearch.com/

Online job postings for those in search of or recruiting for health care positions.

Miscellaneous Medical Education Page

http://www.fcm.missouri.edu/medical/mismed.htm

Lots of valuable links to discussion groups, indexes, tools, and more for medical school and pre-medical school students.

Pre-Medical School

Alpha Epsilon Delta Pre-Medical Honor Society

http://jhunix.hcf.jhu.edu/~scheel/aed/aed.html

American Medical College Application Service

http://www.aamc.org/stuapps/admiss/amcas/start.htm

Find-O-Rama

http://www.review.com/medical/find/med_schools_search.html

Princeton Review Online's medical school search engine. Enter your specific criteria and receive statistics and a description of schools which may fit your profile.

Premed Engine P.A.G.E.

http://premed.imagiware.com/

P.A.G.E. = Premed Advisor Goes Electronic.

WWW Med School Lists

http://premed.edu/medschls.html

Helpful information and support for pre-medical school students.

Residency

Family Practice Residency Program Web Guide

http://www.geocities.com/CapeCanaveral/Lab/1775/fp.htm

Residency Page

http://www.webcom.com/~wooming/residenc.html

A list of medical residencies available on the web. Select specialty.

ResidentNet

http://www.residentnet.com/

Surgical resident's home page.

MEN'S HEALTH

Circumcision

Circumcision Information and Resource Pages
http://www.cirp.org/CIRP/
> Technical, medical and patient material on circumcision.

Circumcision Issues
http://www.eskimo.com/%7egburlin/circ.html

Fertility
See also: Sexual & Reproductive Health - Fertility.

Ask NOAH about: Vasectomy
http://www.noah.cuny.edu/wellconn/vasectomy.html
> Good information and responses to important questions about vasectomies.

How to Enhance Your Fertility
http://www.coolware.com/health/joel/malefertility.html
> Information and advice for men.

Male Infertility Factor
http://www.ivf.com/male.html

Patient's Guide to Vasectomy Reversal
http://cait.cpmc.columbia.edu/dept/urology/vasr0000.html

Planned Parenthood: All About Vasectomy

http://www.igc.apc.org/ppfa/vasecpub.html

General Topics

Cosmetic Surgery for Men

http://www.phudson.com/male.html

EZ Connect: Men's Health Links

http://ezconnect.web.aol.com/mensh.htm

Fathering Magazine

http://www.fathermag.com/

This magazine includes mental and physical health topics.

Gay Men's Health Crisis

http://www.thebody.com/gmhc/gmhcpage.html

Home Page for this AIDS advocacy and support group.

Healthtouch: Men's Health

http://www.healthtouch.com/level1/leaflets/101529/101529.htm

Includes information for men on nutrition, abuse, sexually transmitted diseases, cancer and prostate problems.

Male Health Center Internet Education Site

http://www.malehealthcenter.com/

Information for men on exercise, erections, and guidelines regarding regular physical examinations.

Man's Life

http://www.manslife.com/

Health and fitness articles for men, along with other columns and news slanted to men's interests.

Medic: Men's Health Issues

http://medic.med.uth.tmc.edu/ptnt/00000391.htm

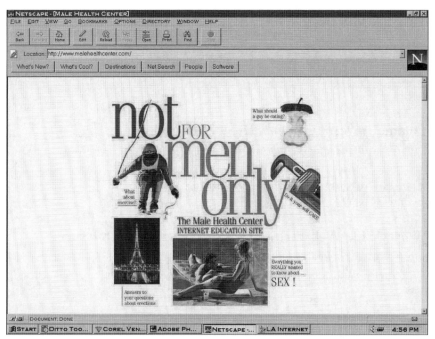

The Male Health Center. http://www.malehealthcenter.com/

Men's Fitness

http://www.mensfitness.com/

Online journal covering fitness, nutrition, health and sex, for men.

Men's Health Consulting

http://www.menshealth.org/

Site's mission is to promote better health in men by offering services that help them to understand and address how ideals of masculinity can damage their health.

Men's Health Index

http://menshealth.com/mens_index.html

Online magazine.

Men's Health Issues

http://h-devil-www.mc.duke.edu/h-devil/men/men.htm

Topics covered include erectile dysfunction, premature ejaculation, testicular self-examination, and urinary tract infections.

Men's Health Section

http://www.doctors-10tv.com/alt/men/men.htm

This section of the Doctor's Hospital Home Page addresses concerns about prostate cancer and treatment, impotence, testicular cancer, vasectomy and hair loss.

Tulane University: Men's Health Issues

http://www.tulane.edu/~health/text/mhi.html

Urologic and Male Genital Diseases

http://www.mic.ki.se/Diseases/c12.html

World Wide Web Virtual Library: Men's Health Issues

http://www.vix.com/pub/men/health/health.html

Articles, studies and links to issues related to men's physical and mental health.

Gynecomastia

Gynecomastia

http://www.surgery.uiowa.edu/surgery/plastic/gyneco.html

Information on male breast enlargement.

Gynecomastia - Correction of Enlarged Male Breasts

http://www.plasticsurgery.org/surgery/gyne.htm

Hair Loss

See also: Skin & Connective Tissue/Dermatology - Hair Loss.

Bald Is Beautiful

http://www.thoughtport.com/budobear/

Bald Man's Home Page

http://www.thebaldman.com/

Includes the Bald Man's Live Hair Chat Room, The Baldman's Forum ("ask a doctor"), research and articles, horror stories, jokes and commercial products.

Regrowth! *http://www.regrowth.com/*

Bosley Medical Institute

http://www.bosley.com/

This site allows you to click on the baldness pattern similar to your own to find out about hair restoration options. Learn about the history of coping with hair loss, how to choose the best option for you, and how to find a good doctor.

Hair Today

http://www.hairtoday.com/

Hairloss Information Center

http://hairloss.com/index.htm

Includes free evaluation and pamphlets, and consumer information about hair loss.

International Hair Transplant Center

http://www.ispace.com/hair/

More information about the medical restoration of hair.

Male Pattern Baldness FAQ

http://www2.xstar.com/html/mpbfaq.htm

Regrowth!

http://www.regrowth.com/

Hair loss headlines, frequently asked questions (FAQs), discussion group and mailing list.

Impotence

Impotence Information Center

http://www.medic-drug.com/impotence/impotence.html

A lot of information on impotence.

Impotence: It's Reversible

http://www.cei.net/~impotenc/

Basic but reassuring information.

Impotence Resource Center

http://www.impotence.org/

This site is for both patients and medical professionals provides information and basic facts on the causes and treatment of impotence. A women's perspective is offered and participation in an online survey is invited.

On-Line Guide to Impotence

http://www2.impotent.com/caverject/caverject/guide.html

Successfully Treating Impotence

http://www2.impotent.com/caverject/

Facts, myths, and frequently asked questions (FAQs) about impotence. Information on prescription drugs, and a physician referral service.

Penile Surgery

Penile Lengthening and Enlargement Surgery Center for Men

http://www.2020tech.com/mensurg/

Penis Enlargement Surgery

http://www.SURGEON.org/penis.htm

Information and referrals about penile lengthening and augmentation. Includes size statistics and art gallery.

Reed Centre for Ambulatory Urological Surgery

http://www.webcom.com/reed/

Includes penile enlargement, penile prosthetic implants, vasectomy, vasectomy reversal, circumcision, male breast reduction, and Peyronie's disease information.

Prostate Cancer

Articles on Prostate Cancer

http://www.cancer.med.umich.edu/prostcan/articles.html

Articles on prostate cancer from medical journals and other sources.

CaP CURE

http://www.capcure.org/Welcome.htm

The Association for the Cure of Cancer of the Prostate.

My Prostate and Me: Dealing with Prostate Cancer

http://pmadt.com/prostate/

Introduction to and overview of a book of the same name by William Martin. Includes information on how to order the book, and links to related sites.

OncoLink's Basic Information on Prostate Cancer

http://oncolink.upenn.edu/disease/prostate/index.htm

News, reports and links to sites addressing prostate cancer.

Prostate Cancer

http://www.cancer.org/prostate/prmenu.html

General prostate cancer information from the American Cancer Society. Includes the "Man to Man Prostate Cancer Education and Support Program" which offers group education, one-on-one visitation and telephone support, a quarterly newsletter and free patient education information.

Prostate Cancer Fact Sheet

http://www.cancer.org/prostate.html

Fact sheet on prostate cancer from the American Cancer Society.

Prostate Cancer Health Zone

http://www.prostate-cancer.com/

Information for patients and families about prostate cancer treatment options, stages, recovery, support groups and a glossary of terms. In addition, professional resources and information are provided.

Prostate Cancer InfoLink

http://www.comed.com/Prostate/index.html

Site provides information and support for men with prostate cancer.

"Real Men Cook" to Fight Prostate Cancer

http://www.cinenet.net/~prostate/awareness/

This is the site for a non-profit educational and support organization whose goal is to fight prostate cancer and promote early detection. Find information about the organization, prostate cancer, prevention guidelines and further links.

Prostate Health

Anatomical Radical Retropubic Prostatectomy

http://prostate.urol.jhu.edu/surgery/surg/

Educational brochure and audiovisual presentation for surgeons. Detailed anatomical drawings provided.

Center for Men's Health: Prostate Disease and Sexual Dysfunction

http://www1.drive.net/_allhealth/pages/mens-center.htm

Male Health Centres

http://www.malehealth.com/

Information on erectile dysfunction and prostate disease.

Prostate Dictionary

http://www.comed.com/Prostate/Glossary.html

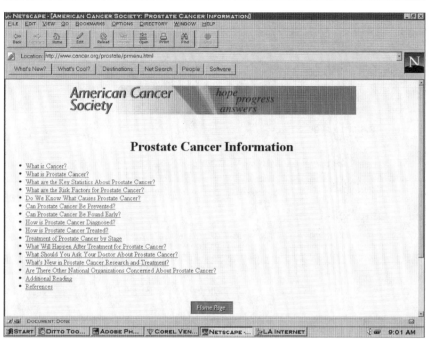

American Cancer Society Prostate Cancer Information.
http://www.cancer.org/prostate/prmenu.html

Prostate Pointer

http://rattler.cameron.edu/Prostate/

Prostatitis Home Page

http://www.msn.fullfeed.com/~prosfnd/

Home page for the Prostatitis Foundation. Provides clinical and patient information on treatment and research, as well as links, pointers, and information about a prostate e-mail list.

Prostatitis Home Page

http://www.prostate.org/

Testicular Cancer

Testicular Cancer

http://www.noah.cuny.edu/cancer/nci/cancernet/201/21.html

Information intended for physicians, but of interest to anybody concerned about testicular cancer.

Testicular Cancer Resource Center

http://www.acor.org/diseases/TC/

Testicular Self-Exam

http://h-devil-www.mc.duke.edu/h-devil/men/tse.htm

Mental health

Anxiety

Anxiety Disorders Association of America
http://www.adaa.org/

Attacking Anxiety
http://www.sover.net/~schwcof/
   Video documentary, booklets, newsletters and pamphlets about overcoming anxiety. Also deals with post-traumatic stress disorder and the "false traumatic memory" controversy.

Basic Guidelines for Coping with Stress and Anxiety
http://www.net-dot-com.com/midwest/stress.htm/

Center for Anxiety and Stress Treatment
http://www.stressrelease.com/
   Books and audio tapes, anxiety symptom checklist and stress busters.

CyberPsych: Anxiety Disorders on the Internet
http://www.cyberpsych.org/anxiety.htm

Managing Your Anxiety
http://www.vh.org/Patients/IHB/FamilyPractice/AFP/December/DecFour.html
   Symptoms, tips and bibliography.

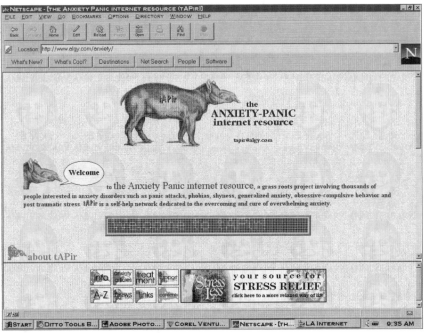

tAPir. http://www.algy.com/anxiety/

Meditation/Relaxation Exercises

http://members.tripod.com/~Aquamoon/medit.html

National Panic/Anxiety Disorder Newsletter

http://206.13.127.230/NPADNews/

Noodles' Panic-Anxiety Page

http://www.algy.com/anxiety/anxiety.html

Online Screening for Anxiety Test

http://www.med.nyu.edu/Psych/screens/anx.html

Professional Life Stress Scale

http://www.hcc.hawaii.edu/hccinfo/facdev/StressTest.html
　　Take a test measuring the amount of stress in your life.

Progressive Relaxation or Jacobsen's Technique

http://23.maine.com/pictureyourself/progress.htm

Stress Education Center
http://www.dstress.com/

Articles and other publications about stress and stress management; links, seminar registration, and products such as audio tapes.

tAPir: The Anxiety Panic Internet Resource
http://www.algy.com/anxiety/

Treatment of Panic Disorder
http://text.nlm.nih.gov/nih/cdc/www/85txt.html

Text of Treatment of Panic Disorder Statement issued by the 1991 National Institutes of Health Consensus Development Conference.

Counseling/Therapy

Finding Help: How to Choose a Psychologist
http://www.apa.org/pubinfo/howto.html

The American Psychological Association discusses when you should consider psychotherapy, what you should look for in a therapist, what questions to ask, and related issues.

Marriage Builders
http://www.marriagebuilders.com/

Therapy FAQ
http://abulafia.st.hmc.edu/~mmiles/faq.html

Written for people who may be interested in trying out psychotherapy.

Depression

Clinical Depression Screening Test
http://sandbox.xerox.com/pair/cw/testing.html

Depression and Mental Health Links
http://drycas.club.cc.cmu.edu/~maine/depress.html

Depression and Mental Health Sources on the Internet
http://stripe.Colorado.EDU/~judy/depression/

Depression FAQ

http://avocado.pc.helsinki.fi/~janne/asdfaq/index.html

This "Depression Primer" includes causes, treatment and resources.

Depression Home Page - Index

http://greed.isca.uiowa.edu/users/david-caropreso/depression.html

User groups, educational, commercial and miscellaneous sites related to depression.

Depression: Uni/Bipolar Disorders Page

http://www.duke.edu/~ntd/depression.html

Many links and lots of information on major depression.

Documents Concerning Depression

http://www.blarg.net/~charlatn/Depression.html

Dr. Ivan's Depression Central

http://www.psycom.net/depression.central.html

Clearinghouse for information on depression and other mood disorders, divided helpfully by topic. Includes an area with a large introduction to depression, especially how it is defined, how it is treated and frequently asked questions (FAQs). Links to material on depression in Spanish is also provided, as well as a special section devoted to women and depression.

Internet Depression Resources List

http://www.execpc.com/%7Ecorbeau/

Melatonin and Seasonal Affective Disorder

http://members.aol.com/mindbend2/index.htm

Online Depression Screening Test

http://www.med.nyu.edu/Psych/screens/depres.html

Serotonin: The Neurotransmitter for the 90's

http://www.fairlite.com/ocd/articles/ser90.shtml

Women (and Girls) and Depression

http://members.aol.com/depress/womendep.htm

Emotional Support

Emotional Support Guide
http://asa.ugl.lib.umich.edu/chdocs/support/emotion.html

Links to support resources on the internet for those experiencing physical loss, bereavement or chronic illness, as well as for their families and caregivers.

Emotional Support on the Internet
http://www.cis.ohio-state.edu/hypertext/faq/usenet/support/emotional/resources-list/faq.html

Bi-monthly posting of different resources with addresses and instructions on how to reach them or post a listing. Everything from newsgroups addressing abuse issues to listservers relating to gay parenting. Links to suicide prevention and intervention counseling.

False Memory Syndrome

False Memory Syndrome Foundation
http://iquest.com/~fitz/fmsf/

FAQ about False Memory Syndrome
http://www.csicop.org/~fitz/fmsf/faq.html

General Topics

American Academy of Child and Adolescent Psychiatry
http://www.aacap.org/web/aacap/

This site includes fact sheets to help children and their families and is available in English, Spanish and French. Includes issues such as adoption, bedwetting, abuse, divorce, TV violence, grief, medications, and suicide. Also covers the Academy's activities and publications, legislative and clinical updates, practice guidelines and research.

Community Access Information Resource Network
http://www.cairn.org/

A non-profit agency that provides funding and advocacy for people with psychiatric disabilities.

Dr. Bob's Mental Health Links

http://uhs.bsd.uchicago.edu/~bhsiung/mental.html

Also known as "Dr. Bob's Virtual En-psych-lopedia," this site contains psycho-pharmacology and prescription tips, web links on mental health, and a limitless number of related organizations, academic sites, publications, hardware and software.

Dream Central's Dream Analysis Pages

http://www.sleeps.org/analysis.html

Basics of dream analysis, interpretation and dream dictionary of symbols.

Drugs for Treating Mental Health

http://pharminfo.com/disease/mental_db.html#drgs

Internet Mental Health

http://www.mentalhealth.com/

An encyclopedia of mental health information. Look up disorders and medications, and find links to magazines, software demos, and other mental health sites.

Internet Mental Health Resources

http://fiona.umsmed.edu/~sturges/stock.html

Broken down by category, this site includes an area on the psychological effects of AIDS, as well as issues of abuse-recovery, autism, cults, depression, hypnosis, mood disorders, men's issues, schizophrenia, suicide and more.

Madness

http://www.io.org/madness/

A web site of internet resources and information about the Madness Mailing List, which is an online discussion group where users of mental health services join in dialogues about how to improve community service systems. To subscribe, send e-mail to: LISTSERV@sjuvm.stjohns.edu and in the body, type "SUBSCRIBE MADNESS Yourfirstname Yourlastname." Or, to obtain a list of internet resources, for people who experience mood swings, fear, or hear voices or see visions, in the body of the e-mail type: GET MADNESS PSYCHRC.

Madness.
http://www.io.org/
~madness/

Mental Health Education Page

http://www.metrolink.net/~jquimby/mh.htm

Dedicated to removing the stigma of mental illness. Includes cyber-psychotherapy survey for mental health professionals and consumers, information on where to go for help online, a description of the therapeutic process, real accounts of therapy and additional links.

Mental Health Information

http://www.mhsource.com/

Search engine for mental health issues on the internet. Also includes regular columns, chat rooms, mail lists, and links to patient advocacy groups, information on different mental disorders, and a professional directory.

Mental Health Net

http://www.cmhc.com/

Over 4,200 mental health resources covering depression, anxiety, panic attacks, chronic fatigue syndrome and substance abuse. Professional resources in psychology, psychiatry and social work, including journals and online magazines. Search engine provided.

National Institute of Mental Health

http://www.minh.nih.gov/

Offers public information on specific mental disorders, a report titled "Mental Illness in America," educational programs on depression and panic disorder, as well as information for scientists on grants and research activities, news and events.

National Mental Health Services Knowledge Exchange Network (KEN)

http://www.mentalhealth.org/

Information about mental health resources. Prevention, treatment and rehabilitation services for mental illness offered. Lots of information about the children's campaign, online databases, emergency services, events and statistics.

Psych Central

http://www.coil.com/~grohol/

Maintained by Dr. John Grohol, Psych Central strives to be a one-stop index for psychology, support and mental health issues, resources, and people on the internet. Features newsgroups, mailing lists, web sites, books, articles, surveys, and checklists, as well as a Suicide Helpline. Good place to browse or start to search for support groups, newsgroups and mailing lists on mental disorders.

Psychology Around the World
http://sage.und.nodak.edu/org/BAT/psyches.html
Long alphabetical list of academic and organizational mental health sites.

Psychology in Daily Life
http://www.apa.org/pubinfo/
Several online brochures on mental health issues: abuse, sexual harassment, anger control, violence, sexual orientation, depression and panic attacks.

Self-Injury: You are Not the Only One
http://www.palace.net/~llama/psych/injury.html

Shyness Home Page: An Index to Resources
http://www.shyness.com/

Specifica
http://www.realtime.net/~mmjw/
Find a lot of mental health information links sorted by the broad categories of General Mental Health, Specific Problem Areas, and General Information for Professionals. The site doesn't confuse browsers by listing all of the resources available, but suggests one or two carefully selected sites.

Substance Abuse and Mental Health Services Administration
http://www.samhsa.gov/

Grief and Bereavement
See also: Death & Dying - Grief and Bereavement.

Bereavement Self-Help Resources Guide
http://www.inforamp.net/%5Ebfo/d_2800.html

Emotional Support Guide
http://asa.ugl.lib.umich.edu/chdocs/support/emotion.html
Links to support resources on the internet for those experiencing physical loss, chronic illness and bereavement, as well as for their families and caregivers.

Sands (Vic)

http://www.vicnet.net.au/~sands/sands.htm

A support group for parents who have experienced miscarriage, stillbirth, or neonatal death.

Homelessness and Mental Illness

Mental Illness and Homelessness

http://nch.ari.net/mental.html

Fact sheets on mental health issues related to homelessness and other information. From the National Coalition for the Homeless.

Mood Disorders

Bipolar Disorder

http://www.frii.com/~parrot/bip.html

Good information.

Bipolar Disorder: The Artist Formerly Known as Manic Depression

http://www.i1.net/~juli/bipolar.html

A lot of information about creativity and its relation to bipolar disorder. Includes medical links and more.

Bipolar Planet

http://www.tcnj.edu/~ellisles/BipolarPlanet/

Llama Central

http://crystal.palace.net/~llama/

Depression, self-injury, Prozac and related topics are addressed with honesty. Also find poetry and other forms of creative expression. An attractive site.

Mood Disorders

http://avocado.pc.helsinki.fi/~janne/mood/mood.html

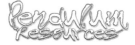

The Pendulum Pages.
http://www.pendulum.org/

Moodswing.Org

http://moodswing.org/

    Online resources for people with bipolar disorder. Includes advocacy groups, frequently asked questions (FAQs), books, support groups, and internet links.

Pendulum Pages

http://www.pendulum.org/

    Site offers information and support for bipolar (manic-depression) and other mood disorders. Articles, books, support groups, alternative therapies, discussion area, mailing list, medication, links and humor.

Walkers in Darkness

http://www.primenet.com/~jtp/walkers.html

    This is a support list for depression, bipolar disorder and related mental illnesses. To subscribe, send e-mail to: majordomo@world.std.com and type "subscribe walkers" in the body.

Wings of Madness

http://users.aol.com/depress/index.htm

    This page discusses clinical uni- and bipolar depression, as opposed to "feeling down." An attractive site.

Obsessive Compulsive Disorder

Obsessive Compulsive Anonymous

http://members.aol.com/west24th/index.html

Obsessive Compulsive Disorder

http://www.fairlite.com/ocd/

    Contains a bulletin board, abstracts, articles, information on medications, and links to mental health sites related to obsessive compulsive disorder. Includes advice on how to deal with OCD, personal accounts, and web links.

Obsessive-Compulsive Disorder

http://www.psyc.memphis.edu/students/abramowitz/ocd.htm

General description and bibliography for self-help and for professionals.

Obsessive Compulsive Disorder Resource Center

http://www.ocdresource.com/

Introduction to the causes, symptoms and treatment of obsessive compulsive disorder (OCD); OCD resources.

Obsessive-Compulsive Foundation

http://pages.prodigy.com/alwillen/ocf.html

Visit this site to discover what obsessive compulsive disorder (OCD) is, support groups, events, newsletters and publications, book reviews and Foundation information.

Organizations

National Mental Health Association

http://www.nmha.org/

The NMHA is a citizen volunteer advocacy organization dedicated to improving the mental health of all. This site has news about NMHA activities, advocacy efforts (including public policy and legislative alerts), community outreach and prevention issues. Jumplist includes a good description of helpful web sites to visit. Direct e-mail links to the President, Vice President, Senate, House of Representatives, and First Lady.

PsychNET

http://www.apa.org/

The American Psychological Association page for members and the public includes information for the general public, media, and updates in public policy issues. Also available is the *APA Monitor Online*, practice and educational information, books and databases.

World Federation of Mental Health

http://ssw.ab.umd.edu/wfmh.html

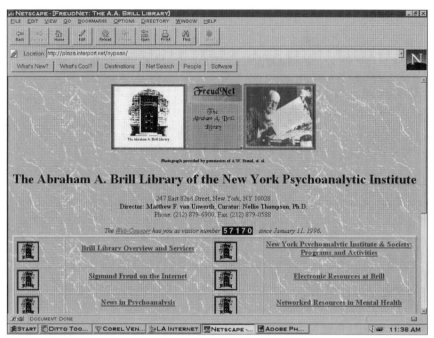

The Brill Library. *http://plaza.interport.net/nypsan/*

Personality Disorders

Alt.Support.Dissociation FAQ
http://www.tezcat.com/~tina/asd.html

Astraea's Unorthodox Multiple Personality Resources
http://www.asarian.org/~astraea/household/

Avoidant Personality Disorder
http://www.mentalhealth.com/dis/p20-pe08.html

Borderline Personality Disorder Information
http://www-leland.stanford.edu/~corelli/borderline.html
    Description, symptoms, etiology, and treatment.

BPD Central
http://members.aol.com/BPDCentral/Index.html

BPD Experiences

http://members.aol.com/BPDCentral/bpdexp.html

Dissociation and Beyond

http://www.netrail.net/~swiggins/alterego.html

Dissociation Resources, Mental Health Links, and Other Fun Stuff

http://www.suba.com/~wheezer/resource.html

Divided Hearts: DID/MPD Info and Support

http://www.dhearts.org/

Essential Information on Trauma and Dissociation

http://www.mcs.net:80/~kathyw/trauma.html

Firewheel Vortex

http://www.geocities.com/SoHo/Lofts/6140/vortex.htm

Addresses multiple personality disorder and dissociative identity disorder. It uses the "multiple" metaphor by providing links to all kinds of interesting, scary, weird, funny and useful information, to give an idea of what being a multiple is like. Includes information and links with MPD/DID and abuse recovery sites.

Frequently Asked Questions about Dissociative Disorder

http://www.tezcat.com/~tina/asd/asd-faq1.htm#

Information on Dissociation

http://www.tezcat.com/~tina/dissoc.shmtl

International Society for the Study of Dissociation

http://www.issd.org/

Kaleidoscope

http://www.geocities.com/SoHo/Lofts/1488/kaleid.html

Laura's Home Page

http://huizen.dds.nl/%7Elaura_d/

Personal account and theories about Borderline Personality Disorder.

MPD/DID FAQ
http://netdesigns2000.com/mpd/faqmpd.html

Mr. Kohen's Abnormal Psychology Project
http://www.chs.chico.k12.ca.us/Staff/kohencla.htm

Multiple Personality Disorder and Dissociation Resources
http://www.vuw.ac.nz/~anita/dissociation.html

Online Screening for Personality Disorders
http://www.med.nyu.edu/Psych/screens/pds.html

Overview of Dialectical Behaviour Therapy in the Treatment of Borderline Personality Disorder
http://www.cityscape.co.uk/users/ad88/dbt1.htm

This site describes the methodology behind this therapeutic method of treating personality disorder.

Paranoid Conditions: A Guide for Families
http://www.mentalhealth.com/book/p42-gpar.html

Personality and Personality Disorders
http://www.geocities.com/HotSprings/2836/paper1.html

Personal account and numerous links.

Spectrum of Dissociative Disorders: An Overview of Diagnosis and Treatment
http://www.voiceofwomen.com/centerarticle.html

When Someone You Love Is a Multiple
http://www.freenet.edmorton.ab.ca/~spratz/mpd.htm

Psychiatry/Psychology

American Psychoanalytic Association
http://apsa.org/index.htm/

Professional organization of psychoanalysts. Offers information describing psychoanalysis, and information for members about organization activities, meetings and programs. Literature search, newsletter, journal information and access are provided, along with list of additional related links.

Keirsey Temperament Sorter
http://sunsite.unc.edu/personality/keirsey.html

Take an online personality test that sorts results according to the Myers-Briggs method.

Online Psychiatric Tests
http://www.med.nyu.edu/Psych/public.html

PSALMS
http://www.az.com/~bipolar/PSALMS.html

The Psychiatric Survivors Advocacy/Liberation Movement.

Psych Web
http://www.gasou.edu/psychweb/

Psychology-related information for students and teachers of psychology. Includes a browsable web version of Freud's *The Interpretation of Dreams*, as well as other books, brochures and articles; commercial sites, journal links, discussion groups for students and a psychology quiz. Many links to further resources, broken down by topic.

Psychiatry and the Law
http://ua1vm.ua.edu/~jhooper/index.html

Psychiatry and Psychotherapy
http://www-leland.stanford.edu/~corelli/

PsycINFO
http://www.apa.org/psycinfo/

Information service on psychology issues.

Shoshanna's Psychiatric Survivor's Guide

http://www.harborside.com/home/e/equinox/

Psychoanalysis

American Psychoanalytic Foundation

http://www.cyberpsych.org/apf.htm

This no-nonsense site describes the mission and programs of the APF, provides links to organizations and publications on the internet, and offers a listing of all its members as well as a literature search engine.

Brill Library of the New York Psychoanalytic Institute

http://plaza/interport.net/nypsan/

Also known as "Freudnet," this site describes the program and activities of the Institute, as well as provides access to its library, which consists of over 40,000 books, articles and reprints dealing with psychoanalysis and related fields. Contains the Freud Archives, a collection of internet resources related to Sigmund Freud's life and works.

Sigmund Freud - Father of Psychoanalysis

http://www.austria-info.at/personen/freud/index.html

Includes a brief biography of Freud, a description of the significance of his work and some of the influence he had on contemporary theory. Site is maintained by the Austrian National Tourist Office.

Publications

Medscape's Mental Health

http://www.medscape.com/Medscape/MentalHealth/public/journal.MH.html

Peer-reviewed, clinical journal on the diagnosis and treatment of mental illness.

Psychiatry On-Line

http://www.cityscape.co.uk/users/ad88/psych.htm

From the *International Journal of Psychiatry*. This site presents the latest journal articles, papers, and news. Also provides forensic psychiatry online, child and adolescent psychiatry online and transcultural mental health online. Information on other World Wide Web psychiatry resources is provided.

Schizophrenia

Schizophrenia
http://www.psy.med.rug.nl/0012/

The Department of Psychiatry at the University of Groningen's site on schizophrenia.

Schizophrenia Digest
http://www.vaxxine.com/schizophrenia/

Schizophrenia Home Page
http://www.schizophrenia.com/

Resource and education center for schizophrenia. Includes current news and events, newsletter, online discussion groups, information for individuals with schizophrenia, their friends and family, professional health care providers and the general public. General information, causes, coping, recovery stories, physical disturbances, diagnosis, types, medications, family issues, denial, legal issues, homelessness, managed care, recommended resources, volunteer opportunities, journals, and additional internet links.

Schizophrenia in Children
http://www.psych.med.umich.edu/web/aacap/

Schizophrenia Newsletter
http://www.schizophrenia.com/help/NewsL2.html

Weekly e-mail on schizophrenia. To subscribe, send e-mail to: brianc@infomaniac.com and include your e-mail address in the body of the message.

Schizophrenia Pages
http://www.mentalhealth.com/dis/p20-ps01.htm

Internet Mental Health's schizophrenia pages.

Schizophrenia: Questions and Answers
http://www.psy.med.rug.nl/0031/

Schizophrenia Treatment Research

http://199.45.66.207/dis-rs2/p25-ps0.html

Abstracts of recent research on schizophrenia.

VA-Yale Schizophrenia Biological Research Center

http://www.yale.edu/vayale/

Self-Help and Support Groups

National Mental Health Consumer's Self-Help Clearinghouse

http://www.libertynet.org/~mha/cl_house.html/

All about the electronic mailing list discussing consumer's self-help movement and related issues. To subscribe, send e-mail to: majordomo@philadelphia.libertynet.org and in the body type: "subscribe thekey Yourname." This site also provides public policy alerts, recent journal articles, and related web links.

Psychology Self-Help Resources on the Internet

http://www.gasou.edu/psychweb/resource/selfhelp.htm

Links to non-commercial sites providing information and help about specific disorders related to psychology.

Self-Help and Psychology Magazine

http://cybertowers.com/selfhelp/

Offers numerous "zones" to reflect on, learn about, discuss and investigate self-help and psychology issues. Written by mental health professionals for the discussion of general psychology as applied to everyday life. Articles, news, reviews, books, professional resources and links.

Starting a New Online Support Group

http://www.coil.com/~grohol/howto.htm

This site is a friendly and informative "how-to" about starting a new online support group. It provides examples and a step-by-step guide. First, make sure there isn't a group out there already; next, decide what format is best (mailing list, newsgroup); and then follow instructions on how to create it.

Suicide

Archives of Suicide Research

http://www.priory.com/journals/kluwer.htm
Online journal.

Canadian Association for Suicide Prevention

http://idirect.com/~casp/tmplocx.html/

Samaritans

http://www.mhnet.org/samaritans/
The Samaritans is a volunteer, non-religious group that offers emotional support to suicidal and despairing individuals via e-mail, phone, personal visit and letter. It is confidential, and e-mail may be sent anonymously to: samaritans@anon.twwells.com or directly (not anonymously) to: jo@samaritans.org.

San Francisco Suicide Prevention

http://www.sfsuicide.org/

[Suicide]

http://www.paranoia.com/~real/suicide/
Frequently asked questions (FAQs), resources, facts and prevention, links and internet resources.

Suicide Awareness/Voices of Education

http://www.save.org/
Informative site discussing the link between depression and suicide. Questions and answers, common misconceptions, symptoms of depression, suicide danger signals, how to help friends or yourself, and list of recommended books. Additional text files may be e-mailed to interested individuals.

Suicide Chat IRC

http://www.4-lane.com/supportchat/pages/suicidechat.html
Information about the Internet Relay Chat on suicide.

Suicide - FAQ

http://www.lib.ox.ac.uk/internet/news/faq/archive/suicide.info.html

Suicide Prevention

*http://wonder.cdc.gov/WONDER/static|^SYSTEM=PREVGUID^LEVEL=topics
.htm^URL=tp_00873.htm*

Guidelines from the Centers for Disease Control and Prevention.

Suicide Resources - How to Find Help in a Crisis

http://rtfm.mit.edu/pub/usenet/news.answers/suicide/resources/

Trauma

David Baldwin's Trauma Information Pages

http://gladstone.uoregon.edu/~dub/trauma.htm

Nate's Traumatology Page

http://dolphin.upenn.edu/~prentice/trauma.html

Post Traumatic Stress Resources Web Page

http://www.long-beach.va.gov/ptsd/stress.html

Information and links on post traumatic stress syndrome occurring from any
cause. Includes links for veterans of different military conflicts.

TimePassages - Discussion Forum

http://www.timepassages.com/Intro.html

Trauma Resources

http://gladstone.uoregon.edu/~dvb/pg3.htm

Warning Signs of Trauma-Related Stress

http://www.apa.org/ptsd.html

MUSCLES & MUSCULOSKELETAL DISORDERS

Arthritis

Ah! (Arthritis Help)
http://rheuma.bham.ac.uk/primer.html
> Primer on rheumatic diseases for those with no prior knowledge.

Arthritis and Joint Reconstruction Associates
http://www.intergate.com/~ajira/

Arthritis Information and Resources: Doctor's Guide
http://www.pslgroup.com/ARTHRITIS.HTM
> Medical news and drug information, discussion groups and newsgroups.

Arthritis Source
http://orthop.washington.edu/Bone%20Joint%20Sources/zzzzzzzz5_1.html

Elfstrom's Arthritis and Rheumatology
http://elfstrom.com/arthritis/

Intramural Clinical Studies
http://www.nih.gov/miams/clinic/
> Clinical studies undertaken by the National Institute of Arthritis, Musculoskeletal and Skin Diseases.

Multipurpose Arthritis and Musculoskeletal Disease Center
http://hacuna.ucsd.edu/ra/

National Arthritis Foundation
http://www.arthritis.org/

A great deal of information and links relating to arthritis. Includes advocacy and support organizations, public information and fact sheets, news and research updates as well as access to the medical journal *Arthritis Today*, and a listing of treatment centers.

National Institute of Arthritis and Musculoskeletal and Skin Diseases
http://www.nih.gov/niams/

This site describes the research of this NIH branch, and offers fact sheets, brochures, reports and other information about the many forms of arthritis and diseases of the musculoskeletal system and the skin.

Types of Arthritis
http://204.92.87.170/types/

Carpal Tunnel Syndrome

See also: Repetitive Strain, later in this section.

Carpal Tunnel Syndrome Page
http://www.netaxs.com/%7Eiris/cts/welcome.html

Early Intervention for Carpal Tunnel Syndrome and Repetitive Stress
http://www.tpcorm.com/macmorran/resources.html

Patient's Guide to Carpal Tunnel Syndrome
http://www.sechrest.com/ming/cts/ctsintro.html

Anatomy, diagnosis, treatment and frequently asked questions (FAQs).

True Carpal Tunnel Syndrome
http://concentric.net/~Orthodoc/carpaltunnel.shtml

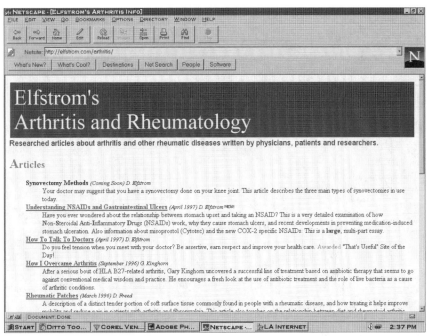

Elfstrom's Arthritis and Rheumatology. http://elfstrom.com/arthritis/

Fibromyalgia

Fibromyalgia Information

http://www.cais.com/cfs-news/fibro.htm

Fibromyalgia Page

http://www.pendulum.org/Fibro/

Writings, information, resources and links about fibromyalgia, a disorder related to depression and chronic fatigue syndrome, but thought to be linked to a sleep disorder.

Fibromyalgia Resources

http://www.hsc.missouri.edu/fibro/fibrotp.html

Maintained by the Missouri Arthritis Rehabilitation Research and Training Center.

Joy's World's Best Sites for Fibromyalgia Survivors
http://home.earthlink.net/~fotojoy/index.html

Information on fibromyalgia, suggestions on what to do if you have just been diagnosed, bibliography and links.

Physician's Guide to Fibromyalgia Syndrome
http://www.hsc.missouri.edu/fibro/fm-md.html

General Topics

CliniWeb: Musculoskeletal Diseases
http://www.ohsu.edu/cliniweb/C5/C5.html

Here, find resources and information on bone and cartilage diseases; fascitis and foot deformities; hand, jaw, joint and muscular diseases; musculoskeletal abnormalities; rheumatic disease; and tennis elbow.

Musculoskeletal Diseases
http://www.mic.ki.se/Diseases/c5.html

This site provides a great number of links, maintained by Sweden's Karolinska Institute.

Knees

Cyberportal
http://www.imparcial.com.mx/orthonet/

Addresses arthroscopy and knee surgery. Available in both English and Spanish.

Patient's Guide to Artificial Knee Replacement
http://www.sechrest.com/mmg/tkr/index.html

Patient's Guide to Knee Problems
http://www.sechrest.com/mmg/knee/knees.html

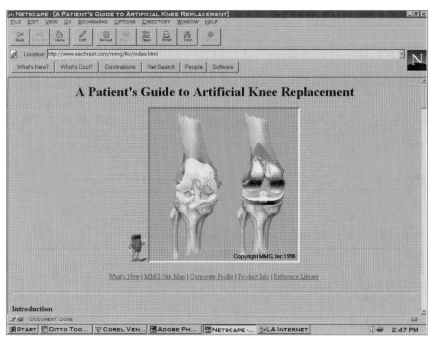

A Patient's Guide to Artificial Knee Replacement.
http://www.sechrest.com/mmg/tkr/index.html

Repetitive Strain Injuries

See also: Carpal Tunnel Syndrome, earlier in this section.

Amara's RSI Page

http://www.amara.com/aboutme/rsi.html

Text of an article that describes repetitive strain injury, what causes it, how to avoid it, and how to treat it.

Computer-Related Repetitive Strain Injury

http://engr-www.unl.edu/ee/eeshop/rsi.html

Site describes what computer-related repetitive strain injury is, how to prevent it and how to treat it. Also offers books and links to related internet sites, and information about products to reduce repetitive strain.

Correct Posture

http://www.mindspring.com:80/~metaguy/

Site describes the correct posture one should have when stationed in front of a computer.

Repetitive Strain Disorders FAQ

http://www.impaccusa.com/impacc9b.html

Repetitive Strain Injuries

http://dragon.acadiau.ca/~rob/rsi/rsi.html

Repetitive Strain Injuries: The Hidden Cost of Computing

http://webreference.com/rsi.html

Repetitive Strain Injury Home Page

http://members.aol.com/tmcrouch/rsi/rsi.htm

Repetitive Stress Injuries Article Series

http://planet-hawaii.com/~billpeay/TECHT08.html

RSI Network Newsletter

To subscribe, send e-mail to: majordomo@world.std.com and in the message type: "subscribe rsi."

Typing Injury FAQ: General Information

http://www.cs.princeton.edu/dwallach/tifaq/general.html

Typing Injuries/Repetitive Stress Injury Archives (Caltech)

http://alumni.caltech.edu/~dank/typing-archive.html

Rheumatology

American College of Rheumatology

http://www.rheumatology.org/

Composed of physicians, health professionals and scientists who are educators, researchers, and advocates of the care of people with arthritis and rheumatic and musculoskeletal diseases.

HealthWeb: Rheumatology

http://www.medlib.inpui.edu/hw/rheuma/home.html

Links to rheumatology resources on the internet.

MedWeb's Rheumatology

http://www.gen.emory.edu/medweb/medweb.rheumatology.html

Like all of MedWeb's indexes, this site offers a well-organized and extensive list of links.

Patient Information: American College of Rheumatology

http://www.rheumatology.org/patient/patient.htm

Shoulder/Spine/Back Problems

Back Be Nimble

http://www.backbenimble.com/

Ergonomics site.

Back - FAQ

http://www.impaccusa.com/impacc9a.html

Common questions about back pain.

Clinical Trials of Cervical Manipulation

http://www.mbnet.mb.ca/~jwiens/research.txt

Patient's Guide to Common Shoulder Problems

http://www.sechrest.com/mmg/shoulder/index.html

Patient's Guide to Low Back Pain

http://www.sechrest.com/mmg/back/backpain.html

Scoliosis

http://www.rad.washington.edu/Books/Approach/scoliosis.html

Spinal Cord Injury Information Network

http://www.sci.rehabm.nab.edu/

Search engine for medical, psycho-social topics and equipment related to spinal cord injuries. Includes SCI organizations, audiovisual materials, magazines, publications, and information about vocational training.

Spinal Manipulation Research Group

http://www.cchs.su.edu.au/Academic/BIO/biomech/smrg/smrg.html

Spine Surgery

http://www.spine-surgery.com/

Includes articles, information and online consultation about spine surgery.

SpineInfo

http://www.hscsyr.edu/~haiy/spine.htm

Links to academic and organizational sites, spine clinics, references and additional materials related to the spine. Contains many links.

Texas Back Institute

http://www.texasback.com/

Site claims that the TBI is the largest spine specialty clinic in the United States.

Syringomyelia

Syringomyelia: Do You Have These Symptoms?

http://wwww.syringo.org/

Symptoms include back pain, headache, weakness, shoulder and/or leg pain, and numbness in the hands. Description and frequently asked questions (FAQs).

Syringomyelia Fact Sheet

http://www.ninds.nih.gov/healinfo/disorder/syringo/syringfs.htm

Syringomyelia occurs when a cyst forms on the spinal cord, eventually destroying the center of the spinal cord and resulting in pain, weakness, and stiffness.

NEUROLOGICAL DISORDERS

Epilepsy

Andrew Patrick's Epilepsy Resources
http://debra.dgbt.doc.ca/~andrew/epilepsy/resources.html

Epilepsy Discussion Forum
http://neuro-www.mgh.harvard.edu/webx?14@^6386@.ee6b6c5

Epilepsy Discussion Group with FAQ
http://www.neuro.wustl.edu/wwwboard/wwwboard.html

Epilepsy Foundation of America
http://www.efa.org/indexf.htm

Includes epilepsy information, research, advocacy and news features. Also includes links, a page for kids with epilepsy and an online journal.

Epilepsy in Young Children
http://www.geocities.com/HotSprings/1000/

Epilepsy Legal Rights/Legal Issues
http://www.efa.org/what/advocacy/legal.html

Epilepsy-List and Epilepsy-Pro Mailing Lists
http://debra.dgbt.doc.ca/~andrew/epilepsy/Epilepsy-Pro/

Discussions about epilepsy and seizure disorders. To subscribe to either list, send e-mail to: listserv@calvin.dgbt.doc.ca. Epilepsy-List is for people living with epilepsy, their friends and family. To subscribe, in body of e-mail, type: "subscribe epilepsy-list Firstname Lastname." Epilepsy-Pro is for health care professionals. To subscribe this list, send e-mail to same address and in body of message type: "subscribe epilepsy-pro Firstname Lastname."

Ketogenic Diet

http://www-leland.stanford.edu/group/ketodiet/ketobinder.html

Information on the high fat/low sugar and low carbohydrate diet that has been used to help control seizures in children with intractable epilepsy. Guidelines for checking if diet is appropriate, and how to follow it.

Mike's Epilepsy Home Page

http://www.sgh.gov.sg/gnr/people/gnrchmh.html

Medical information for epileptics and those interested in the scientific and medical aspects of this disorder. Links.

TBI, ABI and Epilepsy Home Away From Home

http://canddwilson.com/tbi/tpiepil.htm

Washington University Comprehensive Epilepsy Program

http://www.neuro.wustl.edu/epilepsy/

Find information about epilepsy medications and surgery. Connect with epilepsy internet links, publications, support groups and services, and epilepsy discussion groups.

General Topics

Central Nervous System Diseases

http://www.mic.ki.se/Diseases/c10.228.html

Large list of links to articles and web-sites, courtesy of the Karolinska Institute of Sweden.

Fact Sheets: Neurological Conditions

http://www.aan.com/public/fact.html

National Institute of Neurological Disorders and Stroke. http://www.ninds.nih.gov/

National Institute of Neurological Disorders and Stroke
http://www.ninds.nih.gov/

News and neurological health information, including guides to stroke, epilepsy and Parkinson Disease; general interest information on neurological conditions and publications available from the NINDS; clinical alerts and advisories. Part of the National Institutes of Health.

Other Specific Neurological Diseases
http://www.healthouch.com/level1/leaflets/104947/105154.htm

Guillain-Barre Syndrome

Acute Immune Polyneuropathies (Guillain-Barre) Syndrome
http://www.neuro.wustl.edu/neuromuscular/antibody/gbs.htm

Classification of neuropathies and GBS-like syndromes.

Guillain-Barre Association

http://www.ozemail.com.au/~guillain/

Guillain-Barre Syndrome Fact Sheet

http://www.ninds.nih.gov/healinfo/disorder/guillain/guillain.html

Information from the National Institute of Health, National Institute of Neurological Disorders and Stroke.

Guillain-Barre Syndrome Foundation International

http://www.adsnet.com/jsteinhi/html/gbs/gbsfi.html

Information about this rare, paralyzing disease of the peripheral nerves.

Huntington Disease

Caring for People with Huntington's Disease

http://www.kumc.edu/hospital/huntingtons/

Facing Huntington's Disease: A Handbook for Families and Friends

http://neuro-chief-e.mgh.harvard.edu/mcmenemy/facinghd.html

Huntington Disease

http://www3.ncbi.nlm.nih.gov:80/htbin-post/Omim/dispmim?143100

Clinical information about Huntington Disease.

Huntington's Disease

http://www.interlog.com/~rlaycock/2nd.html

News, information and links.

Huntington's Disease Fact Sheet

http://www.kumc.edu/instruction/medicine/neurology/hd.html

Huntington disease is a neurodegenerative disorder that affects motor, mood and cognition.

Huntington's Disease Research Highlights

http://www.ninds.nih.gov/healinfo/disorder/huntingt/hdreport.htm

Huntington's Disease Society of America

http://neuro-www2.mgh.harvard.edu/hdsa/hdsamain.nclk

Information about the disease and the Society. Includes information on genetic testing, HD research, support groups and internet links.

Hydrocephalus

Hydrocephalus: HYCEPH-L E-Mail Discussion Group

http://neurosurgery.mgh.harvard.edu/hyceph-l.htm

To subscribe, send e-mail to: listserv@listserv.utoronto.ca and in the message, type: "subscribe HYCEPH-L Yourfirstname Yourlastname."

Steve's Hydrocephalus Page

http://web.syr.edu/~sndrake/hyd1.htm

Individuals with hydrocephalus suffer from the abnormal accumulation of cerebrospinal fluid in the brain. Find out more about it and what can be done for it on Steve's page.

Multiple Sclerosis

Drug Infonet's Multiple Sclerosis Sites

http://www.druginfonet.com/ms.htm

Jooly's Joint

http://www.mswebpals.org/realind.htm

Group which shares personal experiences with MS and seeks to give and receive support; for people with multiple sclerosis and their families.

MS Direct

http://www.aquila.com/dean.sporleder/ms_home/

Lots of links are listed with a brief description of each site.

MS from the Horse's Mouth

http://stripe.colorado.edu/~leonarm/ms/

Support and personal stories.

MS News

http://www.medlib.arizona.edu/~sumption/indexa.htm

MS-Stuff

http://www.helsinki.fi/~ahalko/ms.html

Links to MS information sites, personal pages, research, treatment and helpful software.

Multiple Sclerosis

http://www-medlib.med.utah.edu/kw/ms

An introduction to MS for medical students and physicians in training. The site provides a guide to the disease and includes a patient video.

Multiple Sclerosis Foundation

http://www.icanect.net/msf/

Information about the services offered by this foundation, frequently asked questions (FAQs) and newsletter.

National Multiple Sclerosis Society

http://www.nmss.org/home.html

MS information, resources, links, and information about the Society.

World of Multiple Sclerosis

http://www.ifmss.org.uk/

Neurofibromatosis

Neurofibromatosis, Inc.

http://www.nfinc.org/

Neurofibromatosis Online Service

http://nf.org/

The neurofibromatoses 1 and 2 are a group of genetic disorders causing tumors to grow along various types of nerves. They may affect bones and skin, and sometimes lead to mental disability. This site provides information for patients, their families and health care professionals about the disease, its diagnosis and

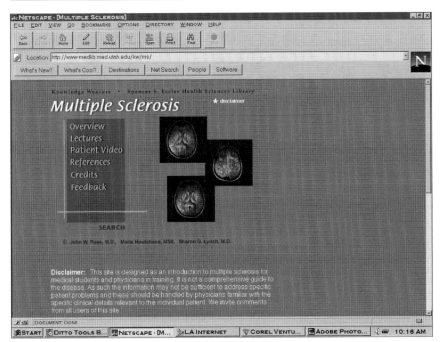

Multiple Sclerosis. *http://www-medlib.med.utah.edu/kw/ms/*

genetic management. Also provided are counseling and support groups, literature references and online resources.

Neurofibromatosis - von Recklinghausen's Disease - Acoustic Neuroma
http://www.geocities.com/HotSprings/8494/

General information on neurofibromatosis and related disorders. Also includes links to related sites and photographs which demonstrate the visible aspects of the disease.

Parkinson Disease

European Parkinson Information Site
http://users.glo.be/~jeepees/index.html

More Links to Parkinson's
http://neuro-chief-e.mgh.harvard.edu/parkinsonsweb/Main/Other/More2.html

Parkinson's Digest
http://www.harfordweb.com/pd/

    This site aspires to be a worldwide support group and information exchange regarding Parkinson disease. Find everything from personal pages, to information on drug treatments and surgery, to research updates and ways to cope with symptoms. This site doesn't seek to be the hot-spot for dissemination of medical information; rather, it hopes to share how individuals with this disease and their families and friends cope.

Parkinson's Discussion Group
http://www.crpht.lu/SANTEL/html/diseases/maillists/parkinsn.html

    To join, send e-mail to: listserv@vm.utcc.utoronto.ca and in the body of the message, type: "subscribe PARKINSN Yourfirstname Yourlastname."

Parkinson's List Information
http://neuro-chief-e.mgh.harvard.edu/parkinsonsweb/Main/Other/listserv.html

    Read for instructions on how to search the Parkinson archives.

Parkinson's Web
http://neuro-chief-e.mgh.harvard.edu/parkinsonsweb/Main/PDMain.html

    Information about Parkinson disease, how to cope with it, where to find support, recent research updates and publications, surgical procedures, advocacy efforts and links.

Rett Syndrome

International Rett Syndrome Association
http://www2.paltech.com/irsa/irsa.htm

Profile: Rett Syndrome
http://www.dircsa.org/au/pub.docs/factrett.txt

    This neurological diseases affects girls and results in severe retardation and physical problems.

Rett Syndrome
http://www.icondata.com/health/pedbase/files/RETTSYND.HTM

    Clinical information about this neurological disorder.

Swedish Rett Center

http://www.jll.se/rett/start.htm

> Soon available in English and Swedish.

Tourette Syndrome

Guide to the Diagnosis and Treatment of Tourette Syndrome

http://www.mentalhealth.com/book/p40-gtor.html

National Tourette Syndrome Association, Inc.

http://neuro-www2.mgh.harvard.edu/tsa/tsamain.nclk

Nova Scotia Tourette Syndrome Site

http://www.ccn.cs.dal.ca/Health/Tourette/TS.html

> Includes Tourette syndrome frequently asked questions (FAQs), articles, mailing lists, and internet links.

Tourette Syndrome

http://www.ninds.nih.gov/healinfo/disorder/tourette/tourette.htm

> Information from the National Institute of Neurological Disorders and Stroke.

Tourette Syndrome Home Page

http://www-personal.umd.umich.edu/~infinit/tourette.html

> To subscribe to the Tourette Syndrome Mailing List, send e-mail to: majordomo@igc.apc.org and in the body, write: "subscribe pov-twitch."

Tourette Syndrome Primer

http://www.chadd.org/tsprime.htm

Tourettes on the Net

http://caffeine.mindport.net/ts-links.html

Tuberous Sclerosis

Lisa's Tuberous Sclerosis Page

http://www.title14.com/ts/

Luke's Tuberous Sclerosis Page

http://marlin.utmb.edu/tsc/

National Tuberous Sclerosis Association

http://www.ntsa.org/

Tuberous Sclerosis International

http://crystal.feo.hvu.nl/Groepen/TSI/TSI.htm

Tuberous Sclerosis Talk

http://www.title14.com/tsctalk/

Tuberous sclerosis occurs when benign tumors appear on various organs. It is often accompanied by seizures and retardation. This site provides frequently asked questions (FAQs), news, archives and chat line. To subscribe to the mailing list, e-mail: majordomo@aura.title14.com and in body, type: "subscribe tsctalk."

NEUROMUSCULAR DISORDERS

Covered in this section: Amyotrophic Lateral Sclerosis; General Topics; Muscular Dystrophy; Myasthenia Gravis.

Related sections: Disabilities; Muscles & Musculoskeletal Disorders; Neurological Disorders; Rare Diseases.

Amyotrophic Lateral Sclerosis

ALS Association
http://www.ALSA.org/

Amyotrophic lateral sclerosis (a.k.a. Lou Gehrig's disease) is a fairly common disorder of the nervous system. Life expectancy upon diagnosis is usually two to four years, but many with this disease live much longer.

Beat ALS!
http:/www.phoenix.net/~jacobsen/beatals.html

What is ALS?
http://www.vcn.bc.ca/als/what_is/

General Topics

Muscle Power
http://www.disabilitynet.co.uk/groups/musclepower/

National organization of people with neuromuscular impairments.

MuscleNet
http://www.bio.unipd.it/~telethon/muscle.html

Nerve-Muscle Connection
http://www.allabouthealth.com/Current/News/Items/news423.htm

Neuromuscular Disease Center

http://www.neuro.wustl.edu/neuromuscular/

Neuromuscular disorders, neuromuscular evaluation, autoantibody testing, patient information, links to related sites and additional references.

Neuromuscular Disease Database

http://disability.ucdavis.edu/database/

Includes information about amyotrophic lateral sclerosis (Lou Gehrig's disease), muscular dystrophy, polio, spinal muscular atrophy, and Charcot-Marie-Tooth syndrome.

Neuromuscular Diseases

http://www.mic.ki.se/Diseases/c10.668.html

Neuromuscular Disorders: Official Journal of the World Muscle Society

http://www.elsevier.nl.inca/publications/store/9/7/3/973.pub.shmtl

Muscular Dystrophy

Duchenne Muscular Dystrophy

http://users.neworld.net/woliver/md.html

One of the most common types of muscular dystrophy, Duchenne's is a rare, inherited neuromuscular disorder characterized by rapid progression of muscle degeneration.

Duchenne Muscular Dystrophy Research Center

http://www.mgen.pitt.edu/dmdrc.htm

Family services and research.

Haynes Family's Duchenne Muscular Dystrophy Home Page

http://www.geocities.com/CapeCanaveral/8676/

Muscular Dystrophy Association - USA

http://www.mdausa.org/

Neuromuscular Disease Center. http://www.neuro.wustl.edu/neuromuscular/

Muscular Dystrophy Association of Australia

http://www.mda.org.au/

Muscular Dystrophy by Giovanni Naso

http://www.rtmol.stt.it/users/gnaso/muscdyst.html

Parent Project for Muscular Dystrophy Research, Inc.

http://www.parentdmd.org/

Discusses Duchenne muscular dystrophy and Becker muscular dystrophy.

Ryan's Page: The Place to Meet for People with Muscular Dystrophy

http://www.mda.org.au/ryansrag.html

This site was created and is maintained by a boy with muscular dystrophy.

Myasthenia Gravis

Life with Myasthenia
http://pages.prodigy.com/lifewithmg/

Myasthenia Gravis Links
http://pages.prodigy.com/myasthenia/

Myasthenia Gravis Medical Information
http://pages.prodigy.com/myasthenia/medical.htm

Myasthenic Crisis: Diagnosis and Management
http://www.geocities.com/HotSprings/4357/myasthenia.html

Practical Guide to Myasthenia Gravis
http://www.med.unc.edu/mgfa/mgf-prac/

Myasthenia gravis is an autoimmune disease in which important receptors on the muscle cells are destroyed, leading to paralysis.

NURSING

General Topics

American Journal of Nursing
http://www.ajn.org/ajn/page1.html

AND/RN Concepts
http://www.azstarnet.com/~jlichty/
rn.htm

    Forum for current issues related to nursing, including education, health reform and other topics.

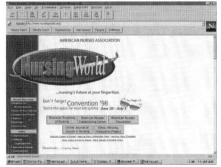

Florence Nightingale
http://www.dnai.com/~borneo/
nightingale/

    Country Joe McDonald's tribute to Florence Nightingale.

Nursing World. *http://www.nursingworld.org/*

HealthWeb Nursing Page
http://www.lib.umich.edu/tml/nursing.html
    Provides excellent information, discussion and resources.

Home Care Web Page
http://www.silcom.com/~peter/nurse.html
    For home care nurses.

Idea Nurse
http://www.silcom/~peter/nurse.html
Links to sites and articles by and about nurses and nursing.

Lippincott's Nursing Center
http://www.ajn.org/
For nurses, researchers and educators.

NetNurse Home Page
http://www.wp.com/NetNurse/

NURSENET
http://www.ualberta.ca/~jrnorris/nursenet/nn.html
Collections of different discussions on nursing topics.

NurseWIRE: Nurse Entrepreneurs on the Internet
http://www.callamer.com/itc/nursewire/

Nursing and Health-Related Internet Resources
http://www.access.digex.net/~nurse/website.htm

Nursing Lists
http://www.callamer.com/itc/nurse/nrslist.html

Nursing Net
http://www.communique.net/~nursgnt/

Nursing Theory Page
http://www.ualberta.ca/~jrnorris/nt/theory.html

Nursing World
http://www.nursingworld.org/
All about the American Nurses Association.

Thomas Moll's Cool Nursing Site of the Week
http://www.odyssee.net/~fnord/nurselink.html

"Virtual" Nursing Center
http://www-sci.lib.uci.edu/HSG/Nursing.html

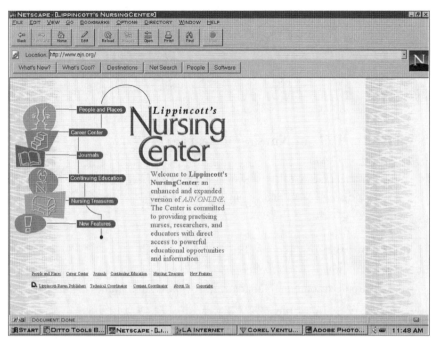

Lippincott's Nursing Center. *http://www.ajn.org/*

Virtual Nursing College
http://www.langara.bc.ca/vnc/

WEBster's Fine Art of Nursing
http://ally.ios.com/~webster/nurse.html

WholeNurse
http://www.wholenurse.com/

Nursing Humor

Home Health Humor
http://www.whidbey.com/ihn/humor.html

Journal of Nursing Jocularity
http://www.jocularity.com/

Weird Nursing Tales
http://users.twave.net/texican/

Research

National Institute of Nursing Research
http://www.nih.gov/ninr/

Site contains research, news, events, fact sheets, frequently asked questions (FAQs) and further resources about nursing research. Part of the National Institutes of Health.

Registry of Nursing Research
http://www.stti.iupui.edu/mr/about.html

An electronic resource of nursing research programs, studies, and results.

ORGANIZATIONS

Academic Orthopaedic Society
http://ortho1.uth.tmc.edu/

The Acoustic Neuroma Association Home Page
http://neurosurgery.mgh.harvard.edu/ana/

Agency for Toxic Substances and Disease Registry
http://atsdr1.atsdr.cdc.gov:8080/

American Academy of Allergy, Asthma and Immunology
http://www.aaaai.org/

American Academy of Child and Adolescent Psychiatry
http://www.aacap.org/web/aacap/

American Academy of Hospice and Palliative Medicine
http://www.aahpm.org/

American Academy of Medical Acupuncture
http://www.medicalacupuncture.org/

American Academy of Orthopaedic Surgeons
http://www.aaos.org/

American Academy of Pediatric Dentistry
http://www.aapd.org/

American Academy of Pediatrics
http://www.aap.org/

American Academy of Podiatric Sports Medicine
http://www.clark.net/pub/aapsm.html

American Association for the Surgery of Trauma Webnet
http://www.aast.org/

The American Association of Clinical Endocrinologist
http://www.ace.come/

American Association of Colleges of Osteopathic Medicine
http://www.aacom.org/

American Association of Immunology
http://www.scienceXchange.com/aai/

American Association of Blood Banks
http://www.aabb.org/

American Association of Kidney Patients
http://cybermart.com/aakpaz/aakp.html

American Association of Naturopathic Physicians
http://www.infinite.org/Naturopathic.Physician/Welcome.html

American Association of Pediatric Dentistry Online
http://aapd.org

American Association of Poison Control Centers
http://198.79.220.3/aapcc/aapcc.htm

American Association of Retired Persons
http://aarp.org/

American Association on Mental Retardation
http://www.aamr.org/

The American Cancer Society
http://www.cancer.org/

American Chiropractic Association
http://www.cais.com/aca/

American College of Healthcare Executives
http://www.ache.org/

American College of Legal Medicine
http://execpc.com/~aclm/

American College of Nurse-Midwives
http://www.acnm.org/

American College of Physicians
http://www.acponline.org/

American College of Rheumatology
http://www.rheumatology.org/

American Council for Headache Education
http://www.achenet.org/index.html

American Council of the Blind
http://www.acb.org/

American Cryonics Society, Inc.
http://www.jps.net/cryonics/

American Dental Association Online
http://www.ada.org/

American Diabetes Foundation
http://www.diabetes.org/custom.asp/

The American Foundation for the Blind
http://www.igc.apc.org/afb/

American Gastroenterological Association
http://www.gastro.org/

American Heart Association
http://www.amhrt.org/

American Holistic Medical Association
http://www.doubleclickd.com/about_ahma.html

American Hyperlexia Association Home Page
http://www.hyperlexia.org/

American Institute of Ultrasound in Medicine
http://www.well.com/user/aium/

American Liver Foundation
http://sadieo.ucsf.edu/alf/alffinal/homepagealf.html

American Lung Association
http://www.lungusa.org/noframes/index.html

American Lyme Disease Foundation, Inc.
http://www.w2.com/docs2/d5/lyme.html

American Medical Association
http://www.ama-assn.org/

The American Medical Women's Association
http://www.amwa-doc.org/

American Physical Therapy Association: Geriatrics Section
http://geriatricspt.org/

American Porphyria Foundation
http://www.enterprise.net/apf/

The American Psychoanalytic Association
http://apsa.org/index.htm

The American Psychoanalytic Foundation
http://www.cyberpsych.org/apf.htm

The American Psychological Association
http://www.apa.org/

American Public Health Association
http://www.apha.org/

American Social Health Association
http://sunsite.unc.edu/ASHA/

American Society for Aesthetic Plastic Surgery
http://surgery.org/

American Society for Clinical Nutrition
http://www.faseb.org/ascn/

American Society of Cataract and Refractive Surgery
http://www.ascrs.org/

American Society of Health-System Pharmacists
http://www.ashp.org/

American Society of Transplant Physicians
http://www.astp.org/

American Thoracic Society
http://www.thoracic.org/

American Trauma Society
http://www.amtrauma.org/index.htm

The American Yoga Association
http://members.aol.com/amyogassn/index.htm

Anorexia Nervosa and Bulimia Association
http://qlink.queensu.ca/~4map/anabhome.html

The Arc of the United States Home Page
http://TheArc.org/welcome.html

Association of American Medical Colleges
http://www.aamc.org/

Association of Emergency Physicians

http://www.aep.org/index.html

The Association for the Study of Dreams

http://www.outreach.org/gmcc/asd/

Autism Society of America

http://www.autism-society.org/asa_home.html

The Brain Tumor Society

http://www.tbts.org/

Canadian Association for Suicide Prevention

http://idirect.com/~casp/tmplocx.html/

Cardiovascular Institute of the South

http://www.cardio.com/

CARE

http://www.care.org/

Centers for Disease Control and Prevention

http://www.cdc.gov/

Crohn's and Colitis Foundation of America

http://www.ccfa.org/

Cystic Fibrosis Foundation

http://www.cff.org/

Directory of Digestive Diseases Organizations for Patients

http://www.niddk.nih.gov/DigDisOrgPat/DigDisOrgPat.html

The Endocrine Society

http://www.endo-society.org/

Endometriosis Association

http://www.ivf.com/endoassn.html

The Epilepsy Foundation of America

http://www.efa.org/indexf.htm

Federal Emergency Management Agency

http://www.fema.gov/

Glaucoma Research Foundation

http://www.glaucoma.org/

Health Care Financing Administration

http://www.hcfa.gov/

Health Organizations

http://www.social.com/health/nhic/data/index.html

Includes approximately 1,000 health organizations throughout the United States. Browse by state or alphabetically.

Healthcare Financial Management Association

http://www.hfma.org/

Helicobacter Foundation

http://www.helico.com/

The Hemlock Society

http://www.irsociety.com/hemlock.htm

Holistic Dental Association

http://simwell.com/hda/

Hospice Foundation of America

http://www.hospicefoundation.org/

Huntington's Disease Society of America

http://neuro-www2.mgh.harvard.edu/hdsa/hdsamain.nclk/

Hydrocephalus Association

http://neurosurgery.mgh.harvard.edu/ha/

Institute for Child Health Policy

http://mchnet.ichp.ufl.edu/

Institute of Medicine

http://www2.nas.edu/iom/

International Association of Physicians in AIDS Care

http://www.iapac.org/

International Committee of the Red Cross

http://www.icrc.ch/

International Diabetic Athletes Association

http://www.genet.com/~idea/

The International Foundation for Bowel Dysfunction

http://incontinet/adscopy/ads_nfpo/ifbd.htm

International Society for Child and Adolescent Injury Prevention

http://weber.u.washington.edu:80/~hiprc/iscaip.html

International Society of Nephrology

http://synapse.uah.ualberta.ca/isn/000i0000.htm

Internet Dermatology Society

http://www.telemedicine.org/ids.htm

Joint Commission on Accreditation of Healthcare Organizations

http://www.jcaho.org/

The Juvenile Diabetes Foundation

http://www.bcm.tmc.edu/chrc/

Life Extension Society

http://www.clark.net/pub/kfl/les/les.html

Lupus Association

http://www.ttsh.gov.sg/lupus/lupus.html

Maternal and Child Health Bureau

http://www.os.dhhs.gov/hrsa/mchb

Medical Protection Society

http://www.mps.org.uk/medical/

Medical Research Council of Canada

http://www.hinetbc.org/information/2fmed.html

National Academy of Sciences/National Academy of Engineering/Institute of Medicine/National Research Council

http://www.nas.edu/

National Arthritis Foundation

http://www.arthritis.org/

National Association of Developmental Councils

http://www.igc.apc.org/NADDC/

National Association to Advance Fat Acceptance

http://www.naafa.org/

The National Association of Women's Health Professionals

http://www.nawhp.org/

National Ataxia Foundation

http://www.nwwin.com/ATAXIA.htm

The National Cancer Institute

http://www.nci.nih.gov/

National Center for Health Statistics

http://www.cdc.gov/nchswww/nchshome.htm

The National Coalition for Birthing Alternatives

http://www.ptw.com/~troytash/

National Coalition for the Homeless
http://nch.ari.net/

National College of Naturopathic Medicine
http://www.ncnm.edu/

National Committee for Quality Assurance
http://www.ncqa.org/

National Enuresis Society
http://www.peds.umn.edu/Centers/NES/

National Eye Institute
http://www.nei.nih.gov/

The National Federation of the Blind
http://www.nfb.org/default.htm

National Foundation for Infectious Diseases
http://www.medscape.com/NFID

National Health Information Center
http://nhic-nt.health.org/

National Heart, Lung and Blood Institute
http://www.nhlbi.nih.gov/nhlb/nhlbi.htm

National Hospice Organization
http://www.nho.org/

National Institute of Allergy and Infectious Diseases
gopher://gopher.niaid.nih.gov/1

National Institute of Arthritis and Musculoskeletal and Skin Diseases
http://www.nih.gov/niams/

National Institute of Child Health and Human Development
http://www.nih.gov:80/nichd/

National Institute of Deafness and Other Communication Diseases
http://www.nih.gov/nidcd/

National Institute of Dental Research
http://www.nidr.nih.gov/

National Institute of Environmental Health Sciences
http://www.niehs.nih.gov/

National Institute of General Medical Sciences
http://www.nih.gov/nigms/

National Institute of Mental Health
http://www.minh.nih.gov/

National Institute of Neurological Disorders and Stroke
http://www.ninds.nih.gov/

National Institute on Aging
http://www.nih.gov/nia/

National Institute on Alcohol Abuse and Alcoholism
http://www.niaaa.nih.gov/

National Institutes of Health
http://www.nih.gov/

National Kidney Foundation
http://www.kidney.org/index.html

National Lymphedema Network
http://www.wenet.net/users/lymphnet/

National Mental Health Association
http://www.nmha.org/

The National Organization for Rare Disorders, Inc.
http://www.pcnet.com/~orphan/

National Organization for Women
http://www.now.org/

National Osteoporosis Foundation
http://www.nof.org/

National Psoriasis Foundation
http://www.psoriasis.org/

The National Science Foundation
http://www.nsf.gov/

The National Sleep Foundation
http://www.sleepfoundation.org/

National Stroke Association
http://www.stroke.org/

National Vitiligo Foundation
http://pegasus.uthct.edu/Vitiligo/index.html

Obsessive-Compulsive Foundation
http://pages.prodigy.com/alwillen/ocf.html

Organizations Offering (Diabetes) Support
http://www.demon.co.uk/diabetic/orgs.html

Overeaters Anonymous
http://www.overeaters.anonymous.org/

PBC Foundation
http://www.nhtech.demon.co/uk/pbc/index.html

Planned Parenthood Federation of America
http://www.igc.apc.org/ppfa/

Radiological Society of North America
http://www.rsna.org/edu/internet/launchpad.html

Renal Physicians Association
http://kdp-sparc.kdp-baptist.louisville.edu/rpa.

Royal National Institute for the Blind, UK
http://www.trib.org.uk

Scholarly Societies Project
http://www.lib.uwaterloo.ca/society/healthsci_soc.html

Sjogren's Syndrome Foundation
http://www.sjogrens.com/

Society for Clinical Trials
http://www.members.aol.com/sctbalt/index.htm

The Spina Bifida Association of America
http://www.infohiway.com/spinabifida/

Thyroid Foundation of Canada
http://www.io.org/~thyroid/canada.html

United Cerebral Palsy Association
http://www.ucpa.org/

UNICEF
http://www.unicef.org/

United Scleroderma Foundation
http://www.sceleroderma.com/

U.S. Department of Health and Human Services
http://www.os.dhhs.gov/

U.S. Environmental Protection Agency
http://www.epa.gov/

The World Association for Disaster and Emergency Medicine
http://www.pitt.edu/HOME/GHNet/wadem/wadem.html

World Federation of Mental Health
http://ssw.ab.umd.edu/wfmh.html

World Health Organization
http://www.who.ch/

Xeroderma Pigmentosum Society, Inc.
http://www1.mhv.net/~xps/

OSTEOPATHY

Access AOA

http://www.am-osteo-assn.org/

Information for the general public and professionals about osteopathy and osteopathic resources, from the American Osteopathic Association

American Association of Colleges of Osteopathic Medicine

http://www.aacom.org/

Informative and professional site.

Cranial Osteopathy Page

http://www.users.dircon.co.uk:80/~med-man/

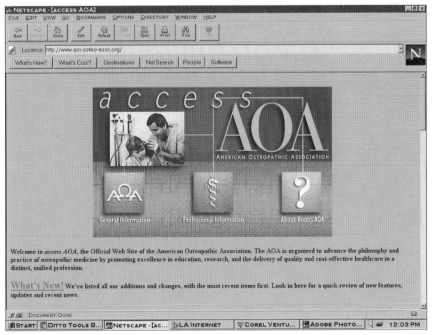

Access AOA. *http://www.am-osteo-assn.org/*

Osteopathic Medicine International WWW Resource Website
http://www.rscom.com/osteo/

Osteopathic Net
http://osteopathic.net/index.shtml

Still Alive
http://www.rscom.com/osteo/journal/intro.htm

Journal about the science and art of osteopathic manipulative medicine and naturopathic medicine.

What is a D.O.?
http://dale.hsc.unt.edu:80/~brent/whatisado.html

PAIN & PAIN MANAGEMENT

Chronic Pain

Chronic Pain: Questions and Answers
http://www.asri.edu/neuro/brochure/pain1.html

Information about Chronic Pain
http://gamma132.s-online.com/clsolutions/paininfo.html

PAIN.USA
http://www.genesisnetwork.net/users/keithd/index.html-ssi
    Articles related to chronic pain and links to other web sites.

General Topics

American Society for Pain Relief, Research and Education
http://www.cris.com/~jgupta/ASPRRE.htm

Institute for the Study and Treatment of Pain
http://www.istop.org/istop/

Pain Resources for Patients and Their Families
http://weber.u.washington.edu/~crc/CRCpage/patients.html

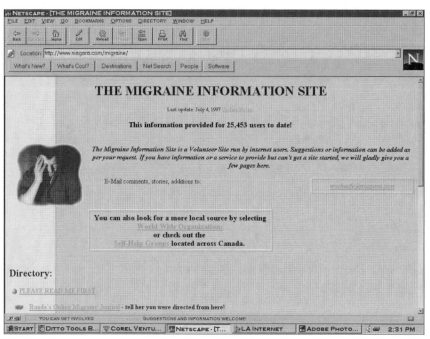

The Migraine Information Site. *http://www.niagara.com/migraine/*

Partners Against Pain

http://www.partnersagainstpain.com/index.html

Divided into resources intended for medical professionals and non-professionals, this site provides information and advice about caring for people in pain. It includes news, books, pain control guides, support groups, and suggestions for controlling side-effects. Information for the medical professional includes education, management, prescription and patient education.

Questions and Answers about Pain Control

http://nysernet.org/bcic/nci/adult/pain.4518/pain.control.html

Online book about managing pain.

Talaria: The Hypermedia Assistant for Cancer Pain Management

http://www.stat.washington.edu/TALARIA/TALARIA.html

Headaches/Migraines

American Council for Headache Education (ACHE)
http://www.achenet.org/index.html

Understanding, preventing and treating headaches; and information about ACHE.

Glaxol Wellcome's Migraine Resource Center
http://www.migrainehelp.com/

Lots of information about migraines, including diagnosis, how to cope, news, support and related internet links.

Migraine Headaches
http://www.med.upenn.edu/~ophth/migraine.html

Migraine Information Site
http://www.niagara.com/migraine/

Lots of information and links for migraine sufferers.

Migraine: The Non-Pharmaceutical Medical Magazine
http://www.etonhall.com/mig1.htm

Newspaper Articles and Other Information on Migraines
http://www.niagara.com/migraine/newsdir.html

On-Line Migraine Journal
http://www.msn.fullfeed.com/~ronda/history/history.html

Personal stories of migraine sufferers.

Ronda's Migraine Page
http://www.msn.fullfeed.com/~ronda/

Palliative Care

Palliative Care FAQs
http://www.mol.com.my/cancare/pcfaq.htm

Palliative Care for Children

http://www.wwdc.com/death/iwg/children.html

University of Ottowa Institute of Palliative Care

http://www.ochin.on.ca/pallcare/

WHO Definition of Palliative Care

http://www.mol.com/cancare/pallidef.htm

Surgery Pain

Pain Control After Surgery: A Patient's Guide

http://pain.roxane.com/library/AHCPR/apmp1.html

This electronic pamphlet contains advice on assessing and managing pain felt after surgical procedures.

PATHOLOGY

Covered in this section: *Blood/Hematology; Cancer/Oncology; General Topics; HIV/AIDS; Kidneys/Nephrology & Urology; Liver/Hepatology.*

Blood/Hematology

American Journal of Pathology

http://www.at-home.com/PATHOLOGY/

From the American Society for Investigative Pathology.

Histology Lessons: An Outline of Blood

http://www.mc.vanderbilt.edu/histo/blood/

Cancer/Oncology

Pathology Simplified

http://www.erinet.com/fnadoc/path.htm

Good information for patients about lung cancer, breast cancer, and Pap smear tests. Includes photo archives and hotlinks.

General Topics

Internet Resources for Pathology and Laboratory Medicine

http://www.pds.med.umich.edu/users/amp/Path_Resources.html

Includes pathology departments on the web, listservers and databases, usenet, commercial and regulatory links, as well as sub-specialty resources.

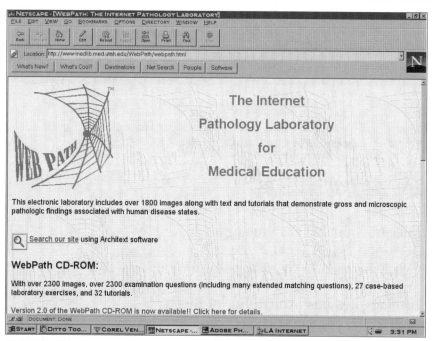

Web Path. *http://www-medlib.med.utah.edu/WebPath/webpath.html*

PathIT Pathology Online

http://www.pathit.com/

Includes images and text on anatomic, clinical, veterinary, forensic and quantitative pathology, as well as morphometrics (the measurement of forms or structures of organisms) and pathology informatics.

Pathology Hypermedia Archive

http://scarlett.wustl.edu/path/images/

This is an image archive of lectures. Great site with lots of information.

Slice of Life

http://www-medlib.med.utah.edu/sol/

Urbana Atlas of Pathology

http://www.med.uiuc.edu/PathAtlasf/titlepage.html

PathIT. http://www.pathit.com/

Web Path: The Internet Pathology Laboratory for Medical Education

http://www-medlib.med.utah.edu/WebPath/webpath.html

Electronic laboratory of over 1800 images with text and tutorials demonstrating gross and microscopic pathologic findings associated with human disease states.

HIV/AIDS

AIDS Pathology Images

http://www-medlib.med.utah.edu/WebPath/AIDSPATH.pdf

Requires Acrobat Reader.

Large Images: Pathology of AIDS

http://scarlett.wustl.edu/path/images/l09.htm

Kidneys/Nephrology & Urology

Renal Pathology Index
http://www-medlib.med.utah.edu/MedPath/RENAHTML/REALIDX.html

Renal Pathology Tutorial
http://www.gamewood.net/rnet/renalpath/tutorial.htm

Demonstrates normal glomerular histology and some of the diseases that cause the nephrotic syndrome.

Liver/Hepatology

Atlas of Liver Pathology
http://indy.radiology.uiowa.edu/Providers/Textbooks/LiverPathology/

A multimedia textbook of liver pathology by Frank A. Mitros, M.D., of the University of Iowa College of Medicine. Includes text, tables and images.

Hepatic Pathology Index
http://www-medlib.med.utah.edu/WebPath/LIVEHTML/LIVERIDX.html

Over 60 images of normal and diseased livers and liver cells.

Hepatitis A to E
http://www.cdc.gov/nicdod/diseases/hepatitis/slideset/httoc.htm

An overview of the epidemiology and prevention of viral hepatitis A through E is presented in slide show format with accompanying text. Bibliography also provided.

PREGNANCY & CHILDBIRTH

Covered in this section: *Birth Defects; Breastfeeding; Cesarean Section; General Topics; Homebirth/Birthing Alternatives; Midwifery; Miscarriages; Premature Birth.*

Related sections: Children's Health/Pediatrics; Sexual & Reproductive Health; Women's Health.

Birth Defects

Neonatal Diseases and Abnormalities

http://www.mic.ki.se/Diseases/ c16.html

This extensive collection of links assembled by the Karolinska Institute includes organizations, indexes and research facilities dealing with genetic, neonatal and developmental disorders, from jaundice and fetal alcohol syndrome, to cystic fibrosis and Down syndrome.

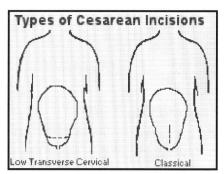

Cesarean Childbirth.
http://www.cmhc.com/factsfam/cbirth.htm

Preventing Birth Defects and Developmental Disabilities

http://www.cdc.gov/nceh/pubcatns/1994/cdc/brosures/surv-epi.htm#surv-epi

The Centers for Disease Control and Prevention's brochure provides online surveillance and epidemiology data, as well as links to related sites.

Wide Smiles: Cleft Lip and Palate Resources

http://www.widesmiles.org/

Breastfeeding

Breastfeeding Advocacy Page
http://www.clark.net/pub/activis/bfpage/bfpage.html

Breastfeeding Articles and Resources
http://www.parentsplace.com/readroom/bf.html

Breastfeeding Page
http://www.islandnet.com/~bedford/brstfeed.html
   Information, discussion, issues and resources.

FAQ about Breastfeeding
http://www.lalecheleague.org/FAQ/FAQMain.html

Cesarean Section

Cesarean Childbirth
http://www.cmhc.com/factsfam/cbirth.htm
   General information on cesarean sections in frequently asked question (FAQ) format.

Cesarean Section Homepage
http://www.childbirth.org/section/section.html
   This site provides a long list of web links and fact sheets on cesarean sections and pregnancy in general.

International Cesarean Awareness Network Homepage
http://www.childbirth.org/section/ICAN.html

Understanding Cesarean Birth
_http://www.noah.cuny.edu/pregnancy/march_of_dimes/birth/csection.html_
   Site addresses basic questions about C-sections, including indications for, benefits, risks and effects of this procedure.

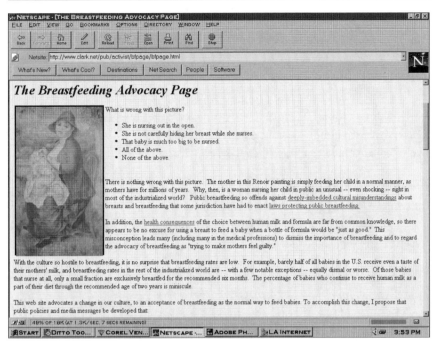

The Breastfeeding Advocacy Page. http://www.clark.net/pub/activist/bfpage/bfpage.html

General Topics

American Institute of Ultrasound in Medicine

http://www.well.com/user/aium/

Center for Human Reproduction

http://www.centerforhumanreprod.com/

Dr. Pranikoff's Ob/Gyn Web Library

http://www.uc.edu/~pranikjd/

Maternal and Child Health Network Gopher Server

gopher://mchnet.ichp.ufl.edu/

MotherStuff

http://www.teramonger.com/dwan/mother.htm

Internet resources on birthing, miscarriage, premature babies, breastfeeding and midwifery.

Neonatology on the Web
http://www.csmc.edu/neonatology/

OB/Gyn Toolbox
http://www.cpmc.columbia.edu/resources/obgyntools/

Includes "tools" such as: body surface area calculator, birth weight conversions, creatinine clearance estimation, endometriosis scoring, gestational age calculator, and OB ultrasound analyzer.

Obstetric Ultrasound
http://home.hkstar.com/~joewoo/joewoo2.html

Addresses basic questions about this technology and how it works, with hypertext links and an image gallery.

Plus-Size Pregnancy Website
http://www.vierday.com/~rvireday/plus/

Pregnancy and Birth Center Reading Resources
http://www.parentsplace.com/genobject.cgi/readroom/pregnant.html

Pregnancy Calculator
http://fox.nstn.ca/~rgiffen/PregnancyCalculator.html

Pregnancy Institute
http://www.preginst.com/

Site for the Pregnancy Institute, a non-profit organization that studies normal pregnancies.

Pregnancy Links
http://www.childbirth.org/articles/preglinks.html

Prenatal Diagnosis
http://www.fetal.com/

Signs of Pregnancy
http://www.ausoft.com/pregnancy/

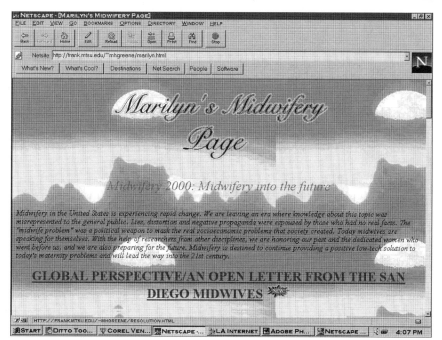

Marilyn's Midwifery Page. http://frank.mtsu.edu/~mhgreene/marilyn.html

Yahoo: Birth

http://www.yahoo.com/Society_and_Culture/Birth/
   Loads of links.

Homebirth/Birthing Alternatives

Homebirth

http://www.islandnet.com/~browns/homebirth/homebirth.html

   Describes home birth, offers stories from individuals who have chosen this method, and provides links.

National Coalition for Birthing Alternatives

http://www.ptw.com/~troytash/

Water Birth Information

http://www.well.com/user/karil/

Midwifery

American College of Nurse-Midwives
http://www.acnm.org/

Marilyn's Midwifery Page
http://frank.mtsu.edu/~mhgreene/marilyn.html

Midwifery Today
http://www.efn.org/~djz/birth/MT/Mtindex.html

Miscarriages

Hygeia
http://www.connix.com/~hygeia/
Journal for pregnancy and neonatal loss.

For People Who Know Someone Who Has Recently Miscarried
_http://www.hcc.cc.fl.us/services/staff/dawn/mc_do's.htm_
Suggested "do's" and "don'ts."

Frequently Asked Questions about Miscarriage
http://scalos.mc.duke.edu/~brook006/miscarriage.html

Sands(Vic)
http://www.vicnet.net.au/~sands/sands.htm
A support group for parents who have experienced miscarriage, stillbirth, or neonatal death.

Premature Birth

ABC's of Resuscitation of Infants
http://www.ozemail.com.au/~karlat/abcs.htm

After the NICU

http://home.earthlink.net/~gbangs/advice.html

Advice to parents after they bring home their child who has been in the neonate intensive care unit.

For Parents of Preemies

http://www.medsch.wisc.edu/childrenshosp/Parents_of_Preemies/index.html

Answers to commonly asked questions about premature infants.

Preemie Resources

http://www.vicnet.net.au/~garyh/preres.htm

Preemie-L Home Page

http://www.vicnet.net.au/~garyh/preemie.htm

Information about this e-mail discussion list.

Tommy's CyberNursery Preemie Web

http://www.flash.net/~cyberkid/

PUBLIC HEALTH

General Topics

Advisory Committee on Human Radiation Experiments
http://www.seas.gwu.edu/nsarchive/radiation/

American Public Health Association
http://www.apha.org/

This site is a resource for public health professionals. It provides information about the Association, as well as a description of legislative affairs and advocacy efforts, news and publications, practice and policy, and public health resources.

BioSites: Public Health Sites
http://www.library.ucsf.edu/biosites/bin/showByTopic.pl?PublicHealth/

A long list of links with important descriptive material.

CDC Home Page
http://www.cdc.gov/cdc.htm

Home page of the Centers for Disease Control and Prevention. The CDC includes 11 centers, institutes and offices, and they can all be accessed from this site. Information includes help about ill children abroad, diseases, injuries and disabilities, health risks, demographic information, prevention guidelines and strategies. In addition, it provides information about vaccines, disease outbreaks, data and statistics.

CDC Prevention Guidelines Database

http://wwwonder.cdc.gov/wonder/prevguid/prevguid/prevguid.html

The Centers for Disease Control and Prevention's recommendations and guidelines for the prevention of diseases, injuries and disabilities.

Center for Healthcare Information

http://www.healthcare-info.com/

Foundation for Informed Medical Decision Making, Inc.

http://www.dartmouth.edu/dms/cecs/fimdm/

Healthfinder

http://www.healthfinder.gov/

The U.S. government's friendly gateway consumer health and human services information web site. It includes links to selected online publications, clearinghouses, libraries, databases, web sites, and support and self-help groups, as well as the government agencies and not-for-profit organizations that produce reliable information for the public. A number of tours help you to navigate through the web site and the enormous amount of information available. Audio and visual files also provided.

HealthWeb: Public Health Page

http://www.lib.umich.edu/hw/public.health.html

Index of Occupational Safety and Health

http://turva.me.tut.fi/~oshweb/

Medicine/Public Health Initiative

http://www.sph.uth.tmc.edu/mph/

National Health Information Center

http://nhic-nt.health.org/

Health information referral services. Includes resources database of over 1,100 organizations and government offices, containing contact information, abstracts and other information. Also includes a number of referral documents and a search engine.

Centers for Disease Control and Prevention. http://www.cdc.gov/cdc.htm

National Institutes of Health

http://www.nih.gov/

This site offers an overview of the NIH, news and events, and information about the institutes' health resources including CancerNet, AIDS information and Clinical Alerts. Also offers grant and contract information, scientific resources and links to the various (24) separate institutes, centers and divisions that make up the NIH. It is one of the eight health agencies that comprise the federal government's Public Health Service.

Office of Public Health and Science

http://www.os.dhhs.gov/progorg/ophs/

Information on disease prevention, HIV/AIDS policy, international refugee health watch, minority and women's health issues, the Surgeon General, and physical fitness and health.

Public Domain Software and Electronic Resources

http://www.sph.jhu.edu/org/Delta/Omega/software/

For public health professionals.

Sites with Health Services Research and Public Health Information

http://weber.u.washington.edu/~larsson/hsic94/resource/phlinks.html

State of New York Department of Health

http://www.health.state.ny.us/

U.S. Department of Health and Human Services

http://www.os.dhhs.gov/

This site describes DHHS activities. It also has links to research, policy and administration divisions, and offers consumer information on a large number of physical and mental health topics, ranging from adolescent to women's health issues.

U.S. Department of Labor/Occupational Safety and Health Administration

http://www.osha.gov/safelinks.html

OSHA's list of safety and health internet sites.

"Virtual" Public Health Center

http://www-sci.lib.uci.edu/HSG/Phealth.html

Multimedia information resource center.

Global Health Resources & Aid

CARE

http://www.care.org/

International development and relief organization.

DHS: Demographic and Health Surveys

http://www2.macroint.com/dhs/

Conducts national surveys in Africa, Asia, Latin America and the Caribbean on fertility, family planning, maternal and child health, and household living conditions. Funded by the United States Agency for International Development (USAID).

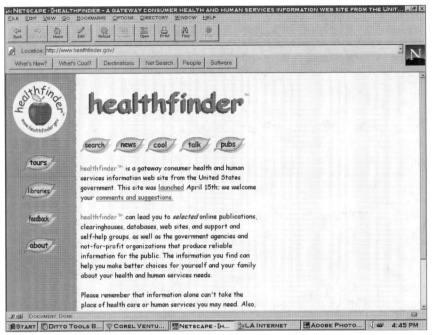

Healthfinder. *http://www.healthfinder.gov/*

Emergency: A Guide to the Emergency Services of the World

http://www.catt.citri.edu.au/emergency/

Flying Samaritans

http://www.geocities.com/Heartland/Plains/1134/

Volunteer organization that operates free medical clinics in Baja, Mexico. Doctors, dentists, translators, pilots and support personnel travel to the clinics and work as invited teachers. The site provides information about the group, its chapters and the clinics they visit.

Global Health: Key Resources

http://www.pitt.edu/HOME/GHNet/GHKR.html

Interplast

http://www.worldaccess.com/NonProfitOrganizations/Interplast/

Interplast is an affiliation of volunteer surgeons, pediatricians, anesthesiologists, nurses and support personnel who work with developing nations to support and develop a free reconstructive surgery programs for children and adults with birth defects, burns, and other crippling deformities. The organization performs over 1500 free surgeries annually. Information about the organization and the trips it has scheduled may be found at this site.

MAP International Internet Services
http://map.org/

Web site for this non-profit relief and development organization that helps provide health services to the world's impoverished people.

U.N.'s World Food Programme
http://www.wfp.org/index.html

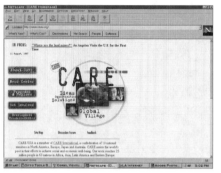

CARE. *http://www.care.org/*

UNICEF
http://www.unicef.org/
United Nations Children's Fund

World Health Organization
http://www.who.ch/
Find out about WHO programs, the World Health Report, public information resources and library.

Home Safety
See also: Children's Health/Pediatrics - Child Safety.

Poison Center Answer Book
http://edison.ucdmc.ucdavis.edu/poison_control/index.html
What to do when you think someone has been poisoned.

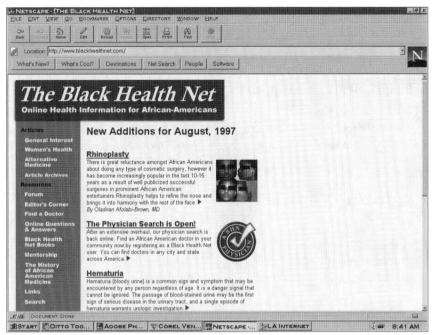

The Black Health Net. *http://www.blackhealthnet.com/*

Safety Related Internet Resources

http://www.mrg.ab.ca/christie/safelist.htm

Includes e-mail addresses, ftp, IRC and gopher sites, electronic publications, mail lists and newsgroups,and a large number of links to WWW sites, alphabetized.

Minority Health Issues

Black Health Care Coalition

http://www.blackhealthnet.com/other/bhcc/default.html

The mission of this coalition is to increase community awareness about health concerns that impact a disproportionate number of minorities.

Black Health Net

http://www.blackhealthnet.com/

Online health information for African-Americans includes articles and resources, online questions and answers, a discussion forum, history of African-American medicine and related links.

Minority Health Listserver

To subscribe, send e-mail to: minhlth-request@family.hampshire.edu and in the body of the message, type: "subscribe minhlth."

Minority Health Network

http://www.pitt.edu/~ejb4/min/

Minority health resources, including listings by minority group, disease, and demographics. Also provides organizations, grant information and education.

Publications

Electronic Journals in Public Health and Health Services Research

http://weber.u.washington.edu/~larsson/hsic94/resource/ejournal.html

NewsFile

http://www.homepage.holowww.com/1V.htm

Includes *AIDS Weekly Plus*, *Antiviral Weekly*, *Blood Weekly*, *Cancer Weekly*, *Disease Weekly*, and several other weeklies covering communicable diseases and public health issues.

University of California at Berkeley Wellness Letter

http://www.enews.com/magazines/ucbwl/

Monthly newsletter from the School of Public Health at Berkeley. It features news about preventive medicine and healthy living. Summaries of articles are available online, and full text comes with a paid subscription.

Research

America's Lifeline Online

http://www.mindspring.com/~hlthdata/lifeline.html

Images and graphs showing public health risks and statistics.

National Center for Health Statistics

http://www.cdc.gov/nchswww/nchshome.htm

Rural Health Network Home Page. http://www.uchsc.edu/sm/sm/rural/index.htm

Outcomes Assessment and Research
http://utsph.sph.uth.tmc.edu/www/utsph/CS/outcome.htm

Rural Health Care

Center for Rural Health and Social Service Development
http://www.siu.edu/~crhssd/

Critical Issues in Rural Health
http://ianrwww.unl.edu/ianr/agecon/rural/center/health/march.htm
Online journal.

Members of the U.S. House of Representatives Rural Health Care Coalition
http://www.nrharural.org/rhccmemb.html
Alphabetical listing of the 111 representatives who are members of the House Rural Health Care Coalition in the 104th Congress.

Research in Action: Improving Health Care for Rural Populations

http://www.ahcpr.gov/research/rural.htm

One-fourth of America's population lives in rural areas which, on the average, have higher poverty rates, a larger percentage of elderly and have fewer doctors hospitals, and other health resources.

Role of Telemedicine in Rural Health Care

http://www.nrharural.org/docs/ipaper7.html

An Issue Paper prepared by the National Rural Health Association in November of 1996.

Rural Health Network Home Page

http://www.uchsc.edu/sm/sm/rural/index.htm

A group of medical students striving to create a central information source for students interested in rural health care.

Travel Recommendations

Emporiatrics: An Introduction to Travel Medicine

http://indy.radiology.uiowa.edu/Providers/Textbooks/TravelMedicine/TravelMedHP.html

Includes advice to travelers with medical conditions. Note that the most common cause of death to travelers is by motor vehicle accidents.

International Travel Clinic

http://www.intmed.mcw.edu/travel/html

Moon Travel Handbooks

http://www.moon.com/staying_healthy

Staying healthy while traveling in Asia, Africa, and Latin America. Includes checklists and health supplies, traveler's aid organizations, advice on what to eat and drink, signs of illness, and how to get medical assistance.

Outdoor Action Guide to High Altitude Acclimatization and Illnesses

http://www.princeton.edu/~rcurtis/altitude.html

Travel Warning and Consular Information Sheets

http://travel.state.gov/travel_warnings.html

Includes the State Department's list of places that Americans are advised to avoid, as well as valuable information on the health situation in hundreds of other countries.

WHO's International Travel and Health Vaccination Requirements and Health Advice

http://jupiter.who.ch/programmes/emc/yellowbook/yb_home.htm

QUIZZES, TOOLS & ONLINE CALCULATORS

> *Covered in this section*: Alcohol Dependency; Fitness; Longevity; Mental Health; Miscellaneous; Pregnancy; Sexuality; Sleep.

Alcohol Dependency

Quizzes to Help Determine Alcohol Dependency

http://www.recovery.org/aa/aa-related/quizzes.txt

Fitness

Calculate Your Body Fat Percentage, Circumference Method

http://www.he.net/~zone/prothd2.html

Coronary Heart Disease Risk Assessment

http://www.amhrt.org/risk/index.html

Finding a Healthy Weight

http://www.amhrt.org/news/fad/fadnews.html

Longevity

Longevity Game

http://www.northwesternmutual.com/games/longevity/longevity-main.html

Input personal information to receive an estimate on how long you will live, based on research done by the life insurance industry.

Mental Health

Clinical Depression Screening Test
http://sandbox.xerox.com/pair/cw/testing.html

Keirsey Temperament Sorter
http://sunsite.unc.edu/personality/keirsey.html
Take an online personality test that sorts results according to the Myers-Briggs method.

Online Depression Screening Test
http://www.med.nyu.edu/Psych/screens/depres.html

Online Screening for Personality Disorders
http://www.med.nyu.edu/Psych/screens/pds.html

Online Screening for Anxiety Test
http://www.med.nyu.edu/Psych/screens/anx.html

Professional Life Stress Scale
http://www.hcc.hawaii.edu/hccinfo/facdev/StressTest.html
Take a test measuring the amount of stress in your life.

Miscellaneous

HDCN Urea Kinetics Calculators
http://www.medtext.com/dzer.htm
This site helps determine a patient's Kt/V, PCRn, and V values by completing a form about the patient and treatment data.

Online Clinical Calculator
http://www.intmed.mcw.edu/clincalc.html
This statistical calculator helps researchers determine the Bayesian Analysis of prevalence, sensitivity and specificity of data. It also aids in clinical calculations of estimated blood level, body surface/body mass ratio, weight and measurement conversions.

Pregnancy

OB/Gyn Toolbox

http://www.cpmc.columbia.edu/resources/obgyntools/

Includes tools such as: body surface area calculator, birth weight conversions, creatinine clearance estimation, endometriosis scoring, gestational age calculator, and OB ultrasound analyzer.

Pregnancy Calculator

http://fox.nstn.ca/~rgiffen/PregnancyCalculator.html

Sexuality

Online Sexual Disorders Screening for Men

http://www.med.nyu.edu/Psych/screens/sdsms.html

Online Sexual Disorders Screening for Women

http://www.med.nyu.edu/Psych/screens/sdsf.html

Sleep

Insomnia Quiz

http://www.healthouch.com/level1/leaflets/sleep/sleep024.htm

Sleep Disorder Tests

http://www.sleepnet.com/links/htm#sleep0

Sleep Questionnaire

http://www.proaxis/~iris/sleep_questionnaire/part_1.html

First part of a six-part, 201-question survey for insomniacs.

RARE DISEASES

Chronic Fatigue Syndrome

American Association for Chronic Fatigue Syndrome
http://weber.u.washington.edu/%7Ededra/aacfs1.html

CFS FAQ
http://www.alternatives.com/cfs-news/faq.htm

CFS-News
http://www.alternatives.com/cfs-news/cfs-news.html
    Electronic newsletter.

CFS-Oriented Discussion Lists
http://www.latrobe.edu.au/Glenn/CFS/MailList.html
    Information on about nine different chronic fatigue syndrome (CFS) online discussion groups and how to join.

Chronic Fatigue Syndrome
http://www.ncf.carleton.ca:80/ freenet/rootdir/menus/social. services/cfseir/CFSEIR.HP.html
    Electronic resources, newsletters, government agencies and articles related to chronic fatigue syndrome (CFS).

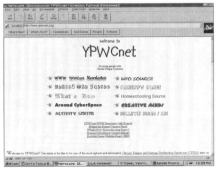

YPWCnet. *http://www.ypwcnet.org/*

Chronic Fatigue Syndrome Guide to Web Resources

http://www.cmhc.com/guide/cfs.htm

Chronic Fatigue Syndrome/Myalgic Encephalomyelitis

http://www.cais.com/cfs-news/

News, information, resources, discussion groups and links.

YPWCnet

http://www.ypwcnet.org/

This is a friendly, creative site for young people with chronic fatigue syndrome.

General Topics

ChronicIllNet

http://www.chronicillnet.org/

Multimedia information source dedicated to chronic illnesses such as AIDS, cancer, Persian Gulf War syndrome, autoimmune diseases, chronic fatigue syndrome, heart and neurological diseases. Offers general and specific information on diseases and research; facilitates discussion; and serves as a vehicle for data exchange. News, scientific articles, references, personal stories, calendar of events, bulletin board, and other web sources on chronic illness are provided.

National Organization for Rare Disorders, Inc. Home Page

http://www.pcnet.com/~orphan/

NORD is devoted to the identification, treatment and cure of rare disorders, which are defined as those affecting less than 200,000 Americans. This site describes NORD programs and events. The NORD database provides general disease information and organizational links based on search items. "NORD Online," a newsletter, describes government activity and legislative news. Action-alerts and medical updates offer research news and articles.

Neonatal Diseases and Abnormalities

http://www.mic.ki.se/Diseases/c16.html

This extensive collection of links assembled by the Karolinska Institute includes organizations, indexes and research facilities dealing with genetic,

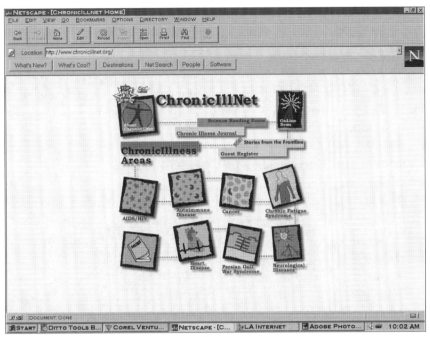

ChronicIllNet. *http://www.chronicillnet.org/*

neonatal and developmental disorders, such as jaundice, fetal alcohol syndrome, cystic fibrosis and Down syndrome.

Office of Rare Diseases

http://cancernet.nci.nih.gov/ord/

Information on more than 6,000 rare diseases by this office of the National Institute of health.

RARE-DIS: St John's University Rare Diseases List

http://tile.net/LISTSERV/raredis.html

To subscribe, send e-mail to: listserv@sjuvm.stjohns.edu with the message: "sub RARE-DIS your name."

Rare Diseases

http://www.richrtm.ok.state.edu/webfiles/raretxt.htm

This site provides information on 15 different rare disorders. Disease descriptions, causes, symptoms, diagnosis, treatment, research and medical support are offered.

Rare Genetic Diseases in Children

http://mcrcr4.med.nyu.edu/~murphp01/support.htm

This is a support-resources directory for parents whose child suffers from rare genetic disorders. Has links to hospice groups, death and dying support sites, parent-to-parent groups, respite care information, mailing lists, numerous newsgroups and bulletin boards. Both disease-specific and more general support links may be found.

Unknown and Rare Disorders/Diseases

http://www.dubuque.net/~manemann/

This site was created to serve those people and their families who suffer from an unknown disorder. Individuals describe their own or their family-member's unusual case history, with the hope that another reader will recognize the symptoms and respond with advice and answers about the unknown affliction.

Sexual & Reproductive Health

Adolescents

Coalition for Positive Sexuality
http://www.webcom.com/~cps/
> Information for teens.

Adoption

Adoption Policy Resource Center
http://www.fpsol.com/adoption/advocates.html
> Legislative news and analysis, adoption and subsidy information, legal resources, and links to related web sites.

AdoptioNetwork
http://207.226.25.92/

Faces of Adoption: America's Waiting Children
http://www.adopt.org/adopt/

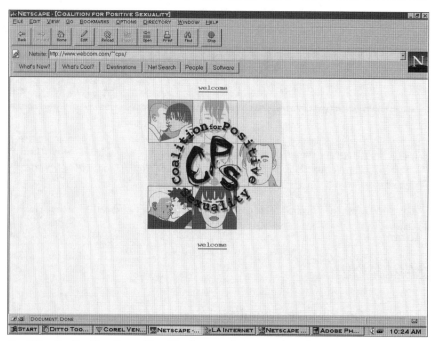

Coalition for Positive Sexuality. *http://www.webcom.com/~cps/*

Condoms

Condom Club International
http://www.webcom.com/~condom/club/club.html

Join Condom Club International to receive practical and novelty condoms through the mail every month.

Condom Country
http://www.condom.com/

Condoms and other items.

Condom Sense
http://www.csense.com/

Condom delivery, offering discreet service and discount name-brands.

Condom Shop

http://geewiz.com/std.html

Frequently asked questions (FAQs) and information from the Department of Health and Human Services.

Condomania Online

http://www.condomania.com/

News, safe sex information and products.

Condoms Express

http://www.webcom.com/~condom/express/express.html

Frequently asked questions (FAQs), products, tips and ordering information.

Official Condom Directory

http://users.deltanet.com/users/agkid/

Contraception

Contraceptive Guide

http://www.mjbovo.com/contracep.htm

Covers various methods of birth control.

Emergency Contraception Website

http://opr.princeton.edu/ec/ec.html

Information on emergency contraception and how to find locations where you can get it. You can prevent pregnancy up to 72 hours after having unprotected sex.

Nature's Method

http://upbeat.com/family/om.html

Calls itself the "ovulation method" and claims to be different from the "rhythm method."

Fertility

Family Helper
http://www.helping.com/family/helper.html
Information on infertility and adoption.

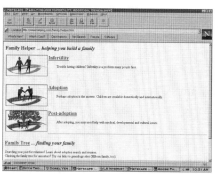

Family Helper.
http://www.helping.com/family/helper.html

Fertilitext
http://www.fertilititext.org/
News and information on fertility and infertility.

Fertility Weekly
http://www.homepage.holowww.com/1f.htm
A weekly digest on fertility and human reproduction.

Ferti.Net
http://www.ferti.net/
Information for health care professionals, researchers and patients interested in assisted fertilization and human reproduction. Infertility and infertility treatment literature and links.

Infertility Resources
http://www.ihr.com/infertility/index.html

MedWeb's Reproductive Medicine
http://www.gen.emory.edu/MEDWEB/keyword/reproductive_medicine.html

Northwestern University Center for Reproductive Science
http://kellye.bmbcb.nwu.edu/KEM.CRS/CRS.html

Spermatology WWW Home Page
http://numbat.murdoch.edu.au:80/spermatology/spermhp.html

Rainbow Query. *http://www.glweb.com/rainbowquery/*

Surrogacy

http://www.surrogacy.com/online_support/
> E-mail discussion lists and support groups on surrogacy topics.

General Topics

ALT.SEX FAQ

http://www.halcyon.com/elf/altsex/longdex.html
> Straightforward answers to sex questions.

American Social Health Association

http://sunsite.unc.edu/ASHA/

Atlanta Reproductive Health Centre WWW

http://www.ivf.com//index.html

HealthGate Healthy Sexuality

http://www.healthgate.com/healthy/sexuality/fs.index.html

Planned Parenthood

http://www.ciserv.com/PlannedParenthood2/

Enter your zip code to get information about local clinics and services.

Planned Parenthood Federation of America

http://www.igc.apc.org/ppfa/

Resources on sexual and reproductive health and education, including contraception, birth control, family planning; pregnancy, sexually transmitted diseases (STDs) and reproductive rights.

Rainbow Query

http://www.glweb.com/rainbowquery/

Features approximately 200 categories of information relating to human sexuality.

ReproLine

http://128.220.176.52/ReproLinerepro.html

Educational, non-profit source of information on reproductive health topics.

Herpes

Cafe Herpe

http://www.cafeherpe.com/

A genital herpes resource. Find information, products and online support groups.

Genital Herpes and Pregnancy Information

http://noah.cuny.edu/pregnancy/march_of_dimes/stds/herpesis.html

Herpes Home Page

http://www.minn.net/racoon/herpes

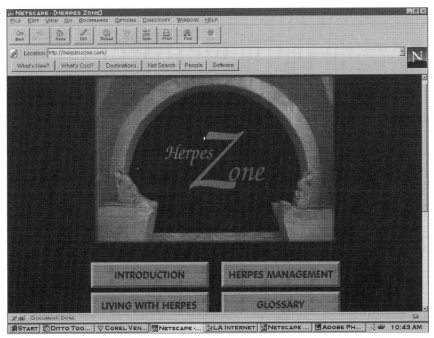

The Herpes Zone. *http://herpeszone.com/*

Herpes IRC Chat Page Information

http://www.power1.net/~budfrog/hpage.html

Features a link to the Dating Page, to meet others with herpes.

Herpes Zone

http://www.herpeszone.com/

All about herpes and how to manage it once you have it. Includes questions and answers, and resources.

Safe Sex

Safer Sex Page

http://safersex.org/

Sexual Disorders

Online Sexual Disorders Screening for Men
http://www.med.nyu.edu/Psych/screens/sdsms.html

Online Sexual Disorders Screening for Women
http://www.med.nyu.edu/Psych/screens/sdsf.html

Sexual Compulsives Anonymous
http://www.sca-recovery.org/

Sexually Transmitted Diseases

Allabout Center: Sexual Diseases
http://www.icemall.com/allabout/sexdis.html

Ask NOAH About: Sexually Transmitted Diseases
http://Noah.cuny.edu/stds/stds.html

AVSC International: Sexually Transmitted Diseases
http://www.avsc.org/stds.html

Access to Voluntary and Safe Contraception information on sexually transmitted diseases (STDs).

Johns Hopkins University STD Research Group
http://www.clark.net/pub/jhustd/

SHAPE: Sexual Health Advocate Peer Education Website
http://www.missouri.edu/~shape/

STD Home Page
http://med-www.bu.edu/people/sycamore/std/std.htm

Information on AIDS, chancroid, chlamydia, gonorrhea, hepatitis B, herpes simplex, public lice and scabies, syphilis, trichomona, and venereal warts. Includes information on what is risky behavior, a quiz, contacts and links.

STD Research Group

http://www.jhustd.org/pub/jhustd/stdpage.htm

From the Johns Hopkins University School of Medicine.

Transgender

FAQ: Hormone Therapy for Transsexuals

http://www.savina.com/confluence/hormones/

Notes on Gender Transition

http://www.avitale.com/

Transgender Forum

http://www.tgforum.com/

Transgender Information

http://www.ren.org/

From the Renaissance Education Association, Inc.

Skin & Connective Tissue / Dermatology

Ehlers-Danlos Syndrome

Ehlers-Danlos National Foundation
http://stgenesis.org/EDS/ednf.html

Ehlers-Danlos Syndrome Home Page
http://www.phoenix.net/~leigh/EDS/

Describes 10 symptoms of Ehlers-Danlos syndrome; offers links to additional resources and mailing list information; features poems and personal stories from patients who suffer from this disease.

General Topics

Contact Dermatitis Home Page
http://www.mc.vanderbilt.edu/vumcdept/derm/contact/

Currently this site lists allergens found in commercial patch-test kits, including synonyms and uses for the allergens, as well as background education and cross reactions.

Department of Dermatology
http://tray.dermatology.uiowa.edu/home.html

The University of Iowa's Department of Dermatology has created a point of access to an impressive number of dermatology-related web sites, image banks, organizations, etc. Also offers an introduction to basic dermatology, a tutorial in diagnosis, and the *Dermatology Online Journal*.

Dermatology Database

http://tray.dermatology/uiowa.edu/DermDB.htm

About 20 different categories of dermatology resources around the world, including career information, clinical images, government agencies, patient support groups and academic dermatology departments. Well-organized site.

Dermatology in the Cinema

http://www.skinema.com/

Dermatologist and film buff Dr. Reese has assembled examples of skin lesions and conditions found in movies to unite his two interests. Entertaining.

Dermatology Internet Server

http://www.derma.med.uni-erlangen.de/index_e.htm

Access to *Dermatology Online Atlas*, courses in dermatology, case reports, statistics, and resources from around the world.

Dermatology Online Journal

http://matrix.ucdavis.edu/DOJ.html

Includes original articles, case reports, commentary, and dermatology news updates. Access recent and past editions.

HealthWeb Dermatology Page

http://www.medlib.iupui.edu/cicnet/derma/derma.html

Includes a list of dermatologic disease resources, including educational resources, electronic publications, online discussion groups, organizations, and miscellaneous dermatological resources. The Dermatological Disease Resources section contains selected chapters and articles from books and journals, related web sites, clinical trial information and contacts, and National Institutes of Health reports.

InfoDerm

http://www.galderma.com/

Internet Dermatology Society

http://www.telemedicine.org/ids.htm

This site is geared to dermatologists worldwide. Its goal is to facilitate communication and share studies by creating an information clearinghouse. Besides society information, this site offers an electronic textbook of dermatology,

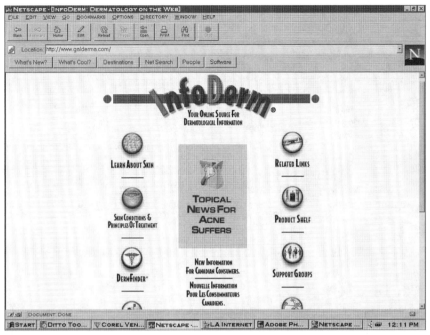

InfoDerm. *http://www.galderma.com/*

global dermatological grand rounds, internet teledermatology triage, dermatology lectures and mailing lists. Has links to the Women's Dermatologic Society and other groups.

Matrix Dermatology Resources

http://matrix.ucdavis.edu/

Contains the *Dermatology Online Journal*, *Atlas of the Skin*, *RxDerm Archives*, and *Tumors of the Skin*. Provides images and accompanying text for medical students and dermatologists.

National Skin Centre, Singapore Skin Web

http://medweb.nus.sg/nsc/nsc.html

Patient information as well as Centre activities and treatment programs for skin diseases. Includes information on laser skin re-surfacing and a "Handbook on Common Skin Disorders." There is also information on the effects ozone depletion, cosmetics and other environmental factors may have on the skin.

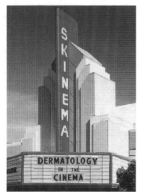

Dermatology in the Cinema. *http://itsa.ucsf. edu/~vcr/index.html*

Project Dermatology Online Atlas
http://www.medic.mie-u.ac.jp/derma/bilddb/db.htm

Goal is to create a hypermedia textbook of dermatology.

Skin and Connective Tissue Diseases
http://www.mic.ki.se/Diseases/c17.html

The Karolinska Institute has provided visitors to this site with a very long list of basic dermatology organizations and resources, as well as links to sites discussing specific skin and connective tissue conditions.

Skin Deep
http://www.grossbart.com/

Contains text from Dr. Ted Grossbart's book of the same name which considers emotions a major factor in skin problems. Chapters include, "Our Skin: Listening and Responding to the World Around You," "Why Me? The Skin Has Its Reasons," "Breaking the Itch/Scratch Cycle," and "The New Psychopsoriasis."

Skin (Diseases) Page
http://www.pinch.com/skin/

Hair Loss (Alopecia)

Alopecia Areata
http://weber.u.washington.edu/~dvictor/alopecia.html

General information and frequently asked questions about alopecia areata, a disease characterized by hair loss suspected to be an autoimmune system disorder. Information about diagnosis, prevalence, research and treatment, along with related web sites.

Alopecia Research and Resources

http://npntserver.mcg.edu/default.htm#npindex-2.1000

This web site is devoted to helping people with abnormal hair loss, also known as alopecia. It offers information and an opportunity to share personal stories, as well as guidelines for managing the disorder. There is a special focus on helping children with alopecia. German language documents also available. A large number of text files are available online through this site.

Hair Loss

http://biomed.nus.sg/nsc/hair.html

Living with Hair Loss

http://www.arcnewmedia.com/hairloss/

Sheila Jacobs lost her hair due to alopecia areata, and has written a book and conducted seminars to help others cope and treat their baldness. This web site lists organizations, articles, books, videos, newsgroups and bulletin boards to which people suffering from alopecia may turn for support and information.

Leprosy

Mycobacterium Leprae

http://www.who.ch/programmes/lep/

The microbiology of the disease and the organism responsible. Transmission and factors determining clinical expression are major sub-topics.

WHO Action Programme for the Elimination of Leprosy

http://www.who.ch/programmes/lep/lep_home.htm

Well-written overview of leprosy and its prevalence worldwide, as well as a description of the WHO program to eliminate the disease. Topics include the disease and its treatment, the global leprosy situation, and other resources such as relevant publications and a link to the leprosy discussion list. Also available in French.

Lupus

Arthritis Information: Lupus

http://ovchin.uc.edu/htdocs/arthritis/lupus.html

Online booklet with basic facts about lupus.

Circle of Friends: Autoimmune Disease and Lupus Support Group

http://members.aol.com//mycircle/index.htm

Colorado Health Net: Lupus Center

http://connect.colorado.edu/health/
_chn/lupus/lupus_main.html_

Information and issues concerning lupus. Includes facts and statistics about the disease, medications and treatment programs, lupus support services and resources, and a free link to ask an expert a lupus-related question. The Lupus Research and Information Library lists books, articles, videos, cassettes and additional web sites related to lupus.

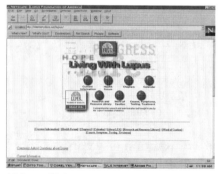

Living with Lupus.
http://internet-plaza.net/lupus/

Living with Lupus

http://internet-plaza.net/lupus/

The home page of the Lupus Foundation of America. Includes frequently asked questions, a research and resource library, and general information about the causes, symptoms, testing and treatment of lupus. Features a calendar of events, chapter activities and contacts. Has a helpful and friendly health forum where you can post questions, help others with answers to their questions, and share experiences, expertise, and/or support.

Lupus Association Home Page

http://www.ttsh.gov.sg/lupus/lupus.html

All about lupus, including patient's perspectives.

Lupus Channel Home Page

http://www.geocities.com/~lupus-channel/

Lupus frequently asked questions (FAQs) and chat group information; additional resources.

Lupus Clinical Overview

http://cerebral.com/lupus/overview.htm

Lupus Home Page

http://www.hamline.edu/~lupus/

For patients and others, this site offers a number of text files on lupus, from both clinical and patient perspectives. The Lupus Foundation of America provides general and clinical information, news briefs, lists of organizations, conferences, and meetings. Two mailing lists are also maintained, LUPUS-L (primarily for patients) and LUPUS-R (primarily for researchers). To subscribe, send e-mail to: listproc@piper.hamline.edu with the message "SUBSCRIBE LUPUS-L Yourfullname" or "SUBSCRIBE LUPUS-R Yourfullname," depending on which list you wish to join.

Systemic Lupus Erythematosus

http://vh.radiology.uiowa.edu/Providers/ClinRef/FPHandbook/Chapter06/ 07-6.html

Systemic Lupus Erythematosus Article

http://www.medicinenet.com/mainmenu/encyclop/ARTICLE/Art_S/ syslupis.htm

Pigmentation

International Albinism Center

http://lenti.med.umn.edu:80/iac/

This site of the International Albinism Center at the University of Minnesota provides a link to an electronic copy of *Facts about Albinism*, as well as links to related web sites.

National Incontentia Pigmenti Foundation
http://medhlp.netusa.net/www/nipf.htm

The NIPF is organized to encourage research and education about incontentia pigmenti, a rare genetic disease for which there is no cure. The disease initially manifests itself in the skin of newborn infants. This web site describes both the disease and Foundation activities.

Porphyria

American Porphyria Foundation Page
http://www.enterprise.net/apf/

The porphyrias are a group of rare metabolic diseases with many symptoms appearing in the skin, as well as in the neurologic system. This site offers in-depth information for patients and the public on porphyria, including information on diet and drug treatment.

Porphyria Web Links
http://darwin.clas.virginia.edu/~rjh9u/aip.html

This site offers about a dozen links to web pages related to this skin and neurologic disease, including an entry about King George III, who was suspected of suffering from this affliction.

Psoriasis

National Psoriasis Foundation On-Line Psoriasis Information Resource
http://www.psoriasis.org/

Offers general information on psoriasis, with statistics, photos and description. Includes psoriasis therapies and case histories, research efforts, Foundation activities, meetings, publications, as well as links to other psoriasis sites on the web.

Psoriasis
http://biomed.nus.sg/nsc/psoriasi.html

General information about the disease; some images.

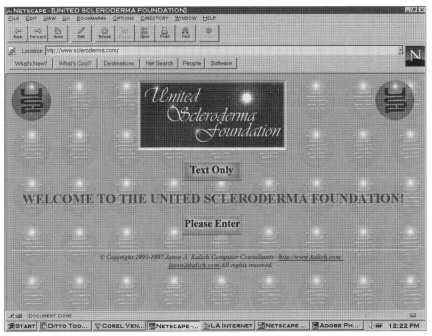

United Scleroderma Foundation. http://www.scleroderma.com/

Psoriasis Research

http://www.tecc.co.uk/psoriasis/

Questions and answers about psoriasis and psoriasis cures, personal accounts, celebrities who suffer from psoriasis, newsgroups about the skin condition and related sites.

Scleroderma

United Scleroderma Foundation

http://www.scleroderma.com/

Provides answers to some basic questions about scleroderma, a disease that results in hardening of the skin and multiple organs due to over-deposit of collagen. Foundation and support group information, scleroderma resources on the internet, and personal stories of patients with the disease are provided.

Sjogren's Syndrome

Sjogren's Syndrome Foundation
http://www.sjogrens.com/

This site acts as an information clearinghouse for Sjogren's Syndrome, an incurable autoimmune disorder where the body attacks its own moisture-producing glands causing dry eyes, mouth, and potentially worse effects.

Sweating (Hyperhidrosis)

Hyperhidrosis
http://www.parsec.it/summit/hyper1e.htm

Hyperhydrosis is excessive sweating in one or more localized portions of the body. This rare affliction has several manifestations and its cause is unknown. The web site offers an overview and description of the disease, its symptoms and treatment options. The page is also available in Italian and German languages.

Vitiligo

National Vitiligo Foundation
http://pegasus.uthct.edu/Vitiligo/index.html

Vitiligo is a spontaneous irregular depigmentation of skin which, while it does not have serious health consequences, does cause much suffering because of social consequences. The National Vitiligo Foundation site describes efforts to promote education and research, and offers support and information for patients and their families. In addition, there are links to other web sites and mail lists related to vitiligo.

V.I.P. - The Vitiligo Information Page
http://goofy.ti6.tu-harburg.de/vitiligo/

Links and information on vitiligo, personal accounts, frequently asked questions and a sample image of this disease. Includes sections on alternative treatments and cosmetics. To subscribe to the vitiligo newsgroup, send e-mail to:

Xeroderma Pigmentosum Society. http://www.xps.org/home.htm

LISTSERV@SJUVM.STJOUHNS.EDU with the message: "SUB VITILIGO Yourfirstname Yourlastname."

Xeroderma Pigmentosum

NORD Information on Xeroderma Pigmentosum
http://www.stepstn.com/nord/rdb_sum/339.htm

General information about this group of rare inherited skin disorders characterized by a heightened reaction to sunlight (photosensitivity).

Xeroderma Pigmentosum
http://www.icondata.com/health/pedbase/files/XERODERM.HTM

Clinical information from the Multimedia Medical Reference Library (MMRL).

Xeroderma Pigmentosum Society, Inc.

http://xps.org/home.htm

This site is devoted to a rare genetic disorder, xeroderma pigmentosum, whose sufferers are unable to tolerate ultraviolet radiation (especially sunlight). The Society seeks to promote awareness of and research into XP, and to support patients and their families. Browsers may obtain a copy of the Society newsletter, and the site provides a list of other publications, organizations, newsgroups and individuals that may be contacted for further information.

SLEEP & SLEEP DISORDERS

Dreams

Association for the Study of Dreams
http://www.outreach.org/gmcc/asd/

Dr. Dream's Resources for People Who Dream
http://www.dr-dream.com/

Dream Lynx
http://www.iag.net/~hutchib/.dream/

Dream Wave
http://www.dreamwv.com/nav.html

Dream Weaver's Web
http://www.webcom.com/dreamwvr/
     Jungian dream analysis.

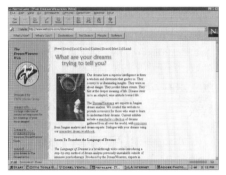

Eclectic Dreams
http://www.phys.unsw.edu.au/~mettw/ edreams/home.html

The Dream Weaver's Web.
http://www.webcom.com/dreamwvr/

Gothic Skywalker's Dream Analysis
http://www.geocities.com/TimesSquare/Dungeon/3913/dream.html

Nightmares, Dreams and Sleep

http://www.proaxis.com/~iris/
    Counseling software and links.

Storyspace Cluster - Dreams

http://www.twine.stg.brown.edu/projects/hypertext/landow/SSPCluster/
Dreams.html

Working (and Playing) with Dreams

http://www1.rider.edu/~suler/dreams.html

General Topics

Diagnosing and Treating Sleep Disorders

http://www.njc.org/MSUhtml/MSU_sleep.html
    Maintained by the National Jewish/University of Colorado Sleep Disorders
Center.

National Sleep Foundation

http://www.sleepfoundation.org/
    Includes information on sleep disorders.

Normal Sleep Cycle

http://www4.umdnj.edu/med/slepsymp.html

On Sleep and Sleeplessness

gopher://gopher.vt.edu:10010/02/39/26/
    Written by Aristotle, in 350 B.C.

Phantom Sleep Page

http://www.newtechpub.com/phantom/

Simmons Company Sleep Information

http://www.simmonsco.com/sleep.info/

Sleep Disorder Centers of America

http://www.sleep-sdca.com/

Sleep Disorder Tests

http://www.sleepnet.com/links/htm#sleep0

Sleep Disorders

http://www.familyinternet.com/peds/scr/00800sc.htm#Prevention

Sleep Home Pages

http://bisleep.medsch.ucla.edu/

Sleep Medicine Home Page

http://www.cloud9.net/%7Ethorpy/

A lot of links to other sites, including sleep-related newsgroups and discussion groups. Alphabetical listing of sleep disorders is available, along with information broken down by the following topics: clinical practice, professional associations, journals, sleep research sites, government information, medications, meetings, centers around the world, book reviews and organizations.

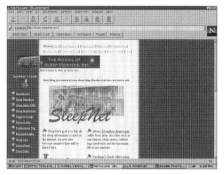

SleepNet. *http://www.sleepnet.com/*

Sleep Well

http://www-leland.stanford.edu/~dement/

SleepDocs Online

http://www.cloud9.net/%7Ethorpy/sleepdoc.html

Sleepnet

http://www.sleepnet.com/

Sleep/Wake Disorders Canada

http://www.geocities.com/HotSprings/1837/

Information about sleep and an introduction to sleeping disorders, including frequently asked questions, diagnosis, books, online and off-line resources.

Humor

Lighter Side of Sleep
http://www-leland.stanford.edu/~dement/sleephumor.html

Insomnia

Insomnia
http://www.saonet.ucla.edu/health/healthed/HANDOUTS/insomnia.htm
This handout offers a brief description of insomnia, its causes, symptoms and treatments.

Insomnia? Just Go to Sleep and Forget About It
http://www.well.com/user/mick/insomnia/
Techniques for insomniacs.

Insomnia Quiz
http://www.healthouch.com/level1/leaflets/sleep/sleep024.htm

Overcoming Insomnia
http://www.hcn.net/au/healthworks/contents/insomnia.htm
Site provides the table of contents for this online book without charge. To read the full text, a user I.D. must be purchased.

Sleep Insomnia Program
http://www.proaxis.com/~iris/sleep.html

Sleep Questionnaire
_http://www.proaxis/~iris/sleep_questionnaire/part_1.html_
First part of a six-part, 201-question long survey for insomniacs.

Melatonin

Melatonin Central
http://www.melatonin.com/

Restless Legs Syndrome Foundation. *http://www.rls.org/*

MIT Study on Melatonin
http://web.mit.edu:1962/tiserve.mit.edu/9000/35029.html

Narcolepsy

Center for Narcolepsy Research
http://www.uic.edu/depts/cnr/index.htm

Cure Narcolepsy Now!
http://www.cloud9.net/~thorpy/NARCO.HTML

Stanford University Center for Narcolepsy
http://www-med.Stanford.EDU/school/Psychiatry/narcolepsy/

Restless Leg Syndrome

Restless Leg Syndrome Support Site
http://www.rls.org/

Restless Legs Syndrome Foundation, Inc.
_http://www.stepstn.com/nord/org_sum/77.htm_

Sleep Apnea

A.W.A.K.E. New York
http://www.bway.net/~marlene/awake.html

Big Apple Support and Education for Sleep Apnea.

Central Sleep Apnea Informational Page
http://members.aol.com/blackcover/csa.html

Sleep Apnea
http://www.i1.net/~sifuchar/apnea.html

Sleep apnea is a breathing disorder during sleep which is often accompanied by loud snoring. Individuals with sleep apnea may stop breathing many times during sleep.

SURGERY

Anesthesiology

Anesthesiology Clinical Manuals and Resources

http://www.anes.ccf.org:8080/lab2.htm

GASNet

http://gasnet.med.yale.edu/

The Global Anesthesiology Server Network (GASNet) is for the anesthesiology community world wide. Abstracts, journals, newsletters, meetings, book reviews, discussion groups, software and video library, further links to anesthesiology organizations and information sites are all provided at this site. Reference area includes the *Global Textbook of Anesthesiology.*

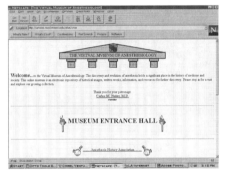

The Virtual Museum of Anesthesiology.
http://umdas.med.miami.edu/aha/vma

SUNY Health Science Center - Syracuse Department of Anesthesiology

http://eja.anes.hscsyr.edu/anes/home.html

Anesthesiology meetings calendar, medical professionals internet registry, and mailing list database. Links and program information.

Virtual Anaesthesia Textbook

http://gasnet.med.yale.edu/vat/VAT.html

Virtual Museum of Anesthesiology

http://umdas.med.miami.edu/aha/vma

Historical images, written works, information and resources regarding the history of anesthesiology. Includes a portrait gallery and images of early anesthetic equipment and devices, as well as written archives.

Wright's Anesthesia and Critical Care Resources on the Internet

http://www.eur.nl/FGG/ANEST/wright/

Site provides a link to the ACCRI discussion group on anesthesiology and critical care topics. Thorough and precise site includes news and a featured internet site of the month, discussion list, FTP sites, peer-reviewed journals, other gopher resources, and an exhaustive list of hundreds of anesthesiology web sites around the world. A bibliography and non-net educational resources (mostly software and CD-ROM) are offered as well.

Cataract Surgery

Cataract Surgery

http://mystic.biomed.mcgill.ca/Medinf/Home/ZSPROJECTS/Opthalmology/OphthHpertext/Contents.html

Interactive tutorials in cataract surgery topics.

Computers and Surgery

Computer Aided Surgery

http://journals.wiley.com/cas/

Journal.

International Society for Computer Aided Surgery

http://www.iscas.org/

Internet Resources of Computer Aided Surgery

http://www.aist.go.jp/NIBH/~b0673/english/cas.html

Medical Robotics and Computer-Assisted Surgery

*http://www.cs.cmu.edu/afs/cs/
project/mrcas/www/mrcas-home/
MRCAS.html*

Video Surgery

*http://www.mindspring.com/
~videosur/*

Video Surgery.
http://www.mindspring.com/~videosur/

Virtual Environments and Real-Time Deformations for Surgery Simulation

http://www.cc.gatech.edu/gvu/visualization/surgsim/

The goal of this project is to explore deformations of organs in a surgery scene while emphasizing real-time interaction.

Dental and Oral Surgery

Columbia-Presbyterian Medical Center School of Dental and Oral Surgery

http://cpmcnet.columbia.edu/dept/dental/

Information about the Columbia program, courses and tutorials in dental ethics, dental informatics, dental trauma, oral pathology and more.

Maxillofacial Surgery Resources on the Web

http://bpass.dentistry.dal.ca/mfsurg.html

Oral Surgery Center

http://cust.iamerica.net/molar/

Links to maxillofacial surgery departments at academic institutes and to related dentistry and medical sites, and to a maxillofacial graphic-of-the-month.

General Topics

Emphysema

http://www.columbia.net/phys/emph.html

The surgical treatment of emphysema is discussed.

General Surgery

http://indy.radiology.uiowa.edu/Providers/ClinRef/FPHandbook/09.html

From the Family Practice Handbook of the University of Iowa, this site discusses wound management, pre-op and post-op care. Some sections include the general surgical treatment of abdominal pain, appendicitis, gall bladder disorders, burns and more. Written in outline form.

Questions to Ask Your Doctor Before You Have Surgery

http://www.ahcpr.gov/consumer/surgery.htm

Checklist of issues that should be addressed and understood before a surgical operation, and the reasons for asking them. Assembled by the Agency for Health Care Policy and Research. Additional sources are also listed.

Neurosurgery

Brain Surgery Information Center

http://www.brain-surgery.com/

"Everything you wanted to know about brain surgery...almost." The goal of this site is to provide usable, non-technical information about the conditions which require brain surgery. It offers a primer on brain tumors, information on aneurysms, hemorrhages, and other sources of "brain attack.' The site also describes the brain surgery patient's experience.

Center for Minimally Invasive Brain Surgery

http://nsi.tjh.tju.edu/MIBS/mibs.html

Major topics include gamma knife radiosurgery, image-guided micro-neurosurgery, restorative neurosurgery, neuroendoscopy, and stereotopic neurosurgery. Updates, news and general information are also offered.

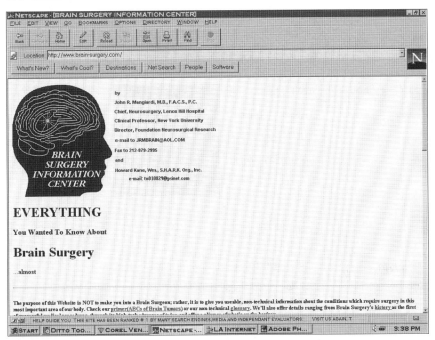

Brain Surgery Information Center. http://www.brain-surgery.com/

Department of Neurosurgery at NYU

http://mcns10.med.nyu.edu/index.html

This site serves as a resource center for patients suffering from neurological disorders, their families and health care professionals. Electronic consultations are invited, and the site also provides access to support groups for individuals who have undergone neurosurgery. The Neurosurgery Internet Grand Rounds includes actual case studies.

Gamma Knife

http://www.elekta.com/gkintro.html

Information about this non-invasive instrument for the treatment of brain tumors, vascular malformations and functional disorders. Information about the technology and procedures for use, as well as information about the technology and procedure, indications treated, patient support, and bibliographical references.

Neurological Surgery: The Center for Spine Surgery at NYU

http://mcns10.med.nyu.edu/spine/spine_main.html

Includes information about some spinal disorders and their treatment.

Topics in Neurosurgery
http://neurosurgeon.com/

Orthopedic Surgery

Orthopedic Surgery Mailing List
http://www.sechrest.com/ortho/index.html

Site provides information on the orthopedic mailing list, but also membership directory, newsgroups, orthopedic surgery grand rounds, FTP site, and numerous related links. To subscribe, send e-mail to: orthopedic-request@weston.com with the following message: "SUBSCRIBE your_first_name your_last_name."

Orthopaedic Surgery on the Web
http://www.swmed.edu:80/home_pages/facultystaff/may/orthosurgeMay/orthosites.html

Colleges, universities, societies, news and discussion groups, educational resources, clinics and institutes related to orthopedics.

Pain Management

Pain Control After Surgery: A Patient's Guide
http://www.roxane.com/Rosane/RPI/HealthcareProfessionalLibrary/AHCPR/apmp1

Advice on assessing and managing pain felt after surgical procedures.

Plastic Surgery

American Society for Aesthetic Plastic Surgery
http://surgery.org/

Describes the most common cosmetic surgery procedures and offers advice on selecting a qualified surgeon. Site is geared to anybody considering a cosmetic surgical procedure, from eye-lid surgery to "body contouring."

Body Space. *http://www.surgery.com/body/topics/body.html*

Best Plastic Surgery Site of the Week

http://www.phudson.com/BESTPS/bestweek.html

Body Space

http://www.surgery.com/body/topics/body.html

Cosmetic Surgery On-Line

http://www.mayo.edu/staff/plastic/Cosmetic/CSOLMain.html

Site discusses who may be a candidate for cosmetic surgery, what the surgery will entail, and a description of all of the specific cosmetic surgical procedures.

E-STHETICS

http://www.phudson.com/

Cosmetic plasctic surgery.

Interplast

http://www.worldaccess.com/NonProfitOrganizations/Interplast/

Interplast is an affiliation of volunteer surgeons, pediatricians, anesthesiologists, nurses and support personnel who work with third world nations to support and develop a free reconstructive surgery programs for children and adults with birth defects, burns, and other crippling deformities. The organization performs over 1500 free surgeries annually. Information about the organization and the trips it has scheduled may be found at this site.

Plastic Surgery Information Service

http://www.plasticsurgery.org/

Site is maintained by the American Society of Plastic and Reconstructive Surgeons and the Plastic Surgery Educational Foundation. It provides news, the latest advances and techniques, professional information, statistics, and a referral service.

Plastic Surgery Link

http://www.nvpc.nl/plink/

Provides numerous links to societies, journals, academic and medical organization, newsgroups, research programs, and more related to plastic surgery.

PRS-Net

http://webmed.com/prs/hotlinks.html

Plastic and reconstructive surgery on the web. This site offers a long list of university programs, journals, societies, and patient and research information.

University of Iowa Plastic Surgery

http://www.surgery.uiowa.edu:80/surgery/plastic/

Information about reconstructive and cosmetic surgery procedures for potential patients and the general public.

TRANSPLANTATION

Covered in this section: Bone Marrow Transplantation; Ethics; General Topics; Heart; Kidney and Pancreas; Liver; Lung.

Bone Marrow Transplantation

See also: Cancer/Oncology - Bone Marrow Transplantation.

BMT (Bone Marrow Transplant) Newsletter
http://nyernet.org/bcic/bmt/bmt.news.html

Bone Marrow Donors Worldwide
http://BMDW.LeidenUniv.NL

Collects information on bone marrow donors from 43 donor and cord blood registries in 30 countries, and seeks to match them up with BMT recipients.

Bone Marrow Transplant and Cancer Treatment
http://137.42.95/BMTCancer/BMT.html

This site offers an overview on bone marrow transplantation for patients, their families, and other interested public. Many images and tables are used to supplement the basic text about cancer treatments, the human immune system, and the bone marrow transplantation process.

Bone Marrow Transplantation
http://oncolink.upenn.edu/specialty/chemo/bmt/

For both physicians and patients, this OncoLink (University of Pennsylvania) site offers a large number of resources about bone marrow transplantation, as well as tutorials, slide shows, news, publications and support organizations. It includes the text of *Bone Marrow Transplants: A Basic Book for Patients*, which offers 12 chapters on many different aspects of BMT. Thorough, but geared to the non-professional.

Bone Marrow Transplants: A Book of Basics for Patients
http://nysernet.org/bcic/bmt/bmt.book/toc.html

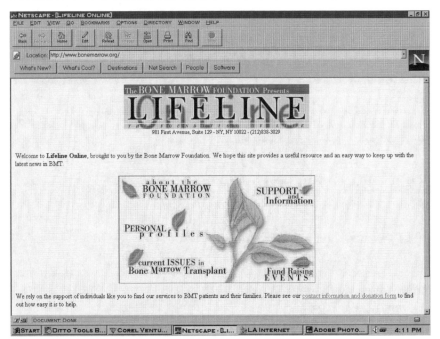

Lifeline Online: The Bone Marrow Foundation. *http://www.bonemarrow.org/*

Lifeline Online: The Bone Marrow Foundation

http://www.bonemarrow.org/

Ethics

Can We Transplant Organs from Animals?

http://whyfiles.news.wisc.edu/007transplant/index.html

Non-Heart Beating Organ Donors - A Medical, Legal and Ethical Overview

http://www.transweb.org/donation_folder/nhbd_text.html

Transplant Ethics

gopher://info.med.yale.edu:70/11/Disciplines/Disease/Transplant/Ethics

General Topics

American Share Foundation
http://www.asf.org/

American Society of Transplant Physicians
http://www.astp.org/

Division of Transplantation
http://www.hrsa.dhhs.gov/bhrd/dot/dotmain.html

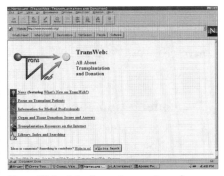

The Division of Transplantation (DOT) of the Health Resources and Services Administration, Department of Health and Human Services, manages the Organ Procurement and Transplantation Network and other organ transplant registries. DOT also provides assistance to organ procurement organizations and

TransWeb. *http://www.transweb.org/*

acts in the area of public education. This site provides facts and statistics about solid organ and bone marrow transplantation, including technical data, health guidelines, a description of the donation and transplantation process, and links to further organizations and publications.

Emory Transplant Center
http://Picasso.eushc.org/transplant/homepage.cgi

Experimental Organ Preservation
http://sapphire.surgery.wisc.edu/preservation/

National Transplant Assistance Fund
http://www.libertynet.com:80/~txfund

Organ and Tissue Coalition on Donation
http://www.infi.net/~donation/

This organization was created to educate the public about organ and tissue donation. The site describes Coalition activities and provides graphs and statistical information on transplantation.

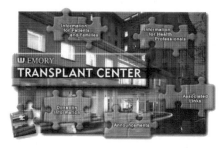

Emory Transplant Center. *http://Picasso.eushc.org/transplant/homepage.cgi*

Surviving Transplantation

http://www.stjosephs.london.on.ca/SJHC/about/programs/mental/survive/

An online guide to coping for persons undergoing major organ transplant.

Tissue Donation

http://quality.red-cross.org/tissue

What is tissue donation? Share the stories of families and patients who have received a donation and learn more about being a tissue donor at this American Red Cross site.

Transplantation on the Web

http://hageman.trnovo.kclj.si/transplant/transweb_e.html

Web sources related to organ and tissue transplantation. Includes not only general resources, but also links to transplantation centers, donor organizations and organ banks, brain death resources, information on histocompatability and bone marrow transplantation.

TransWeb

http://www.transweb.org/

All about organ transplantation and donation. This site includes news, research and patient information, personal stories of transplants, as well as frequently asked questions and answers. Additional resources, organizations and a library search are also available.

United Network for Organ Sharing (UNOS)

http://204.127.237.11/

This site provides facts and statistics about organ transplantation. Information on specific organs, data on survival, prevalence, and a brief history of transplantation are available. Also find UNOS resources and policy proposals, events, publications and related web sites.

Heart

Heart Transplantation at UCLA
http://www.nursing.ucla.edu/Userpages/mwoo/special/htx.htm
> Evaluation and management, and pre- and post-transplant protocols.

Journal of Heart and Lung Transplantation
http://www.mosby.com/Mosby/Periodicals/Medical/JHLT/lt.html

Questions about Heart and Lung Transplantation
http://www.transweb.org/faq/faq_heartlung.html

Transplant
http://www.geocities.com/Heartland/Hills/2571/transplant.htm
> Site addresses basic questions about heart transplantation.

Kidney and Pancreas

Kidney Transplant/Dialysis Association
http://www.ultranet.com/~ktda/index.shtml

My Kidney/Pancreas Transplant
http://members.aol.com/OhLarry922/home.html

Pancreas and Kidney Transplantation
http://www.diabetes.ca/news/trnsplnt.htm

Questions about Kidney Transplant
http://www.transweb.org/faq/faq_kidney.html

Tissot Family Kidney Transplant Stories
http://www.oro.net/~genet/kidney.html
> Personal story to promote living-donor kidney transplantation.

Liver

Facts and FAQ's on Liver Transplantation
http://sadieo.ucsf.edu/alf/alffinal/infoltxfaqs.html

Hepatitis Haven
http://www.tiac.net/users/birdlady/hep.html

Set up for those who have chronic hepatitis, this site contains personal stories and pictures of individuals suffering from the disease, as well as a directory of doctors and support groups, tips for receiving Social Security and liver transplant information.

Liver Transplantation
http://www.livertransplantation.org/

This site was developed to aid the exchange of academic papers and ideas regarding all aspects of liver transplantation.

Lung

Second Wind Lung Transplant Association, Inc.
http://www.arthouse.com/secondwind/

UNOS (United Network for Organ Sharing) Lung Transplant Centers by state, information on financing a transplantation operation, basic organ donation information, transplantation recovery advice, and personal stories.

VIRTUAL MEDICINE & MULTIMEDIA

Anatomy

3D Digital Human Anatomy

_http://www.eai.com/ interactive/dhuman/ dhuman_cdrom.html_

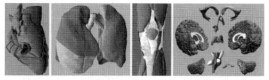

The Digital Anatomist.
http://www1.biostr.washington.edu/DigitalAnatomist.html

This is a demo site for a CD-ROM entitled "Dissectible Human" which contains photographs and movie images of digitally reconstructed systems of the body. Images of the skeletal, muscular, cardiovascular, neural, digestive, respiratory, urinary and reproductive systems have been created from cross-sections of a human cadaver.

Digital Anatomist Program Interactive Atlases

http://www9.biostr.washington.edu/da.html

Interactive atlases of the brain, neuro system, thoracic organs, and knee. With colorful graphics, radiological images and 3-D animations.

Virtual Anatomy Project

http://www.vis.colostate.edu/library/gva/gva.html

Site describes this Colorado State University program to generate a 3-D geometric database of the human body.

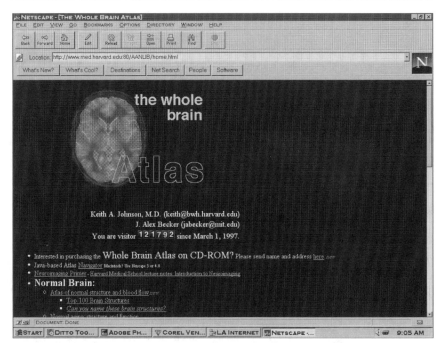

The Whole Brain Atlas. *http://www.med.harvard.edu:80/AANLIB/home.html*

Brain

Human Brain Project
http://WWW-HBP.scripps.edu/Home.html

The Human Brain Project is a long-term research initiative to create a database containing a full range of information about the brain, behavior, and related technological services. Its goal is to help scientists learn how various aspects of the brain function together. The site at Scripps Research Institute is the "master server," and connections to 17 other research institutions which have contributed to the Brain Project Database are provided at this site. Some of the projects currently being undertaken include language/brain mapping, a neural simulation project, a study of the action of drugs on the nervous system, and a 3-D reconstruction of the cerebral cortex.

Structural Information Framework for Brain Mapping
http://www1.biostr.washington.edu/BrainProject.html

This project's goal is to develop a system for organizing, visualizing, integrating and sharing information about human language function.

Whole Brain Atlas

http://www.med.harvard.edu:80/AANLIB/home.html

Computed tomography (CT), magnetic resonance (MR) and other radiographic images of a normal brain and of brains from patients with cerebrovascular disease, neoplastic disease, degenerative disease, and inflammatory or infectious disease. The images may be accessed in sequence, and specific views and anatomic parts of the brain may be selected. The accompanying neuroimaging primer is geared towards those without a technical background. "Tours" and time-lapse "movies" are also provided.

General Topics

Center for Human Simulation

http://www.uchsc.edu/sm/chs/about.html

This site describes the projects going on at the University of Colorado's Center for Human Simulation.

Medical Robotics and Computer-Assisted Surgery

http://www.cs.cum.edu/afs/cs.cmu .edu/project/mrcas/www.mrcas-home/MRCAS.html

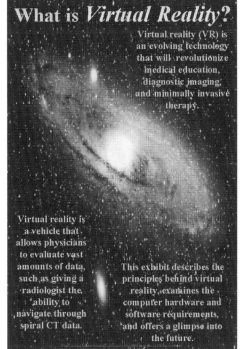

Principles of Virtual Reality Imaging.
http://indigo2.medeng.bgsm.edu/pvri/01vr.html

This site presents several projects concerning medical robotics and computer-assisted surgery. Surgical simulation, image overlay, implant guidance systems and telemedicine projects are described.

Multimedia Medical Reference Library

http://www.med-library.com,

Connect and search this library for software, images, audio files, medical school links, journals and hospitals.

Net Medicine

http://www.netmedicine.com/

Search the internet. Features Cyberpatient Simulator, Medfinder search, EKG of the Month, Radiology Rounds and Pediatric Topics.

Principles of Virtual Reality Imaging

http://indigo2.medeng.bgsm.edu/pvri/

This site offers a dramatic, online exhibit describing the basics of virtual reality, and clinical applications of this technology (e.g., "Drive through Bowels") as well as how it is all done. Modeling software, hardware resources, and additional references are provided.

Project Hippocrates

http://www.cs.cmu.edu/afs/cs/project/mrcas/www/hippocrates.html

This site describes a project whose goal is to develop less invasive, computer-assisted surgical robots, in this case for hip replacement surgery. A biomechanics-based surgical simulator will help surgeons determine the results of a proposed surgical plan which, when combined with the precision of surgical robots, will allow for the ideal surgery.

Slice of Life

http://www-medlib.med.utah.edu/sol/sol.html

Slice of Life is a non-profit project whose goal is to encourage the development of multimedia applications for use in health sciences education. Slice of Life produces and distributes videos, CD-ROMs and computer software. It also offers annual workshops to encourage multimedia sharing of ideas and expertise. Access to a catalog may be found at this site, and demos may be downloaded.

Three Dimensional Medical Reconstruction

http://www.crd.ge.com/esl/cgsp/projects/medical/

A collection of movie clips showing various medical reconstructions, such as colon, lung, brain, torso and skull fly-throughs.. Images were gathered from slice data from medical imaging modalities such as magnetic resonance or computed tomography. The two-dimensional slice data from these scanners was used as input for the three-dimensional reconstructions.

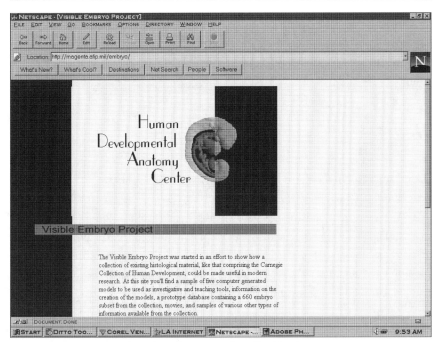

The Visible Embryo Project. *http://magenta.afip.mil/embryo/*

Virtual Environments, 3D Medical Imaging, and Computer Graphics Lab

http://www.afit.af.mil/Schools/EN/ENG/LABS/GRAPHICS/3dmiprojects/
3dmi.html

This site uses somewhat technical language to describe the 3D medical imaging research projects being undertaken by the Air Force Institute of Technology's Graduate School of Engineering. It offers a long reference list of books as well as web links on computer graphics, virtual reality, virtual environments, medical imaging and related resources.

Virtual Hospital

http://indy.radiology.uiowa.edu/VirtualHospital.html

Includes information for health care providers and patients, as well as educational materials, tutors and information about VIDA (Volumetric Imaging Display and Analysis).

Visualization Toolkit

http://www.cs.rpi.edu/~martink/

Computer software for 3D visualization. Used for medical images.

"Whole Frog" Project

http://www-itg.lbl.gov/ITG.hm.pg.docx/whole.Frog/Whole.Frog.Talk.html

This is a project that uses computer-based 3-D visualization to explore the anatomy of a frog.

Heart

The Heart: An Online Exploration

http://sln.fi.edu/biosci/heart.html

This is a great site for the general public and especially children to learn everythingabout the heart: anatomy, development, function and health tips. Images and movies depicting open heart surgery and blood flow are provided, along with recordings of actual heartbeats. Less scientific topics such as the heart in literature and poetry, healthy recipes and exercises are also included.

Interactive Medicine

Cyberounds

http://cyberounds.com/

Online interactive grand rounds and medical conference lectures by and for physicians. Each month, find a new presentation and follow-up discussion.

Interactive Patient

http://medicus.marshall.edu/medicus.htm

Marshall University School of Medicine has created this site to be a teaching tool for physicians, residents and medical students. Simulating an actual patient encounter, the patient's chief complaint is provided, and it is up to the user to ask the proper questions to obtain additional history, physical exam information, tests, and x-rays, then to come up with a diagnosis and treatment plan. The diagnosis and treatment plan are submitted over the web, and feedback is provided.

Outline of the Virtual Hospital

http://indy.radiology.uiowa.edu/Misc/Outline.html

Created by the University of Iowa's Department of Radiology, this site is self-described as a continuously updated digital health sciences library that provides patient care support and distance learning to practicing physicians and other professionals. The Virtual Hospital's search engine allows you to search the entire library database to learn about disorders, symptoms, treatments, and support organizations. Information for patients provides instructional and educational materials by title, organ system, and department. Information for health care providers also includes Continuing Medical Education courses, conferences, a physician consultation and referral center.

Physiological Imaging

http://everest.radiology.uiowa.edu/

Three-dimensional gallery of movies, images, research, tutorials and case studies.

Mental Health

Virtual Reality Exposure Therapy

http://www.ca.gatech.edu/gvu/virtual/phobia/

This site describes research into the use of virtual reality devices in therapy which involves exposing a patient to anxiety-producing stimuli while letting the anxiety fade away in an effort to free the patient from his or her phobia. In this case, the patient is exposed to a virtual environment, which can be controlled more easily. An animation designed to help patients who have a fear of elevators is provided.

Surgery

See also Surgery - Computers and Surgery.

Virtual Environments and Real-Time Deformations for Surgery Simulation

http://www.cc.gatech.edu/gvu/visualization/surgsim/

This project explores deformations of organs in a surgery scene while emphasizing real-time interaction.

Visible Man/Woman

Human Anatomy On Line
http://www.ucar.edu/staffnotes/12.94/vizman.html
> Access to the Visible Man.

Marching Through the Visible Man
http://www.crd.ge.com/esl/cgsp/projects/vm/
> This hypertext paper describes the methodology for using the Visible Male's computed tomography (CT) data to create models of the skin, bone, muscle and bowels.

Marching through the Visible Woman
http://www.crd.ge.com/cgi-bin/vw.pl
> This is a companion paper to Marching Through the Visible Man, and it describes the on-going efforts to process the computed tomography data obtained from the National Library of Medicine's Visible Woman Project, which used the cadaver data of a 59-year-old woman. In contrast with the Visible Man whose cross-section images are 1 mm apart, the Visible Woman's CT slices are .3 mm apart.

Visible Embryo Project
http://magenta.afip.mil/embryo/
> The Human Developmental Anatomy Center's Visible Embryo Project provides computer-generated models and a prototype database containing embryo images for research and teaching.

Visible Human Female Browser
http://www.uchsc.edu/sm/chs/browse_f.html
> Click on any part of the opening coronal view of the Visible Human Female to view the traverse section data.

Visible Human Knee Images
http://www.rad.upenn.edu/rundle/InteractiveKnee.html
> This site provides sagittal and axial radiological views of the human knee. Selecting and clicking on a part of the image pulls up a closer view with descriptive text that describes definitions, location, and activity.

Visible Human Male Browser

http://www.uchsc.edu/sm/ chs/browse_m.html

Clicking anywhere on the opening image of this site, which shows the coronal view of the Visible Human Male, calls up the traverse image that was used to create the coronal view.

Visible Human Male Products

http://www.uchsc.edu/sm/ chs/vhm.html

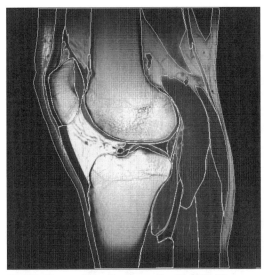

Visible Human Knee Images - Sagittal MR View.
http://www.rad.upenn.edu/rundle/Knee/ kneeMRICONT.html

This site offers sample images, reconstructions and animations of the Visible Human Male, as well as VHM products and specs, and access to the Visible Human Male Browser.

Visible Human Project

http://www.nlm.nih/gov/research/visible/visible_human.html

The U.S. National Library of Medicine project to create complete, anatomically detailed, 3-D representations of the male and female bodies online. Currently, the project includes collecting traverse computed tomography (CT), magnetic resonance (MR) and cryosection images of representative male and female fresh and frozen cadavers. Some collections of images are available at this site, and samples may be found at NLM's FTP site: mlmpubs.mlm.nih.gov. Scaled-down versions are available as *.gif images on the NLM gopher (gopher.nlm.www.nlm.nih.gov), on the Research Projects Page, and in the Visible Human Project Section as *.jpg files. These use CT, MRI, x-rays and photographs of cross slices. The plan is that eventually any anatomical part can be viewed separately from the body. The relationship of organs and other structures can be observed as well. According to one NLM representative, it takes two weeks to download all of the information from the internet and it might take up 15 gigabytes of computer space. However, access to data is free on the internet.

WOMEN'S HEALTH

Covered in this section: ***Breast Cancer; Cervical Cancer; Endometriosis; General Topics; Hysterectomy; Interstitial Cystitis; Menopause; Menstruation; Osteoporosis; Professional Groups.***

Related sections: ***Bones/Orthopedics; Pregnancy & Childbirth; Sexual & Reproductive Health.***

Breast Cancer

Amazon Alternative Therapies for Breast Cancer

http://www.hunter.net/~bedford/curechat.html

Information, bulletin board and real-time chat room.

Avon Breast Cancer Awareness Crusade

http://www.avon.com/about/awareness/frame.html

Information about breast cancer and about Avon's crusade. Includes library and news, support groups, glossary, and answers to common questions.

Breast Cancer

http://www.mediconsult.com/ breast/

Educational material and journal club support information.

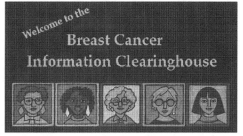

Breast Cancer Answers

http://www.biostat.wisc.edu/bca/

The Breast Cancer Information Clearinghouse.
http://nysernet.org/bcic/

Frequently asked questions (FAQs) and resources, clinical trials and hot topics. Also allows viewers to submit a cancer question via e-mail.

Breast Cancer Discussion Mailing List Information

http://www1.mhv.net/~delaney/owr.htm#oldg

Breast Cancer Forum

http://www.lifetimetv.com/chat/unmoderated_chats.html

Information about this chat group which meets every evening at 8:00 p.m. EST. Most popular nights are Sunday, Wednesday and Friday.

Breast Cancer Information Clearinghouse

http://nysernet.org/bcic/

This site offers information about breast cancer for patients and their families. Maintained by the New York State Education and Research Network.

Breast Cancer Information Service

http://trfn.clpgh.org/bcis/

Information about the diagnosis, treatment and prevention of breast cancer, as well as information on insurance issues and support groups.

Breast Cancer Lighthouse

http://commteclab.msu.edu/CTLProjects/breastcancerlighthouse/index.html

Personal stories of women who have survived breast cancer.

Breast Cancer NCI Statements

http://www.oncolink.upenn.edu/disease/breast/cancernet/

Statements, citations and abstracts on breast cancer from the National Library of Medicine's CANCERLIT database.

Breast Cancer Network

http://www.cancer.org/bcn/bcn.html

The American Cancer Society offers information and resources on breast cancer and breast reconstruction. Site has a glossary of terms, research updates and profiles of research programs. In addition, patient support organizations, advocacy efforts, and awareness campaigns are summarized.

BreastCancer.Net

http://www.breastcancer.net/

Subscribe to receive a free e-mail news summaries, or check out recent headlines and stories on breast cancer.

The Breast Cancer Network. *http://www.cancer.org/bcn/bcn.html*

Common Questions about Breast Cancer

http://www.y-me.org/faq.html

Twenty-five frequently asked questions (FAQs).

Community Breast Health Project

http://www-med.stanford.edu/CBHP/

Experiences of women with breast cancer, medical information, and advice on coping.

Doctor's Guide to Breast Cancer Information and Resources

http://www.pslgroup.com/BREASTCANCER/HTM#DISCUSSIONS

Lots of information and links, including medical news and medical alerts.

Early Detection of Breast Cancer

http://nysernet.org/bcic/subject/early-detection.html

Educare Inc., Breast Health and Breast Cancer Network

http://www.CancerHelp.com/ed/

Patient and clinical resources.

HomeArts Breast Health Center
http://homearts.com/depts/health/00breaf1.htm

Enter through http://homearts.com/ and select the Breast Health Center.

Montana Breast Cancer Resource Guide
http://www2.mbcrg.org/mbcrg/

National Action Plan on Breast Cancer
http://www.napbc.org/

NCI/PDQ Physician Statement: Breast Cancer
http://www.oncolink.upenn.edu/pdq_html/1/engl/100013.html

Information on breast cancer for physicians and other health care professionals.

OncoLink's Breast Cancer
http://www.oncolink.upenn.edu/disease/breast/

Provides general information on cancer, medical care, psychosocial issues and support for breast cancer patients. Information on causes, screening, diagnosis, prevention and treatments available.

Patient's Guide to Breast Cancer
http://www.wp.com/bicbs/gtoc.html

Patient's Guide to Breast Cancer Treatment
gopher://nysernet.org:70/11/BCIC/Sources/strang-cornell/
Patient%27s%20Guide%2010%20Breast%20Cancer%20Treatment

Text of a 14-chapter book that addresses breast cancer. From the New York Hospital Breast Cancer Tumor Board.

Y-Me National Breast Cancer Organization
http://www.y-me.org/

Facts and support for individuals with breast cancer, frequently asked questions (FAQs) and breast self-examination instructions.

Cervical Cancer

Cervical Cancer Tutorial
http://gynoncology.obgyn.washington.edu/Tutorials/Cervical%20tutorial.html

Pap Test
http://www.erinet.com/fnadoc/pap.htm
    Hypertext information about the Pap test which is used to identify cancer signs in cervical cell smears. Claims that the Pap is "the only cancer screening test which has decreased the incidence and mortality... of a cancer."

Endometriosis

Endometriosis: A Painful and Baffling Disease
http://www.dash.com/netro/nwx/tmr/tmr0895/endomet0895.html

Endometriosis Association
http://www.ivf.com/endoassn.html

Endometriosis Care Center
http://www.dunwoodymed.com/endo/question.htm
    Basic information about endometriosis.

Endometriosis Mailing List Information
http://www.ivf.com//witsend.html
    To subscribe, send e-mail to: LISTSERV@listserv.dartmouth.edu and in the first line of the message, write: "subscribe Witsendo Lastname, firstname."

Endometriosis Multimedia Gallery
http://www.ivf.com/galendo.html
    Images and a downloadable video.

Woman's Guide to Overcoming Endometriosis
http://www.ivf.com/endohtml.html

General Topics

Ask a Woman Doctor

http://www.healthwire.com/women/ask.htm

Check out questions that have been asked, or submit your own medical inquiry to a woman physician.

Atlanta Reproductive Health Care WWW: Women's Health

http://www.ivf.com/womhtml.html

CDC Information on Women's Health Risks

http://www.cdc.gov/diseases/women.html

Center for Vulvar Diseases

http://www.med.umich.edu/obgyn/vulva/vulfedu.html

Findings: The Women's Healthcare Advocacy Service

http://www.2cowherd.net/findings/

"Encouraging women to make thoughtful choices about their health by providing them with information and support."

Forum for Women's Health

http://www.healthwire.com/women/

Major areas include the reproductive system, medical issues, social and psychological issues, and wellness (i.e., fitness and nutrition). Lifecycle section includes material for young girls and adolescents; women in their reproductive years; post-reproductive aged women; and senior women.

Gynecological and Reproductive Health

gopher://gopher.cc.columbia.edu:71/00/publications/women/2h14

Text of the first chapter of the *Barnard/Columbia Women's Handbook*. Includes self-care, female sexual and reproductive organs, the menstrual cycle, and examinations.

Harvard Women's Health Watch Online Journal

http://www.med.harvard.edu/publications/Women/index.html

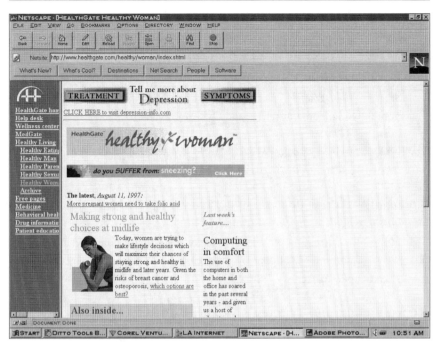

HealthGate Healthy Women. *http://www.healthgate.com/healthy/woman/index.shtml*

HealthGate Healthy Women

http://www.healthgate.com/healthy/woman/index.shtml

Articles on women's health issues.

Links of Interest to Obstetrics and Gynecology

http://www.museum.state.Il.us/isas/oblink.html

MedWeb's Gynecology and Women's Health

http://www.gen.emory.edu/medweb/medweb.gynecology.html

Lots of links by topic.

National Organization for Women

http://www.now.org/

NOW has information on women's abortion rights, other reproductive issues, violence against women, and general, non-medical political issues.

National Women's Health Resource Center

http://www.healthywomen.org/

Natracare Guide to Women's Health Resources on the Internet
http://www.indra.com/natracare/guide.html

ObGyn Educational Resources
http://medweb.nus.sg/kkh/
From the Singapore Obstetrics and Gynecology Web.

Obstetrics and Gynaecology Links
http://www.bris.ac.uk/Depts/ObsGyn/og_links.html

OncoLink's Gynecologic Cancers
http://oncolink.upenn.edu/disease/gynecologic1/
Links and information on cervical cancer; endometrial and uterine cancers; fallopian tube cancer; gestational trophoblastic disease; ovarian cancer; vaginal cancer; and vulvar cancer.

Reproduction and Women's Health
http://www.med.upenn.edu/~crrwh/ScientificSites.html

Web by Women for Women
http://www.io.com/~wwwomen/
Information on pregnancy, contraception, abortion, censorship, sexuality and menstruation. Search engine and links.

WHAM!
http://www.echonyc.com /~wham/
Women's Health Action and Mobilization, a women's rights advocacy group.

Women and Health
http://wellweb.com/WOMEN/WOMEN.HTM
Includes recommended medical tests for women, information on menopause and hormone replacement therapy.

Women and Health Resources
http://www.igc.apc.org/women/activist/health.html

Women of the World

http://www.echonyc.com/~jmkm/wotw/

The subtitle to this site is: "Formal Laws and Policies Affecting their Reproductive Lives."

Women Space

http://www.womencare.com/

Women's Health Hot Links

http://www.soft-design.com/softinfo/womens-health.html

Online newsletter that provides the media with information on women's health.

Women's Health Issues

http://feminist.com/health.htm

Women's Medical Health Page

http://www.best.com/~sirlou/wmhp.html

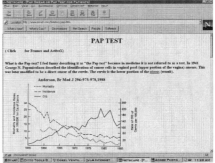

Pap Test information.
http://www.erinet.com/fnadoc/pap.htm

Women's Health Reading Room

http://www.bioscience.peg.apc.org/~awhc/rroom6.htm

Women's Health Weekly

http://www.homepage.holowww.com/1w.htm

Subscribe to either print or e-mail editions. Search their article index and TOC, access summaries of articles.

Yahoo's Women's Health Links

http://www.yahoo.com/Health/Women_s_Health/

Yale Library: Obstetrics and Gynecology

http://info.med.yale.edu/library/resources/obgyn/

Hysterectomy

Hysterectomy

gopher://gopher.health.state.ny.us/00/.consumer/.files/hysterec.txt

Site addresses the question of whether to have a hysterectomy, the possible alternatives, the benefits and risks of these procedures, different kinds of hysterectomies, and post-operation hospitalization and recovery.

Modern Alternatives to Hysterectomy

http://medseek.com/portfolios/reference/modalt.html

While hysterectomy may be a treatment of choice for many women with gynecological problems, there are often alternative procedures which will prevent a woman from losing her uterus. Some of these alternatives are discussed.

Interstitial Cystitis

Information about Interstitial Cystitis

http://www.niddk.nih.gov:80/InterstitialCystitis.html

Interstitial Cystitis Association

http://www.ichelp.com/

Interstitial cystitis is chronic inflammation of the bladder, and it most commonly affects women. This site provides and introduction to IC, self-help, diet information, resources and other related issues.

Interstitial Cystitis Network

http://www.sonic.net/~jill/icnet/icnet.html

Information for patients and professionals.

Menopause

Better Health Profiles: Menopause

http://fbhc.org/Patients/BetterHealth/Menopause/home.html

Better Health Profiles - Menopause.

http://fbhc.org/Patients/BetterHealth/Menopause/home.html

Birthing the Crone: Menopause and Aging through an Artist's Eyes

http://www.birthingthecrone.com/

Meno Times

http://web.aimnet.com/~hyperion/meno/menotimes.index.html

A quarterly journal dedicated to alternative approaches to treating osteoporosis and other effects of menopause.

Menopause Mailing List

http://www.ivf.com/Menopause.html

To subscribe, send e-mail to: LISTSERV@PSUHMC.HMC.PSU.EDU and in the message, write: "subscribe MENOPAUS firstname lastname."

Menopause Matters

http://world.std.com/~susan207/

Menopause: The Journal of the North American Menopause Society

http://www.menopause.org/journal.html

Abstracts of articles, subscription information, and links to NAMS.

Menstruation

Many Faces of P.M.S.

http://www.bairpms.com/

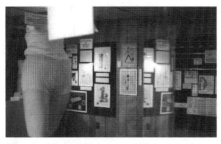

View inside the Museum of Menstruation.
http://www.mum.org/insideMUM.htm

Menstruation

http://users.vnet.net/shae/wissues/menstruate.html

Links to articles and sites on the web dealing with menstruation, cramps, PMS and Toxic Shock Syndrome.

Menstruation Disorders

http://www.ohsu.edu/cliniweb/C13/C13.371.491.html

Museum of Menstruation and Women's Health

http://www.mum.org/

Presents menstrual physiology, customs and products. Also find art related to menstruation. Definitely out of the ordinary.

S.P.O.T.: The Tampon Health Website

http://critpath.org/~tracy/spot.html

Healthier tampons and tampon alternatives.

Women's Health Issues: Menstruation

http://www.stayhealthy.com/hrd/WoHeIs_Meon.htm

Osteoporosis

See also: Bones/Orthopedics - Osteoporosis.

Osteoporosis

http://dpalm2.med.uth.tmc.edu/ptnt/00000767.htm

Bone basics, risk factors, prevention, and good food sources of calcium.

Osteoporosis FAQ

http://text.nlm.nih.gov/nih/cdc/www/43.html

Postmenopausal Osteoporosis-Prevention

http://www.silcom.com/~dwsmith/boned394.html

Professional Groups

American Medical Women's Association

http://www.amwa-doc.org/

Organization of women physicians and medical students dedicated to caring for women patients.

National Association of Women's Health Professionals

http://www.nawhp.org/

INDEX

Disabilities, *continued*
    attention deficit disorder (ADD),
      176-177
    autism, 177-178
    blindness, 199-202
    cerebral palsy, 178-179
    children with, 107-108
    communication/speech, 179-180
    developmental, 180
    Down syndrome, 181-182
    dyslexia, 182
    fragile X syndrome, 183
    hearing, 192-195
    hydrocephalus, 196, 461
    legal issues, 195
    mental retardation, 196
    paralysis, 197
    polio, 197-198
    resources, 183-192
    spina bifida, 198
    visual, 199-202
Disabled children, 107
Disaster preparedness, *see* Emergency
    preparedness, 219
Disaster relief, 217-218
Disease
    Addison, 225
    Alzheimer's, 19-21
    celiac, 147, 165
    Crohn, 165-167
    gastroesophageal reflux
      (GERD), 167-168
    Huntington, 460
    inflammatory bowel, 165-167
    Lou Gehrig's (Amyotrophic
      lateral sclerosis), 467
    Lyme, 321-322
    Ménière's, 211
    Parkinson, 463-464
    polycystic kidney, 339

Disease, *continued*
    Raynaud's, 286
    sickle cell, 68
Diseases, rare, 523-526
Dissociation/dissociative personality
    disorders, 440-442
Domestic violence, 3-4
Donation
    blood, 63-64
    organ, 130
Down syndrome, 181-182
Dreams, 549-550
Drug abuse, 11-14
Drugs/Pharmacology, 203-207, 380
    pharmacology schools, 269
    Phen/Fen, 156
    Prozac, 207
    references, 380
    Ritalin, 207
Dyslexia, 182
Dysphagia, *see* Esophageal disorders,
    167-168
E. coli, 311
Ear/nose/throat (Otolaryngology)
    209-212
    acoustic neuroma, 209
    cochlear implants, 210
    ear infection, 209
    hearing impairments 192-195
    Ménière's disease, 211
    otitis media, 209
    surgery 210
    tinnitus, 211-212
Earthquake preparedness, 219
Eastern medicine, 34-35
Eating disorders, 213-216
    anorexia nervosa, 213
    bulimia, 213
    compulsive eating, 215
    obesity, 215
    weight loss, 161-162